OSCEs in Medicine
A Primer for Postgraduate Students

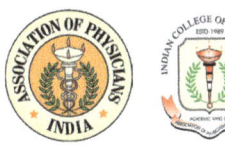

OSCEs in Medicine
A Primer for Postgraduate Students

Editors

Narinder Pal Singh
MD FACP FRCP (Edinburgh) FASN ISHF FISN FAMS FICP MBA
National Vice President
Association of Physicians of India (API)
Dean Research, Eternal University
Baru Sahib, Himachal Pradesh, India
Advisor Research, FMHS—SGT University
Gurugram, Haryana, India
Consultant—Academic Programs
in Nephrology
Max Super Speciality Hospital
New Delhi, India

Jyotirmoy Pal
MD (General Medicine) FRCP FICP FACP WHO Fellow
Dean
Indian College of Physicians (ICP)
President-Elect
Association of Physicians of India (API)
Professor
Department of General Medicine
University College of Medicine and
Sagore Dutta Medical College
Kamarhati, West Bengal, India

Associate Editors

Nandini Chatterjee MD FRCP (London, Glasgow) FICP
Professor, Department of Medicine
Institute of Post Graduate Medical Education and
Research (IPGMER), Kolkata, West Bengal, India

Amit A Saraf
MD FRCP (London, Edinburgh, Glasgow) FACP (Philadelphia) FICP FCPS
Director, Department of Internal Medicine
Jupiter Hospital, Mumbai, Maharashtra, India

Jayanta K Panda MD (Internal Medicine) FICP FACP
Professor and Head, Department of General Medicine
SCB Medical College, Cuttack, Odisha, India

PN Chaudhary MD
Senior Consultant
Department of Internal Medicine
Max Super Speciality Hospital
Ghaziabad, Uttar Pradesh, India

K Mugundhan
MD DM (Neurology) FICP FRCP (Glasgow) FACP (USA)
Professor and Head
Department of Neurology
Government Stanley Medical College
Chennai, Tamil Nadu, India

Technical Editor

Anish Kumar Gupta M Pharm (Pharma Practice)
Consultant (Research and Development)
Faculty of Medicine and Health Sciences
Shree Guru Gobind Singh Tricentenary University
Gurugram, Haryana, India

Forewords
Girish Mathur
Jyotirmoy Pal

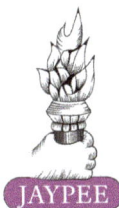

JAYPEE BROTHERS MEDICAL PUBLISHERS
The Health Sciences Publisher
New Delhi | London

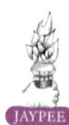 **Jaypee Brothers Medical Publishers (P) Ltd**

Headquarters
Jaypee Brothers Medical Publishers (P) Ltd
EMCA House, 23/23-B
Ansari Road, Daryaganj
New Delhi 110 002, India
Landline: +91-11-23272143, +91-11-23272703
+91-11-23282021, +91-11-23245672
Email: jaypee@jaypeebrothers.com

Corporate Office
Jaypee Brothers Medical Publishers (P) Ltd
4838/24, Ansari Road, Daryaganj
New Delhi 110 002, India
Phone: +91-11-43574357
Fax: +91-11-43574314
Email: jaypee@jaypeebrothers.com

Overseas Office
JP Medical Ltd
83 Victoria Street, London
SW1H 0HW (UK)
Phone: +44 20 3170 8910
Fax: +44 (0)20 3008 6180
Email: info@jpmedpub.com

Website: www.jaypeebrothers.com
Website: www.jaypeedigital.com

© 2024, Jaypee Brothers Medical Publishers

The views and opinions expressed in this book are solely those of the original contributor(s)/author(s) and do not necessarily represent those of editor(s) or publisher of the book.

All rights reserved. No part of this publication may be reproduced, stored or transmitted in any form or by any means, electronic, mechanical, photocopying, recording or otherwise, without the prior permission in writing of the publishers.

All brand names and product names used in this book are trade names, service marks, trademarks or registered trademarks of their respective owners. The publisher is not associated with any product or vendor mentioned in this book.

Medical knowledge and practice change constantly. This book is designed to provide accurate, authoritative information about the subject matter in question. However, readers are advised to check the most current information available on procedures included and check information from the manufacturer of each product to be administered, to verify the recommended dose, formula, method and duration of administration, adverse effects and contraindications. It is the responsibility of the practitioner to take all appropriate safety precautions. Neither the publisher nor the author(s)/editor(s) assume any liability for any injury and/or damage to persons or property arising from or related to use of material in this book.

This book is sold on the understanding that the publisher is not engaged in providing professional medical services. If such advice or services are required, the services of a competent medical professional should be sought.

Every effort has been made where necessary to contact holders of copyright to obtain permission to reproduce copyright material. If any have been inadvertently overlooked, the publisher will be pleased to make the necessary arrangements at the first opportunity.

Inquiries for bulk sales may be solicited at: jaypee@jaypeebrothers.com

OSCEs in Medicine: A Primer for Postgraduate Students

First Edition: **2024**

ISBN: 978-93-5696-519-5

Contributors

EDITORS

Narinder Pal Singh
MD FACP FRCP (Edinburgh) FASN ISHF FISN FAMS FICP MBA
National Vice President
Association of Physicians of India (API)
Dean Research, Eternal University
Baru Sahib, Himachal Pradesh, India
Advisor Research, FMHS—SGT University
Gurugram, Haryana, India
Consultant—Academic Programs in Nephrology
Max Super Speciality Hospital
New Delhi, India

Jyotirmoy Pal
MD (General Medicine) FRCP FICP FACP WHO Fellow
Dean
Indian College of Physicians (ICP)
President-Elect, Association of Physicians of India (API)
Professor
Department of General Medicine
University College of Medicine and
Sagore Dutta Medical College
Kamarhati, West Bengal, India

ASSOCIATE EDITORS

Nandini Chatterjee MD FRCP (London, Glasgow) FICP
Professor
Department of Medicine
Institute of Post Graduate Medical Education and Research (IPGMER)
Kolkata, West Bengal, India

Amit A Saraf
MD FRCP (London, Edinburgh, Glasgow)
FACP (Philadelphia) FICP FCPS
Director
Department of Internal Medicine
Jupiter Hospital
Mumbai, Maharashtra, India

Jayanta K Panda MD (Internal Medicine) FICP FACP
Professor and Head
Department of General Medicine
SCB Medical College
Cuttack, Odisha, India

PN Chaudhary MD
Senior Consultant
Department of Internal Medicine
Max Super Speciality Hospital
Ghaziabad, Uttar Pradesh, India

K Mugundhan
MD DM (Neurology) FICP FRCP (Glasgow) FACP (USA)
Professor and Head
Department of Neurology
Government Stanley Medical College
Chennai, Tamil Nadu, India

TECHNICAL EDITOR

Anish Kumar Gupta M Pharm (Pharma Practice)
Consultant (Research and Development)
Faculty of Medicine and Health Sciences
Shree Guru Gobind Singh Tricentenary University
Gurugram, Haryana, India

CONTRIBUTING AUTHORS

Abraham Ittyachen M MD
Professor and Head
Department of Medicine
MOSC Medical College and Hospital
Ernakulam, Kerala, India

Aminur Rahman
FCPS (Medicine) MD (Neurology) FRCP (Edinburgh) FACP (USA) FINR (Switzerland)
Associate Professor and Head
Department of Neurology
Sir Salimullah Medical College
Mitford, Dhaka, Bangladesh

Amir Hussain MD (Medicine)
Assistant Professor
Department of Medicine
Jawaharlal Nehru Medical College
Aligarh Muslim University
Aligarh, Uttar Pradesh, India

Anuradha Deuri MD (General Medicine)
Professor
Department of Internal Medicine
Gauhati Medical College and Hospital
Guwahati, Assam, India

Arpit Jain DNB (Medicine)
Senior Resident—DrNB (Nephrology)
Department of Nephrology
Sir Ganga Ram Hospital
New Delhi, India

Ashutosh Chaturvedi
MD (Medicine) Certified in Diabetes (Chennai)
Assistant Professor
Department of Medicine
Mahatma Gandhi Medical College
Jaipur, Rajasthan, India

Atul Bhasin
DNB (Internal Medicine, Army Hospital R&R) MNAMS
FIACM FICP FACP (USA) FRCP (London)
Senior Director
Department of Internal Medicine
BLK-Max Super Speciality Hospital
New Delhi, India

Ayan Basu MD DM (Infectious Diseases)
Assistant Professor
Department of Infectious Diseases
Institute of Post Graduate Medical Education and Research
Kolkata, West Bengal, India

Balbir Singh Kohli MD DNB (Medicine)
Head
Department of Critical Care and Emergency
Hira Mongi Navneet Hospital
Consultant Physician, Fortis and Jupiter Hospital
Mumbai, Maharashtra, India

Bhaskar Kanti Nath MD FICP
Associate Professor
Department of Medicine
Dhubri Medical College and Hospital
Dhubri, Assam, India

Bhavin Jankharia MD DMRD
Consultant Radiologist and Partner
Picture This by Jankharia
Mumbai, Maharashtra, India

Bhoomi Angrish MD DNB (Radiology)
Cardiothoracic Fellow, Picture This by Jankharia
Mumbai, Maharashtra, India

Bibhuti Saha MD DTM&H (Kol)
Professor and Head
Department of Infectious Diseases and Advanced Microbiology
School of Tropical Medicine
Kolkata, West Bengal, India

Bidita Khandelwal MD (Medicine)
Professor and Former Head
Department of Medicine
Sikkim Manipal Institute of Medical Sciences
Sikkim Manipal University
Tadong, Sikkim, India

Biswajit Majumder MD DM
Professor and Head
Department of Cardiology
RG Kar Medical College
Kolkata, West Bengal, India

Contributors

Chamila Mettananda
MD MRCP PhD FRCP FRCPE FACP FCCP
Professor and Specialist in General Medicine
Faculty of Medicine, University of Kelaniya
Kelaniya, Sri Lanka

Chayan Mondal MD (Medicine) DNB (Medicine)
Senior Resident
Department of Neurology
Bangur Institute of Neurosciences
IPGMER & SSKM Hospital
Kolkata, west Bengal, India

Deepak Agrawal MD (General Medicine)
Divisional Medical Officer
Central Hospital, North-Western Railway
Jaipur, Rajasthan, India
Senior Faculty: PG Guide

Dilip Kumar Mazumdar
MD (Kol) MRCP (UK) FRCP (London, Edinburgh)
Ex Professor of Medicine
Ramakrishna Mission Seva Pratisthan
Vivekananda Institute of Medical Sciences
Kolkata, West Bengal, India

Dilusha Lamabadusuriya MD MRCP (UK)
Senior Lecturer
Consultant Physician in Internal Medicine
Kotelawala Defence University Hospital
Werahera, Sri Lanka

Dinesh Khullar MD DM (Nephrology)
Chairman and Head
Department of Nephrology and
Renal Transplant Medicine
Max Super Speciality Hospital
New Delhi, India

Dipankar Pal DM (Infectious Disease)
Resident
Department of Infectious Diseases
Christian Medical College
Vellore, Tamil Nadu, India

Gautam Rege MD
Consultant Cardiologist
Jupiter Hospital
Mumbai, Maharashtra, India

Girish Mathur
MD (Medicine) FICP FIACM FACP (USA) FRCP (Glasgow, London, Edinburgh)
Senior Consultant Physician
Alka Diagnostic Centre
Kota, Rajasthan, India
President—Association of Physicians of India

Indranil Thakur MD (Medicine)
Assistant Professor
Diamond Harbour Government Medical College
Kolkata, West Bengal, India

Kaustav Ghosh DNB (General Medicine)
Post Doctoral Trainee Clinical Hematology (DM)
Department of Hematology
Nil Ratan Sircar Medical College and Hospital
Kolkata, West Bengal, India

Kripamoy Das MD (General Medicine)
Professor and Head
Department of General Medicine
IQ City Medical College and Hospital
Durgapur, West Bengal, India

Kumkum Sarkar MD (Tropical Medicine)
Assistant Professor
Department of Tropical Medicine
School of Tropical Medicine
Kolkata, West Bengal, India

Kumudini Jayasinghe MD FRCPE FCCP FACP
Specialist in Internal Medicine
National Hospital
Kandy, Sri Lanka
President, Sri Lanka College of Internal
Medicine-2023

Mainak Mukhopadhyay MD MRCP DM (Cardiology)
Consultant Interventional Cardiologist
Department of Cardiology
AMRI Hospital
Kolkata, West Bengal, India

Mamatha B Patil MD (Internal Medicine)
Professor
Department of Internal Medicine
RRMCH
Bengaluru, Karnataka, India

Manisha Arora
MD MRCP (UK) Diploma in Geriatrics (UK)
Senior Consultant and Unit Head
Department of Medicine
Sri Balaji Action Medical Institute
New Delhi, India

Mohd Aslam MD DM (Nephrology)
Associate Professor
Department of Medicine
Jawaharlal Nehru Medical College
Aligarh Muslim University
Aligarh, Uttar Pradesh, India

Mukunda Prasad Kafle
MD DM (Nephrology) FASN Hon FICP
Assistant Professor
Department of Nephrology
and Transplantation Medicine
Maharajgunj Medical Campus
Institute of Medicine
Tribhuvan University Teaching Hospital
Maharajgunj, Kathmandu, Nepal

N Balamurugan MD DM
Consultant Neurologist
SIMS Chellum Hospital
Salem, Tamil Nadu, India

N Madhuwanthi Hettiarachchi MD
(Colombo) FCCP (SL) FACP (USA) FRCP (Edinburgh)
Specialist Physician in Internal Medicine
Toxicology Unit
Teaching Hospital
Peradeniya, Sri Lanka
Vice President of Sri Lanka College of Internal Medicine

Namal Wijesinghe
MD (Med) MRCP (UK) FRCP FRCPE FRACP FCCP FECS FCSANZ
Professor of Medicine
General Sir John Kotelawala Defence University
Kandawala, Sri Lanka

P Umesh Tharanga De Silva
MD (Medicine, Colombo)
Consultant Physician
Base Hospital Kahawatta
Kahawatta, Sri Lanka

Parveen Gulati MD
Director
Dr Gulati Imaging
New Delhi, India

Pinaki Mukhopadhyay
DM FICP FASN FRCP (London)
Head
Department of Nephrology
Nil Ratan Sircar Medical College
Kolkata, West Bengal, India

Prakas Kumar Mandal
MD DM (Hematology)
Professor
Department of Hematology
NRS Medical College and Hospital
Kolkata, West Bengal, India

Priyamali Jayasekera
MD (Med) MRCP (UK) FRCP (London, Edinburgh)
FACP (USA) FCCP MRCP (Endo & Diabetes UK)
Consultant Physician and Senior Lecturer
Clinical Medicine General
Sir John Kotelawala Defence University
Kandawala, Sri Lanka

Raghav Khullar MD
Department of Medicine
All India Institute of Medical Sciences
New Delhi, India

Rakhi Sanyal
MD DNB MNAMS MRCP (UK) FRCP (Edinburgh)
Associate Professor
Department of Medicine
Jagannath Gupta Institute of Medical Sciences and Hospital
Senior Consultant
Department of Internal Medicine
AMRI Hospitals
Kolkata, West Bengal, India

RK Singal
MD FACP (USA) FRCP (Glasgow) FICP FIAMS
Principal Consultant and Head
Department of Internal Medicine
BLK-Max Super Speciality Hospital
New Delhi, India

Contributors

Saif Quaiser DNB (Medicine) DM (Nephrology)
Assistant Professor
Department of Medicine
Jawaharlal Nehru Medical College
Aligarh, Muslim University
Aligarh, Uttar Pradesh, India

Salil Kumar Pal
MD (Medicine) DM (Endocrinology)
Professor and Head
Department of Medicine
Calcutta National Medical College
Kolkata, West Bengal, India
Chairman, RSSDI, West Bengal Chapter

Sanchita Saha MD
Consultant Physical Medicine and
Neuro-Rehabilitation Specialist
Department of Neurorehabilitation
Institute of Neurosciences
Kolkata, West Bengal, India

Sandhiya Selvarajan
MD DNB DM (Clinical Pharmacology)
Additional Professor and Head
Department of Clinical Pharmacology
Jawaharlal Institute of Postgraduate Medical
Education and Research
Puducherry—Union Territory, India

Sanoop Kumar Sherin Sabu
MD (General Medicine)
Consultant Physician
CSI Hospital
Erode, Tamil Nadu, India

Sathish Kumar M
MD (General Medicine) DM (Neurology)
Assistant Professor
Department of Neurology
Saveetha Medical College
Chennai, Tamil Nadu, India

Saurabh Dutta MD MRCP
Senior Consultants
Department of Internal Medicine
Medica Superspecialty Hospital
Kolkata, West Bengal, India

Shamali Abeyagunawardena
MD MRCP (UK) FRCP (London) FACP (USA)
Professor in Medicine
Faculty of Medicine
University of Peradeniya
Consultant Physician
Professional Medical Unit
Teaching Hospital Peradeniya
Peradeniya, Sri Lanka

Shambo Samrat Samajdar
MD DM (Clinical Pharmacology) PG Dip Endo and Diabetes
(RCP) Diploma in Allergy Asthma and Immunology
Fellowship in Respiratory and Critical Care (WBUHS)
Independent Clinical Pharmacologist and
Consultant
Diabetes and Allergy Asthma Special
Therapeutics Clinic
Kolkata, West Bengal, India

Sharmistha Panja MBBS
Resident
Department of Dermatology,
Venereology, and Leprosy
RG Kar Medical College
Kolkata, West Bengal, India

Shekh Ashraf MD (Medicine)
Senior Resident
Department of Medicine
Jawaharlal Nehru Medical College
Aligarh Muslim University
Aligarh, Uttar Pradesh, India

Sougata Kumar Ghosh MD (Medicine)
Consultant Physician
Serampore Walsh Hospital
Serampore, West Bengal, India

Souren Pal MD (Medicine)
Assistant Professor
Department of General Medicine
Nil Ratan Sircar Medical College
Kolkata, West Bengal, India

SS Dariya MD (Medicine) FACP FGSI FDI FIPA
Senior Consultant Physician
SMS Hospital
Jaipur, Rajasthan, India

Sudip Kumar Ghosh MD DNB MNAMS
Professor and Head
Department of Dermatology, Venereology,
and Leprosy, RG Kar Medical College
Kolkata, West Bengal, India

Sunil Kakkar
Head
Department of Diagnostic Radiology
Deen Dayal Upadhyay Hospital
New Delhi, India

Suranga Manilgama
MD MRCP (UK) FRCPL FRCPE FACP (USA) FCCP MRCP
Endocrinology and Diabetes (UK)
Consultant Physician in Internal Medicine
Colombo North Teaching Hospital-Ragama
Ragama, Sri Lanka

Surya Kant MD (Pulmonary Medicine, Gold Medalist)
Professor and Head
Department of Respiratory Medicine
King George's Medical University
Lucknow, Uttar Pradesh, India

Syed Haider Mehdi Husaini
MD (General Medicine)
Assistant Professor
Department of Medicine
Jawaharlal Nehru Medical College
Aligarh Muslim University
Aligarh, Uttar Pradesh, India

Tapas Bandyopadhyay MD (Medicine) FICP FDI
Senior Consultant
Department of General Medicine
Medica Superspecialty Hospital
Kolkata, West Bengal, India

Thushara Matthias MD (Kol) FRCP (London)
Consultant Physician and Senior Lecturer
Department of Medicine
University of Sri Jayewardenepura
Sri Lanka

Tribeni Sharma MD (General Medicine)
Professor of Medicine
Gauhati Medical College and Hospital
Guwahati, Assam, India

Udas Chandra Ghosh
MD (General Medicine) DNB (General Medicine) DNB
(Respiratory Diseases) DTCD FICP FRCP (Glasgow)
Professor
Department of Medicine and In-Charge of
Rheumatology Division, Medical College Kolkata
Kolkata, West Bengal, India

Uddalak Chakraborty MD (Medicine)
Senior Resident, Department of Neurology
Bangur Institute of Neurosciences
IPGMER and SSKM Hospital
Kolkata, West Bengal, India

Usharani Pingali
DNB (Clinical Pharmacology) MD (Pharmacology)
Professor and Head
Department of Clinical Pharmacology and
Therapeutics
Nizam's Institute of Medical Sciences
Hyderabad, Telangana, India

Vaibhav Gulati MD
Resident
Mercy Catholic Medical Center
Darby, Pennsylvania, USA

Col (Dr) Varghese Koshy
MD (Medicine) Trained in Clinical Immunology and
Rheumatology, EULAR Certified.
Head
Department of Clinical Immunology and
Rheumatology
Command Hospital Southern Command, Pune
Professor, Department of Internal Medicine
Armed Forces Medical College
Pune, Maharashtra, India

Vinant Bhargava
DNB (Nephrology) MNAMS FRCP (London) FASN FACP (USA)
Associate Professor, Department of Nephrology
Sir Ganga Ram Hospital
New Delhi, India

WKS Kularatne MD FCCP (SL) FRCP (London)
Consultant Physician (Internal Medicine)
National Hospital
Kandy, Sri Lanka

Yogesh Godge MD
Consultant Neurologist, Jupiter Hospital
Mumbai, Maharashtra, India

Foreword

In our fast-paced world, the landscape of medical education is constantly evolving, and the Objective Structured Clinical Examinations (OSCEs) has emerged as a pivotal tool for evaluating the clinical competence of medical students.

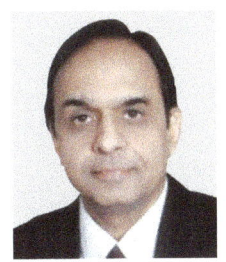

The book OSCEs in Medicine—A Primer for Postgraduate Students adopts a systematic approach, commencing with an insightful introductory chapter on OSCEs, delving into its merits, drawbacks, and the intricacies of the examination process. It then navigates through various OSCE sections tailored to medical specialties, offering a well-rounded perspective on the subject. The inclusion of realistic clinical scenarios is a standout feature, mirroring the diversity of cases encountered in real-world practice. This not only enriches clinical knowledge but also nurtures critical thinking and decision-making skills.

In the dynamic field of medicine, staying abreast of current developments is imperative. I am confident that the author has covered various medical specialties comprehensively, integrating the latest guidelines, evidence-based practices, and emerging trends. This ensures that students are well equipped to tackle the contemporary challenges of healthcare.

I am optimistic that this book will not only empower medical students to excel in OSCEs but also equip them to flourish in their clinical careers, enabling the application of knowledge and skills to provide exceptional patient care.

My heartfelt congratulations go to Dr (Prof) Narinder Pal Singh for eloquently presenting this crucial concept. The entire team deserves commendation for delivering a book that meets the pressing need to acquaint postgraduate students with a broad spectrum of skills and challenges within a concise time frame.

A big shout-out to all contributors for developing a resource that not only mirrors the dynamic landscape of modern medical education but also stands as an indispensable guide for budding healthcare professionals.

Girish Mathur
MD FICP FACP FRCP (London, Glasgow, Edinburgh)
FIACM FRSSDI Fellow Diabetes India
President, Association of Physicians of India (API)

Foreword

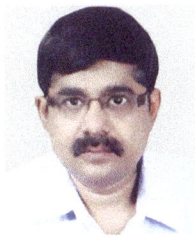

The Objective Structured Clinical Examinations (OSCEs) and Objective Structured Practical Examinations (OSPEs) have become an integral part of both the postgraduate and undergraduate curriculum and there is a scarcity of good guidebooks in this domain.

I congratulate Dr Narinder Pal Singh for compiling such a comprehensive array of OSCEs covering the whole spectrum of disease processes. The whole book is divided into sections containing OSCEs from different systems of the body. It is also a wonderful venture in the sense that these OSCEs have been contributed by our API Member Faculty of Institutions from all over the nation. The associate editors, who have done a great job in selecting and assimilating the OSCEs, also represent various parts of the country.

I am very hopeful and expectant about the response to this book as this is a novel endeavor that is going to be very useful for medical students to pass their exams with flying colors.

Jyotirmoy Pal
MD (General Medicine) FRCP FICP FACP WHO Fellow
Dean, Indian College of Physicians (ICP)
President-Elect, Association of Physicians of India (API)
Professor, Department of General Medicine
University College of Medicine and Sagore Dutta Medical College
Kamarhati, West Bengal, India

Preface

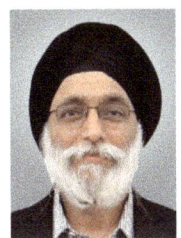

Welcome to a specialized and comprehensive book tailored for postgraduate medical students embarking on the challenging journey of mastering Objective Structured Clinical Examinations (OSCEs). In the dynamic landscape of modern medical education, OSCEs have emerged as a pivotal and mandatory component of assessments in various medical universities. These examinations serve as a critical tool for evaluating the clinical competencies, decision-making skills, and communication abilities of postgraduate medical students.

This book offers specialized insights by dedicating sections to each medical specialty, providing an in-depth exploration of OSCE scenarios tailored to the unique challenges of diverse clinical domains. Real-life clinical scenarios enrich practical understanding, encompassing crucial aspects such as history-taking, examination, diagnosis, and management strategies. The comprehensive review within each section ensures a thorough examination of key concepts and skills pertinent to the respective specialty. Core competencies, including clinical reasoning, evidence-based practice, and interpersonal skills essential for effective medical practice, are seamlessly integrated throughout. Ultimately, the book aims to not only equip medical students for success in OSCEs but also foster their ability to thrive in clinical careers, applying acquired knowledge and skills to provide top-tier patient care.

I thank the esteemed Dr Girish Mathur, President, Association of Physicians of India (API), and Dr Jyotirmoy Pal, Dean, Indian College of Physicians (ICP), for granting us the opportunity to publish the book under their esteemed banner. Your support is invaluable, and we are honored to collaborate with API-ICP dedicated to advancing knowledge.

I extend my heartfelt gratitude to the esteemed Associate Editors Dr Nandini Chatterjee, Dr Amit A Saraf, Dr Jayanta K Panda, Dr PN Chaudhary, and Dr K Mugundhan, and Technical Editor Anish Kumar Gupta for their invaluable contributions to the book. Your dedication, expertise, and collaborative spirit have been instrumental in shaping the content and ensuring the overall success of this book.

I extend sincere gratitude to Jaypee Brothers Medical Publishers for their pivotal role in bringing this book to fruition, showcasing dedication to excellence and support throughout the publishing process.

As OSCEs become an integral part of medical assessments worldwide, this book stands as a testament to the commitment to excellence in medical education. I extend my best wishes for your success in navigating the challenges of OSCEs and in advancing your journey toward becoming a skilled and empathetic medical practitioner.

Warm regards,

Narinder Pal Singh

Contents

1. Infectious Diseases 1
2. Immunology 30
3. Rheumatology 42
4. Endocrinology 60
5. Diabetology 72
6. Hematology 87
7. Oncology 101
8. Nephrology 111
9. Cardiology 139
10. Gastroenterology 165
11. Hepatology 173
12. Neurology 181
13. Respiratory 261
14. Critical Care Medicine 279
15. Poisoning and Toxicology 286
16. Diagnostic Imaging 296
17. Dermatology 307
18. Medical Genetics 320
19. Psychiatry 330
20. Biostatistics 335
21. Test Yourself 341

Index 357

Objective Structured Clinical Examination

Narinder Pal Singh, Anish Kumar Gupta

■ INTRODUCTION

Since its introduction into medical school assessment in 1975 by Haden and Gleeson, the Objective Structured Clinical Examination (OSCE) has become a standard evaluation method for both undergraduate and postgraduate medical students. Initially conceived as a timed assessment involving interactions with simulated patients across stations covering history-taking, physical examination, counseling, and patient management, the OSCE has undergone modifications to adapt to diverse contexts. Globally, reputable medical colleges, including those in the United States, United Kingdom, Canada, and India, consider the OSCE as the primary mode of assessment for evaluating competency and clinical skills. It complements cognitive knowledge testing in essay writing and objective examinations. The OSCE is a versatile tool for assessing healthcare professionals in clinical settings, evaluating competency through direct observation in multiple stations.

What is an OSCE?

- An OSCE, or Objective Structured Clinical Examination, is a method of evaluating a predefined set of clinical competencies.
- This assessment approach involves presenting a case scenario and breaking down each clinical competency into smaller components, such as history-taking, examination performance, interpretation of investigations, and medical management.
- The examination process entails assessing each component individually, and predetermined checklists are used to allocate marks based on the evaluation of each specific aspect.

■ ADVANTAGES AND DISADVANTAGES OF OSCE

The OSCE surpasses traditional clinical examinations by assessing a comprehensive array of competencies, including problem-solving, communication, decision-making, and patient management, beyond the narrow focus of cognitive knowledge and technical skills. Multiple stations allow testing of different subspecialties without the need for patients with clinical findings, eliminating the hassle of procuring patients before examinations. OSCE's advantages lie in its objectivity, reproducibility, and ease of recall, enabling standardized evaluation and teaching audits. Unlike traditional examinations, OSCE involves multiple examiners assessing different stations, eliminating biases, and allowing diverse perspectives to contribute to standards. Despite criticisms, such as the use of unreal subjects, OSCE's efficiency in examining more students across diverse subjects in a shorter time frame makes it a preferred method, though it demands meticulous organization and more resources.

CONTENT AND PROCESS OF OSCE

Objective Structured Clinical Examination consists of a circuit of stations usually connected in series. Each station evaluates one specific competency, with students rotating around the complete circuit. Performance is independently evaluated at each station using a standardized checklist. The number of stations can vary, usually ranging from 12 to 30, with 20 stations being common. Each station is typically allotted 5 minutes. Formulating questions, model keys, and checklists for each station is crucial in preparation.

Setting the standard: Setting the pass mark is a major challenge in OSCE success. Standards can be relative or absolute, with an absolute clear-cut minimum accepted cut-off decided beforehand. For instance, the National Medical Commission of India recommends 50% as the minimum pass marks for all summative examinations in medical specialties.

INDIAN EXPERIENCES WITH OSCE

In India, OSCE has primarily been used for formative assessment of postgraduate medical students. The lack of recognition by the National Medical Commission and the need for faculty training contribute to hesitancy in incorporating it into summative assessments. The National Board of Examination, Ministry of Health and Family Welfare, India, has successfully used OSCE for the summative assessment of postgraduate students for DNB/DrNB certification.

OSCE Component as per the National Board of Examination (NBE), India.

- Candidates seated with at least 1 m apart.
- 20 answer sheets distributed to each candidate.
- Examiners sign on each answer sheet as invigilators.
- All stations run virtually from the NBE command center.
- Questions are shared via video conferencing, and candidates must mention roll number, station number, and sign on each answer sheet.
- 5 minutes of rest after every seven stations.
- Questions of a station may be in two slides (two parts).
- Time allotted for questions displayed on the screen.
- Filled answer sheets kept separately by candidates and collected after each station.
- Only one answer sheet allowed per OSCE station.
- OSCE questions, once completed, will not be shown back or repeated after time has lapsed.
- There is no requirement for the movement of candidates as in traditional OSCE stations.

Some OSCE don'ts.

- Do not pay attention to the examiner's pencil.
- Do not ignore the instructions.
- Do not misinterpret the instructions.
- Do not interrogate the patient.
- Do not talk too much.
- Do not ignore what the patient is telling you.
- Do not assume the examiner can read your mind.
- Do not give generic information.

SUMMARY

The OSCE format for clinical assessment, characterized by its benefits in terms of objectivity, consistency, and adaptability of clinical scenarios, proves to be more advantageous than traditional clinical assessment methods. It facilitates the assessment of postgraduate students at different stages of their training in a relatively brief timeframe, encompassing a wide array of skills and challenges. OSCE eliminates biases in evaluating postgraduates, establishing a standardized framework and criteria for assessment. This renders it a valuable approach in the field of medical practice. The current demand emphasizes the necessity for an integrated multiplanar (three-dimensional) 360° assessment, wherein the OSCE can play a pivotal role.

RECOMMENDED READING

1. Jameson JL, Fauci AS, Kasper DL, Hauser SL, Longo DL, Loscalzo J. Harrison's Principles of Internal Medicine, 20th Edition. New York: McGraw-Hill Education; 2018.
2. Kamath SA, Shah SN, Munjal YP, Nadkar MY. API Textbook of Medicine, 12th edition. New Delhi: Jaypee Brothers Medical Publishers; 2022.
3. Papadakis MA, McPhee SJ, Rabow MW, McQuaid KR. Current Medical Diagnosis and Treatment 2023. New York: McGraw Hill; 2023.
4. Penman ID, Ralston SH, Strachan MWJ, Hobson RP. Davidson's Principles and Practice of Medicine, 24th edition. Philadelphia, PA: Elsevier; 2022.

SECTION 1

Infectious Diseases

QUESTIONS

Q1. A patient presents with a high fever, severe headache, photophobia, and altered mental status. Physical examination reveals generalized petechial rash.
a. What is the likely diagnosis? (3 marks)
b. Explain the significance of the petechial rash. (3 marks)
c. Name two diagnostic tests to confirm this condition. (4 marks)

Q2. A 51-year-old male presented with a 2-week history of fever and overall feeling of unwellness. He had inadequately managed diabetes mellitus (DM) at the time of his visit. His X-ray abdomen is shown below.

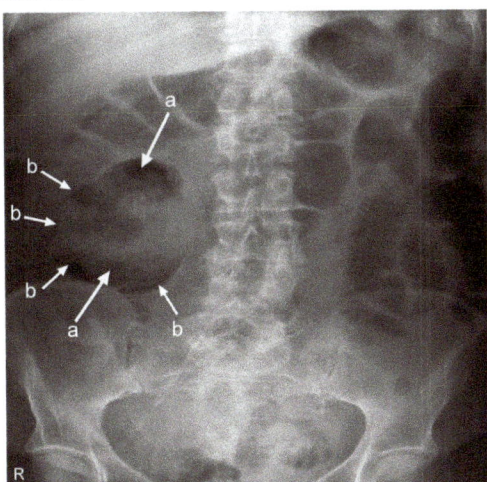

a. Describe the findings. (2 marks)
b. What is your diagnosis? (2 marks)
c. What further investigations should be done? (3 marks)
d. How will you treat? (3 marks)

Q3. A 25-year-old male type 1 DM complained of intermittent dull-aching headache and restricted eye movements. He had neck stiffness. He was able to localize pain and was moving all his limbs equally. He also had facial asymmetry and right upper motor neuron facial palsy.

No seizures or involuntary movements were observed. Both right and left pupils were nonreactive to light. The extraocular movements were restricted, and no doll's eye reflex was noted. A left eyelid swelling was observed with chemosis and discharge. Fundus examination was normal. Neck stiffness and nystagmus were absent. Spasticity of all four limbs was observed with a power of grade 3/5. Deep tendon reflexes at all joints were 2+. Bilateral plantars were equivocal. Sensory examination showed that he was perceiving pain on both sides equally. The cerebellar signs were negative.

MRI brain:

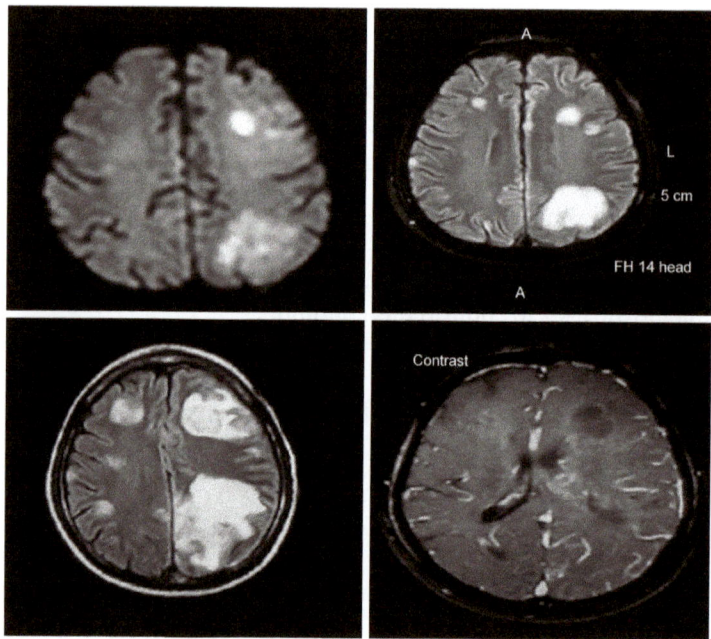

a. What is the diagnosis? (4 marks)
b. What is the etiology? (2 marks)
c. How would you manage? (4 marks)

Q4.

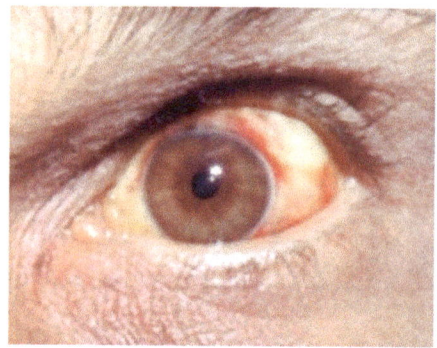

a. Identify the sign. (5 marks)
b. Disease in which it is found. (5 marks)

Infectious Diseases

Q5. A 65-year-old lady presented to the casualty with fever and myalgia. 1 week prior to the onset of her illness she had gone for trekking through a hilly forest area. Physical examination revealed the presence of a lesion on the left part of the chest near her axilla.

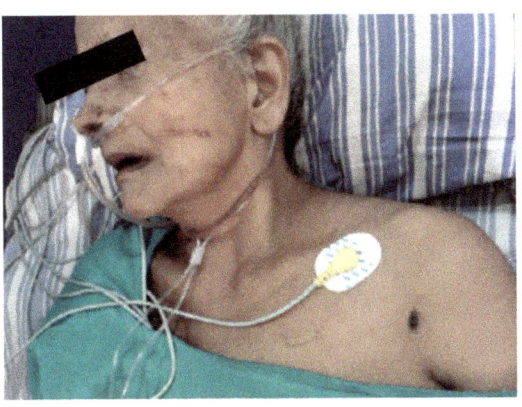
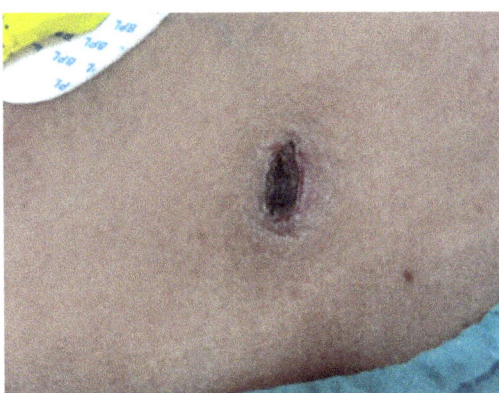

a. Identify the lesion. *(2 marks)*
b. What is the infection she is suffering from? *(2 marks)*
c. Name the drugs used in the treatment of this infection. *(2 marks)*
d. Name the possible complications of this disease. *(4 marks)*

Q6. An 85-year-old female was hospitalized due to vomiting and diminished appetite. Upon clinical examination, numerous nodular lesions were observed in and around the umbilicus.

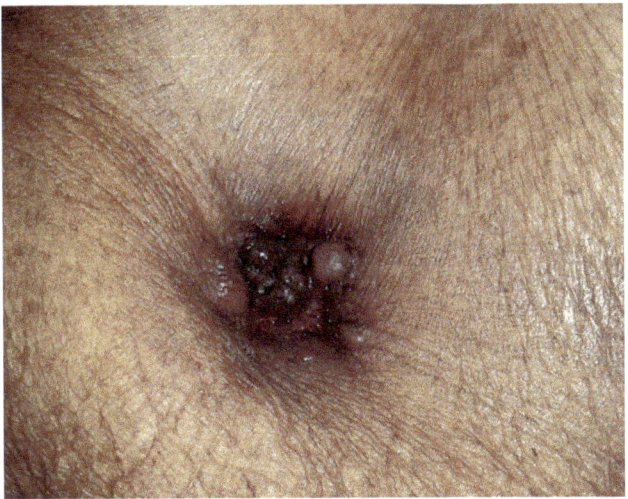

a. Identify the lesion seen in the umbilicus. *(5 marks)*
b. Name two investigations that can be done in this case. *(5 marks)*

Q7. A 52-year-old man presented with cough for 4 weeks. He has lost 3 kg of his weight for last month. His chest X-ray is shown below.

4 Infectious Diseases

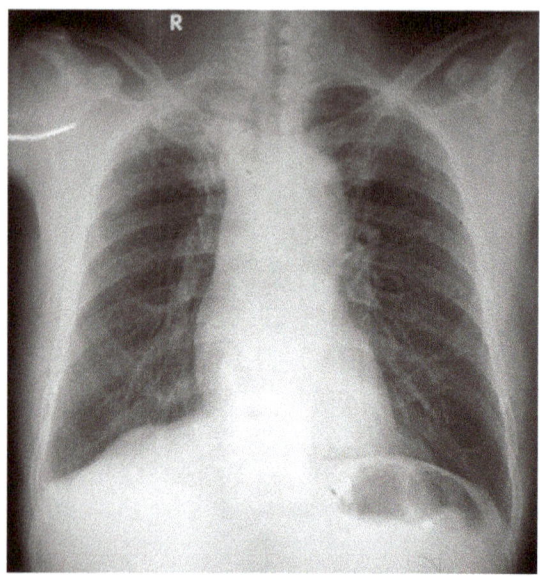

a. List the radiological abnormalities of his chest X-ray. *(3 marks)*
b. What is the most probable diagnosis for the above abnormalities? *(3 marks)*
c. List two important questions you ask in the history to support the diagnosis. *(2 marks)*
d. Enlist investigations to confirm your diagnosis. *(2 marks)*

Q8. Based on Biomedical Waste 2106 guidelines:

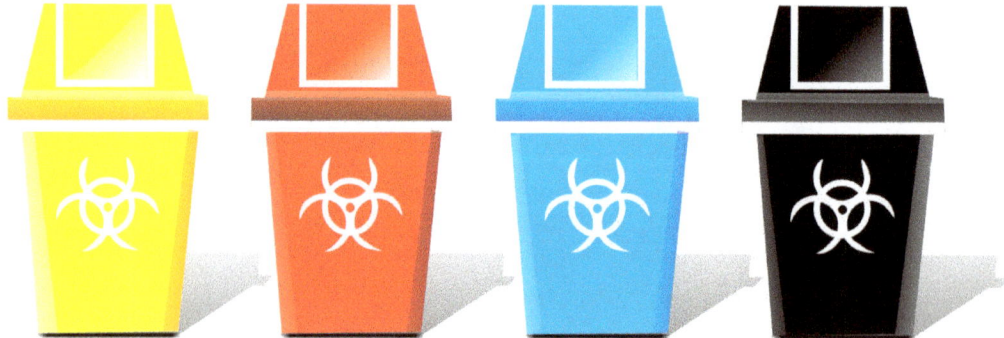

Where do you dispose the following?
a. Paper cover of gloves *(2 marks)*
b. Urine bag *(2 marks)*
c. Vacutainers *(2 marks)*
d. Placenta *(2 marks)*
e. Discarded vials *(2 marks)*

Q9. A 15-year-old female patient presents with pain abdomen. Clinical examination is normal except the following on ophthalmoscopy.

Infectious Diseases

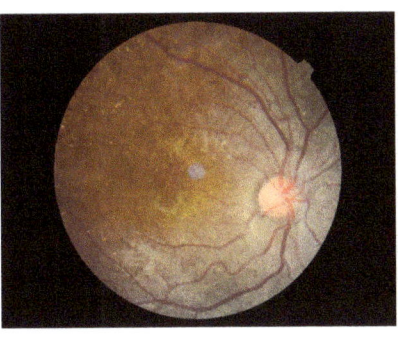
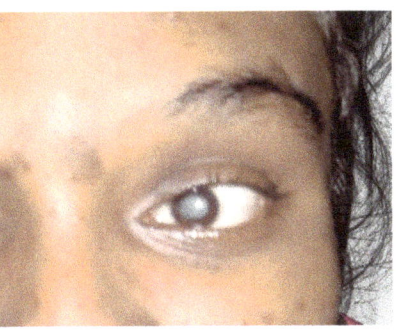

a. What is the diagnosis? (2 marks)
b. What is the classic triad? (2 marks)
c. What are the ophthalmoscopic findings? (2 marks)
d. What are the diagnosis and prevention? (4 marks)

Q10. Mr Sharma, a 55-year-old male with a history of recent surgery for a fractured femur, presents to the emergency department with acute-onset shortness of breath, chest pain, and rapid heartbeat. The patient reports that over the past 24 hours, he has been experiencing increasing shortness of breath, especially upon exertion. He also describes a sharp, stabbing pain in his chest that worsens with deep breaths. The patient denies any recent trauma to the chest.

Chest X-ray showed a wedge-shaped infiltrate, ECG showed right heart strain with S1Q3T3 pattern and laboratories showed elevated d-dimer levels.

a. What is the provisional diagnosis? (3 marks)
b. What is the radiological investigation of choice? (3 marks)
c. What are the drugs used to manage this condition? (4 marks)

Q11. A 22-year-old female diagnosed case of multidrug resistant (MDR) pulmonary TB, taking all-oral longer (AOL) regimen [bedaquiline (Bdq) based] since last 4 months and now patient presented to our side with bilateral lower limb tingling and numbness with Hb—6.2, patient unable to walk properly. Nerve conduction test shows peripheral neuropathy:

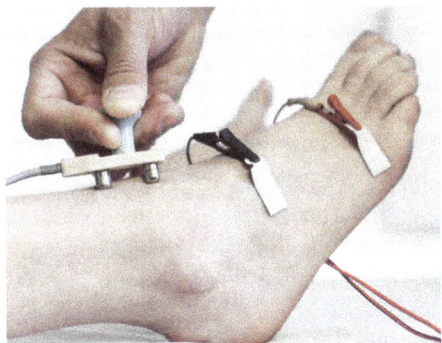

a. What is most likely cause behind this presentation? (2 marks)
b. What drug you should withhold during course of treatment? (4 marks)
c. What is replacement sequence of this drug? (4 marks)

6 Infectious Diseases

Q12. Mr Patel, a 45-year-old male with a history of chronic alcohol consumption, presents to the emergency department with severe abdominal pain that began suddenly after a heavy meal and binge drinking the night before. The patient reports epigastric pain that radiates to his back, worsens after eating, and is associated with nausea and vomiting. He denies any recent trauma or new medications.

a. What is the likely diagnosis? *(3 marks)*
b. What will be the laboratory and USG findings? *(3 marks)*
c. Name two criteria used to diagnose the condition. *(4 marks)*

Q13. Mrs Joshi has a known allergy to shellfish and she accidentally consumed shrimp at a restaurant. Shortly after ingestion, she developed sudden-onset difficulty breathing, generalized hives, and facial swelling. The incident occurred 20 minutes ago.

a. What is the diagnosis? *(3 marks)*
b. What is the drug of choice to manage this condition? *(3 marks)*
c. What is the drug of choice if patient is already on beta-blockers? *(4 marks)*

Q14. Mr Shantanu has a history of hypertension and diabetes. He arrived at the emergency department accompanied by his wife. She reports that he suddenly developed weakness on the left side of his body and slurred speech about 30 minutes ago.

a. What is the diagnosis? *(3 marks)*
b. What is the first radiological investigation to be done? *(3 marks)*
c. Name three differential diagnoses for this condition. *(4 marks)*

Q15. John's parents bring him to the emergency department with a complaint of swelling of his face and legs for the past few days. They also noticed that John's urine output has decreased and he seems more tired than usual. They deny any recent illnesses or infections. However, upon further questioning, the parents mention that John had a sore throat about 3 weeks ago but seemed to have recovered on his own.

a. What is the diagnosis? *(4 marks)*
b. What investigations will you send for workup? *(3 marks)*
c. What should be the expected urinalysis report? *(3 marks)*

Q16. Mr John Smith comes to the emergency department with a complaint of persistent cough, shortness of breath, and fever for the past 5 days. He reports a productive cough with yellow-greenish sputum. He has also experienced pleuritic chest pain and fatigue. Respiratory examination shows decreased breath sounds and crackles heard on auscultation in the right lower lung field; increased tactile fremitus on the right side.

a. What is the provisional diagnosis? *(3 marks)*
b. What is the scoring system used for deciding admission? *(3 marks)*
c. What is the most common microorganism? *(4 marks)*

Q17. A 60-year-old woman presents with dry cough and shortness of breath. Chest X-ray is shown below.

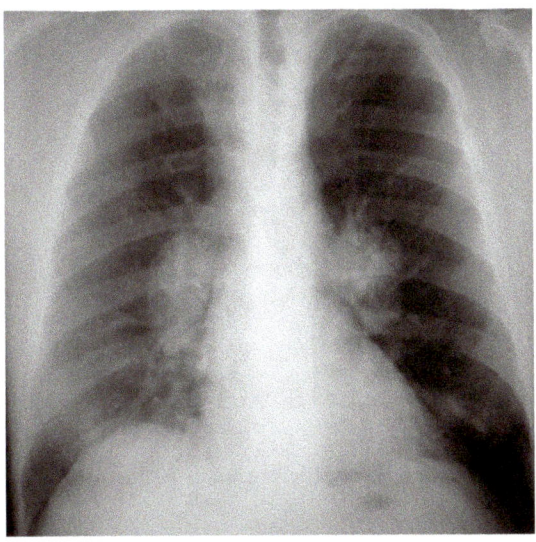

a. What are the four differentials based on X-ray findings? (5 marks)
b. Describe Scadding staging for pulmonary sarcoidosis. (5 marks)

Q18. A 41-year-old female presents with history of fever, cough, and weight loss. Chest X-ray is shown below.

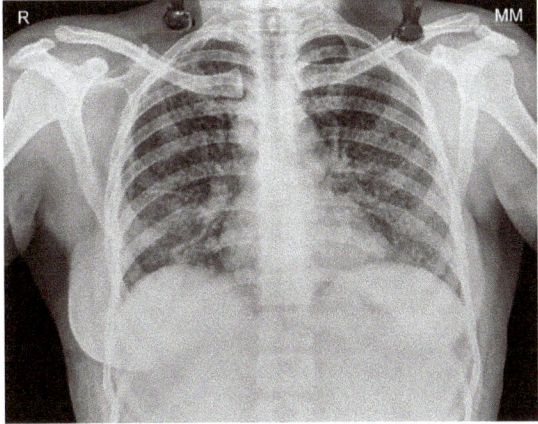

a. Identify the finding seen on the X-ray. (5 marks)
b. What are the causes for this finding? (5 marks)

Q19. A 55-year-old male patient had three episodes of seizures today morning at home. His contrast MRI is done.

Infectious Diseases

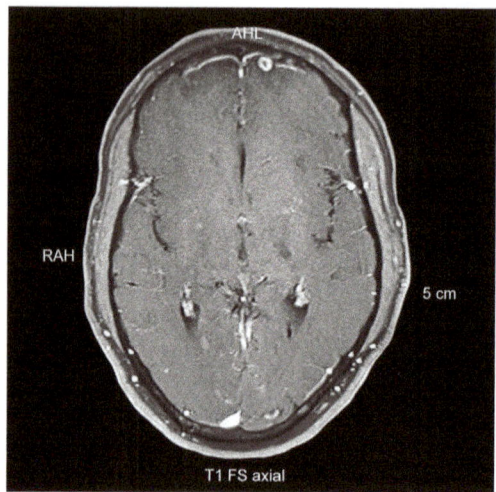

T1 FS axial

a. Identify the finding. (5 marks)
b. What are the two causes for above finding each in immunocompetent and immuno-compromised patient? (5 marks)

Q20. A 30-year-old female presents with complaints of fever and altered sensorium. CSF studies show:
- Mildly elevated opening pressure
- *Proteins:* 80 mg/dL
- *Glucose:* 30 mg/dL
- *Cell count:* 125/μL

a. Interpretation of the CSF studies and diagnosis (5 marks)
b. What is the treatment of the above condition? (5 marks)

Q21. A 25-year-old male presents with complaints of fever and seizures and weight loss. CSF studies show:
- Appearance—cob-web appearance
- Mildly elevated opening pressure
- *Proteins:* 120 mg/dL
- *Glucose:* 10 mg/dL
- *Cell count:* 210/μL
- *Lymphocytes:* 90%

a. Interpretation of the CSF studies and diagnosis. (5 marks)
b. What is the treatment of the above condition? (5 marks)

Q22. A 29-year-old male, known alcoholic, with previous history of jaundice presented with complaints of abdominal distension associated with pain, fever, and altered consciousness. USG abdomen showed gross ascites with hepatosplenomegaly. Ascitic fluid tapping was

done which showed serum ascites albumin gradient (SAAG) >1.1 and elevated total cells with absolute neutrophil count of 500/µL.
a. What is the diagnosis? (5 marks)
b. What is the treatment of the above conditions? (5 marks)

Q23. A 30-year-old male, known case of HIV and DM, presents with complaints of fever, shortness, breath, and cough. Chest X-ray showed cavitation in the middle zone. Bronchoalveolar lavage (BAL) was performed on the patient and the smear is as below.

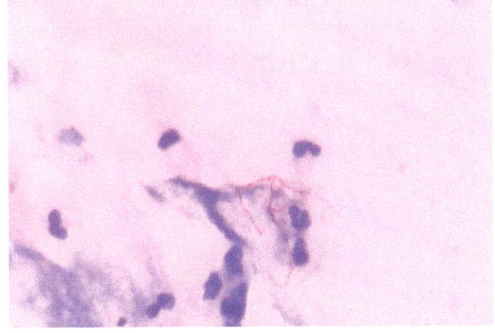

a. What are the differential diagnoses? (5 marks)
b. What are the bedaquiline-based MDR TB regimens? (5 marks)

Q24. A middle-aged men presenting with backache, low-grade fever, and paraplegia since 20 days.

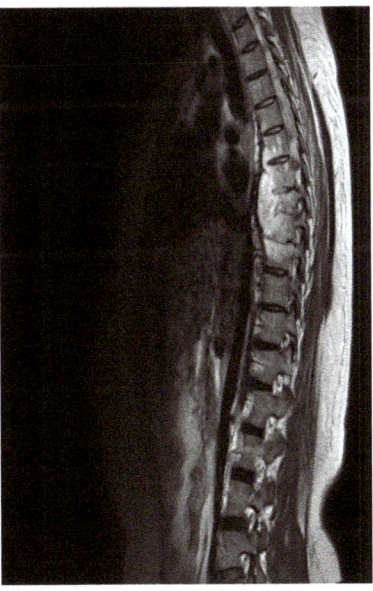

a. What is the most likely diagnosis? (5 marks)
b. What are the indications of surgical treatment of the same? (5 marks)

10 Infectious Diseases

Q25. A diabetic patient presenting with fever with chills, flank pain, hypotension, and altered consciousness.

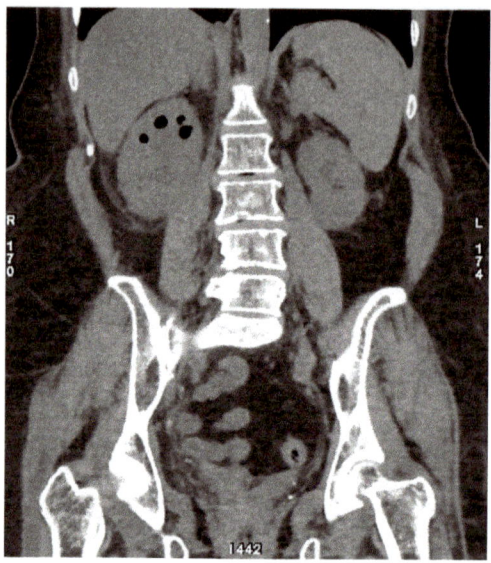

a. Identify the condition with likely causative organism involved. (5 marks)
b. What are the antibiotics used in treatment of uncomplicated cystitis? (5 marks)

Q26. A 26-year-old male, daily wage worker by profession, is having fever for last 4 days associated with productive cough. He presented to the casualty with shortness of breath (SOB) since last 1 day. Patient was tachypneic at admission and SpO_2 was 84% in room air.
A chest X-ray was taken.

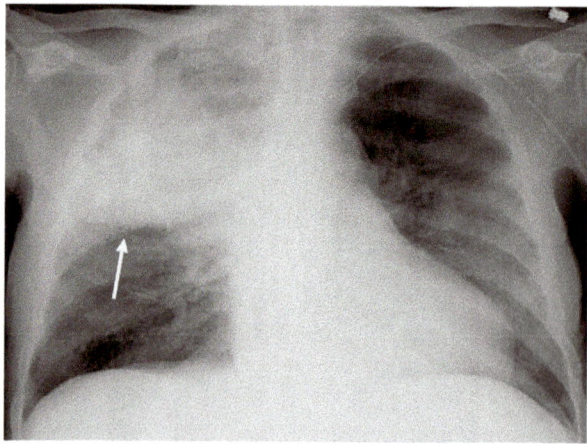

a. Read the X-ray findings. (4 marks)
b. What is provisional diagnosis? (3 marks)
c. What is the most likely causative organism? (3 marks)

Infectious Diseases

Q27. A 32-year-old male patient present with hemoptysis since 8 days admitted in respiratory medicine ward. Tuberculin skin sensitivity was done. After 3 days, the patient's tuberculin skin test (TST) result induration is shown below with measuring size of 15 × 14 mm.

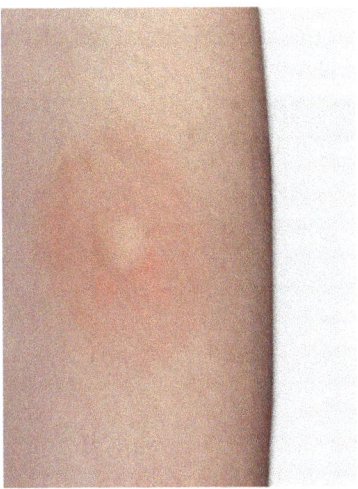

a. What is tuberculin skin testing? (2 marks)
b. How is TST administered? (2 marks)
c. Method of TST interpretation? (2 marks)
d. What are false-positive reactions? (2 marks)
e. What are false-negative reactions? (2 marks)

Q28. A 72-year-old man presented with chronic cough and weight loss for 3 weeks. Chest X-ray is given below.

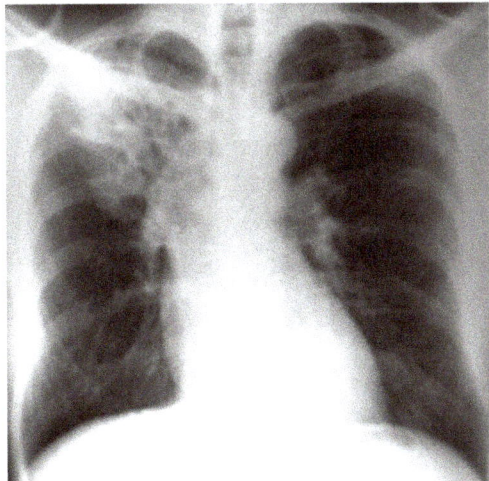

a. State abnormalities in the image. (2 marks)
b. What is the most likely diagnosis? (2 marks)

c. State two other investigations to confirm the diagnosis. *(3 marks)*
d. State the pharmacological treatment of this patient, if it comes out to be sensitive TB, what would be your prescription? *(3 marks)*

Q29. A 45-year-old gentleman presented with cough, dyspnea, fever, and weight loss for 1 month. Chest X-ray is shown below.

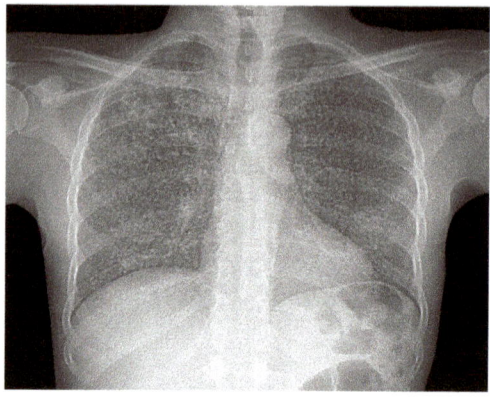

a. What is the disease shown in this X-ray? *(2 marks)*
b. What are the differential diagnoses for this condition? *(2 marks)*
c. What are methods of diagnosis of this disease? *(2 marks)*
d. What are the complications? *(2 marks)*
e. Is steroid required in this condition? If yes what is the dose? *(2 marks)*

Q30. A 25-year-old female presents in TB and chest outpatient department (OPD) with CBNAAT report as advised by PHC medical officer after she had AFB sputum + 3 positive. Sputum CBNAAT report is MTB detected and rifampicin-resistant detected. AOL regimen Bdq, Lzd, Lfx, cycloserine (Cs), clofazimine (Clf) advised. See below image and answer following questions.

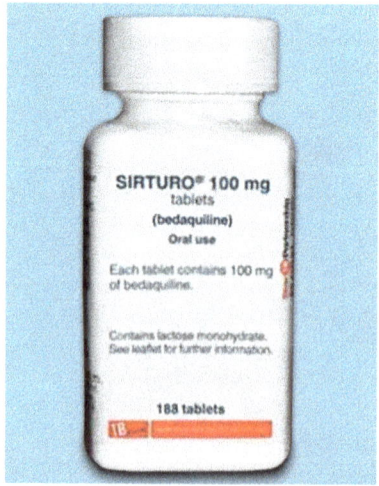

Infectious Diseases

a. What is bedaquiline and how does it works? *(2 marks)*
b. What is dose of bedaquiline? *(2 marks)*
c. What are the side effects of bedaquiline? *(3 marks)*
d. How many pills and calculation of number of pills? *(3 marks)*

Q31. Mr Ramu, a 40-year-old farmer in a village of Maharashtra, presented with episodes of fever, pain in the groin, and swelling of the scrotum for last 1 week. He frequently visits the forest for gathering firewood and often gets bitten by mosquitoes. On examination, his left inguinal lymph node was found to be swollen along with a significant hydrocele and a temperature of 39°C.
a. Which tests can be used to diagnose the patient? *(3 marks)*
b. What are the different clinical presentations of this condition? *(3 marks)*
c. What drugs are used for treating this condition? *(2 marks)*
d. What is the most preferred strategy for drug administration as a method for prevention of this condition? *(2 marks)*

Q32. A 34-year-old HIV positive male resident of Bihar presented in OPD with low-grade fever and weight loss for 1 month. Examination revealed no hepatosplenomegaly. After excluding common causes of fever, we did bone marrow examination which revealed this.

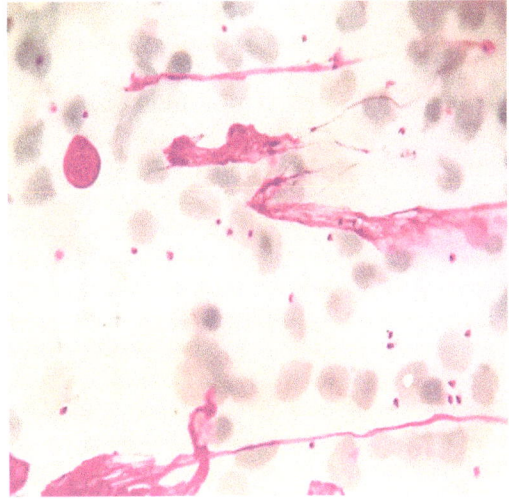

a. Describe the slide findings. *(2 marks)*
b. Any vector needed to transmit the disease. *(1 mark)*
c. Enumerate the other three diseases caused by the organism. *(3 marks)*
d. What peculiar finding was present in this patient? *(1 mark)*
e. How will you manage the case? *(3 marks)*

Q33. A 27-year-old male, migrating carpenter from a village of Malda district of West Bengal, presented with right-sided continuous headache and fever for 2 months. Then, he developed itching in his right eye and the area around the eye became swollen. Half a month later, he developed redness and photophobia and a gradual decrease in visual acuity. On examination, there was conjunctival congestion and mild uveitis. Small worm was found in anterior chamber of the right eye on slit-lamp examination.

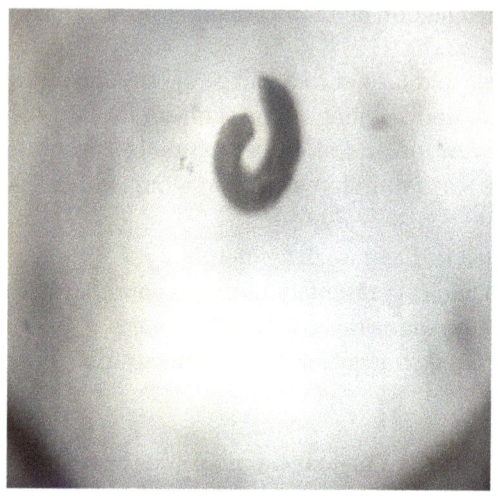

a. What is this worm? (2 marks)
b. What is this condition called? (2 marks)
c. Is there any vector for transmitting this? (2 marks)
d. How will you manage the case? (2 marks)
e. Write two life-threatening complications of this condition. (2 marks)

Q34. The details regarding the usage of drugs in a PHC of population 28,000 from January 2022 to December 2022 are given below. Go through the data carefully and answer the questions given below.

Month	Number of times patients treated (n)	Generics (units)	Antibiotics (units)	Injectable (units)
January	11,688	8,000	4,505	2,078
February	10,888	7,658	4,927	1,996
March	12,997	9,934	4,610	2,573
April	10,847	8,200	3,610	1,898
May	11,340	8,180	4,027	1,992
June	12,100	8,900	4,216	3,008
July	11,540	8,970	3,027	3,277
August	11,764	9,246	3,471	2,800
September	12,898	10,870	3,805	3,898
October	13,876	11,144	4,699	4,100
November	14,008	12,343	5,792	4,388
December	14,784	13,004	6,813	4,566

Antibiotics prescribed during the period with number of units are as given below.

Amoxicillin—8,285; doxycycline—4,022; cefalexin—3,266; cefixime—3,054; metronidazole—2,662; azithromycin—5,472; ampicillin—3,180; cloxacillin—3,519; clindamycin—2,378; cotrimoxazole—4,456; levofloxacin—3,884; and ciprofloxacin—5,064

a. Calculate the usage of antibiotics in this PHC using WHO health indicator. *(2 marks)*
b. Comment and criticize on the use of different class on antibiotics based on AWARE classification. *(2 marks)*
c. Calculate defined daily dose (DDD)/1,000 inhabitants/day for levofloxacin. *(2 marks)*
d. Explain how DDD differs from PDD. *(2 marks)*
e. Mention one effective method to tackle the inappropriate prescribing and use of antibiotic. Which plan can be implemented in your setting? *(2 marks)*

Q35. A 55-year-old man while being evaluated for 20 days fever and headache was diagnosed HIV positive with a CD4 count of 40 cells/mm³.
- On examination (O/E):

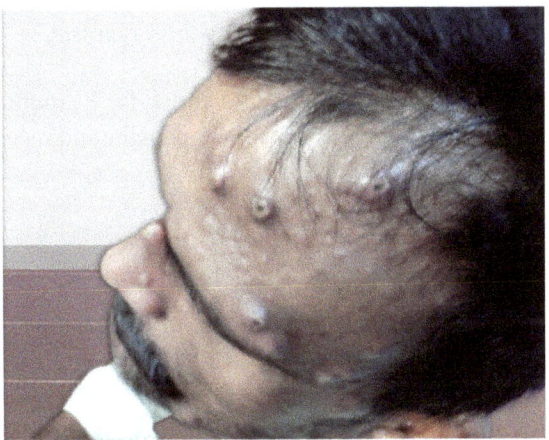

a. Name three differential diagnoses. *(3 marks)*
b. What blood investigation will support your diagnosis? *(2 marks)*
c. How will you confirm the diagnosis? *(2 marks)*
d. What is the preferred treatment option for the most likely diagnosis? *(3 marks)*

Q36. A 24-year-old gym trainer presented with loose watery stool for 4 weeks. He consulted many doctors, took metronidazole and other medicines but his symptoms were not relieved. He is on nutritional supplements since last 4 years but started using some drugs for increasing the muscle bulk for last 6 months.
- Clinical examination was unremarkable.
- Routine blood investigations were normal.
- HIV-1 and 2 (ELISA)—non-reactive
- Stool examination revealed:

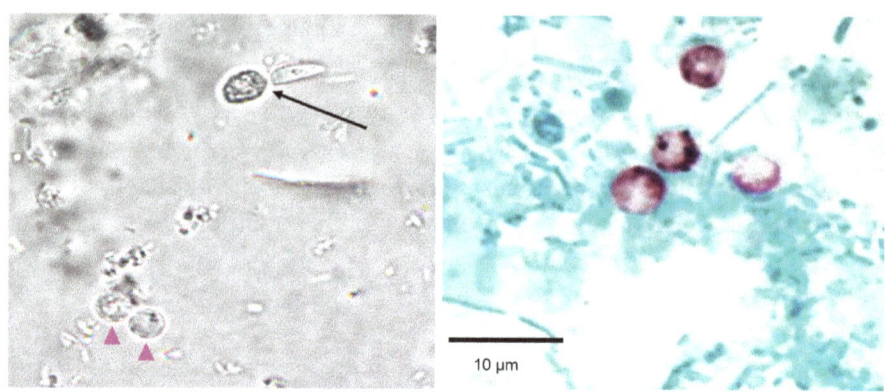

Wet mount Modified Ziehl–Neelsen (ZN) stain

a. What is the most likely diagnosis? (2 marks)
b. What are the differential diagnoses? (2 marks)
c. What could be the possible risk factor in this patient? (1 mark)
d. Write a prescription (drug, dose, and duration). (3 marks)
e. Write two other clinical manifestations caused by this organism. (2 marks)

Q37. A 28-year-old IDU presented with fever and cough for 1 month. He had two episodes of hemoptysis 5 days before admission. He consulted a doctor and received tablet cefuroxime 1 week before admission.

On examination:
- Pallor +
- Chest—bilateral coarse crepitations
- Cardiovascular system (CVS)—systolic murmur along the left lower sternal border
- Hemoglobin (Hb)—9 g/dL, TLC—10,200 (N 75 L 22 M1 B0 E2), platelet 105,000/mm^3 (investigations were done 1 week before admission)
- Anti-hepatitis C virus antibody (anti-HCV Ab) + (done from outside)

Chest X-ray (CXR) PA view and high-resolution computed tomography (HRCT) thorax

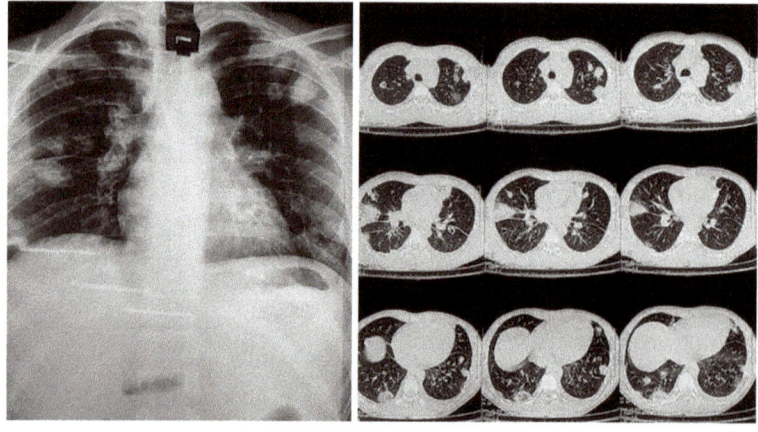

a. What is the most probable diagnosis? *(2 marks)*
b. Which two important investigations would you like to do next to confirm the diagnosis? *(2 marks)*
c. Which is the common organism responsible for this type of presentation in this kind of host? *(2 marks)*
d. What will be the empiric therapy? *(2 marks)*
e. What are the other infections we need to screen in IDU? *(2 marks)*

Q38. A 58-year-old diabetic patient recently diagnosed with sputum positive pulmonary TB (rifampicin sensitive) was started on antitubercular drugs. He stays with his son, daughter-in-law, and his 4-years-old grandson. His daughter in law is pregnant (first trimester). His son is very upset because he has read in Google about the risk of developing TB and wants medicine for his son and pregnant wife to prevent TB.
a. What kind of treatment do you want to give to this family? *(2 marks)*
b. What do you need to rule out before starting any therapy in the family members? *(1 mark)*
c. Would you like to treat this 4-year-old boy? *(1 mark)*
d. Which investigation will you advice for the pregnant lady and her husband before starting therapy? *(2 marks)*
e. What are the treatment options for preventing TB? *(2 marks)*
f. What is the preventive therapy for the pregnant lady? *(2 marks)*

Q39. A 50-year-old male, farmer from West Bengal, presents with fever and weight loss for 2 months duration.

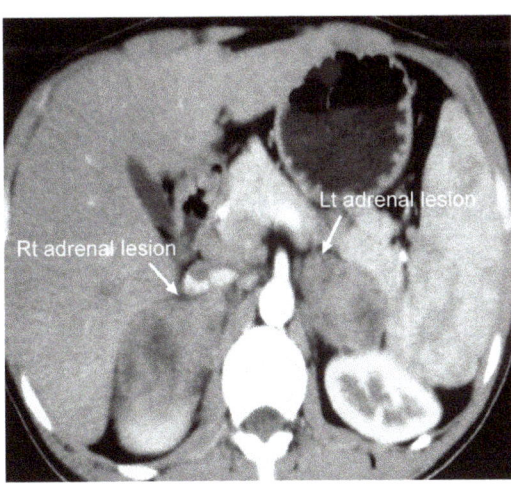
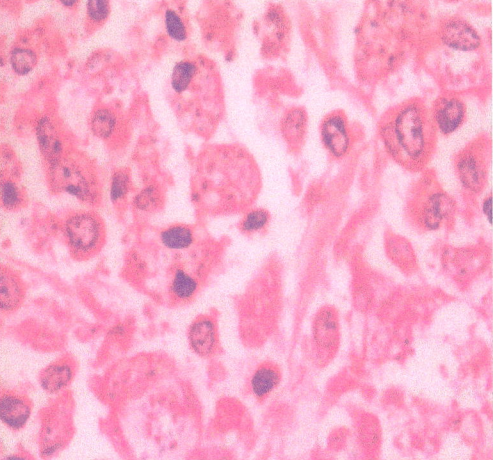

a. Name two differential diagnoses. *(2 marks)*
b. Name one noninvasive test for diagnosis. *(2 marks)*
c. How would you treat this patient? *(4 marks)*
d. Which drugs would you like to add to manage adrenal insufficiency? *(2 marks)*

18 Infectious Diseases

Q40. A 45-year-old man suffering from psychiatric illness presented with multiple discharging nodular skin lesions for 2 months.

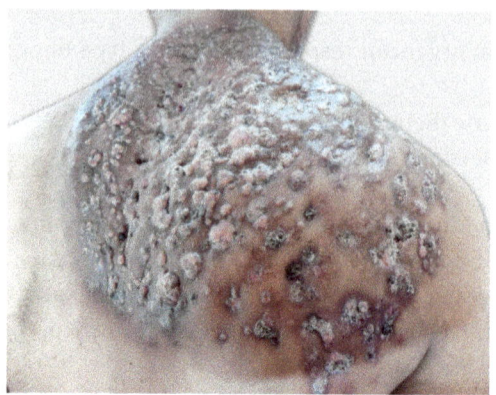

a. Name three differential diagnoses. *(3 marks)*
b. Which investigations will help you to confirm the diagnosis? *(3 marks)*
c. Tissue culture grew methicillin-sensitive *S. aureus*. Which special feature do you expect in histopathological examination (HPE)? *(2 marks)*
d. What are the treatment options in this patient? *(2 marks)*

Q41. A 28-year-old pregnant lady (first trimester) comes to your OPD clinic. She is very upset because the lady who cooks for her family has developed chickenpox and she learnt from Google that if she develops chickenpox her baby will be at high risk of developing infection.

She never had chickenpox before and she is not vaccinated.
a. What are the risks to the mother? *(2 marks)*
b. What are the risks to the baby? *(2 marks)*
c. Discuss the options for postexposure prophylaxis. *(3 + 3 marks)*

Q42. An 18-year-old college student recently came to know about human papillomavirus (HPV) vaccine from one of her friends and comes to the clinic for HPV vaccination.
a. Which serotypes are responsible for causing cervical cancer in women? *(2 marks)*
b. Which vaccines are licensed for use in India? *(2 marks)*
c. What will be the vaccine recommendation for this patient? *(3 marks)*
d. What is the recommendation in immunocompromised persons? *(3 marks)*

Q43. A pregnant mother in second trimester comes to OPD for hepatitis B vaccination. While screening for hepatitis B, she was found to be hepatitis B surface antigen (HBsAg) reactive. No history of jaundice in recent past.
a. What further investigations would you like to do? *(3 marks)*
b. How will you manage this patient? *(3 marks)*
c. What will be the advice for the new born baby? *(4 marks)*

Q44. A 28-year-old lady, dog lover, was recently vaccinated with five doses of rabies vaccine following a category 2 bite 4 months back. She is a known case of immune thrombocytopenic purpura (ITP). This time she got a category 3 bite from a street dog in the left forearm with extensive erythema and swelling.
a. What will be the postexposure prophylaxis for this lady? (4 marks)
b. Does she need immunoglobulin? (2 marks)
c. Name three bacterial infections caused after dog bite? (3 marks)
d. What is the antibiotic of choice in dog bite? (1 mark)

Q45.

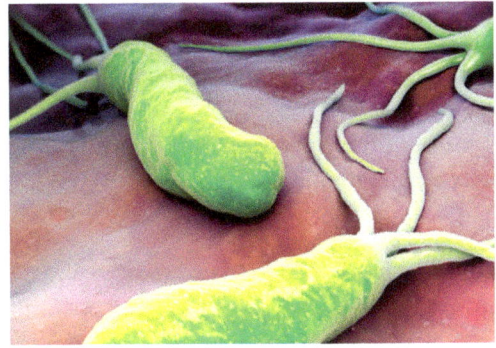

A patient was prescribed a regimen for the above bacteria, following which he complained of frequent urge of urination.
a. Identify the bacteria. (2 marks)
b. Give the regimen. (4 marks)
c. What could be the causative drug of the patient's presenting complaint? (4 marks)

ANSWERS

Ans. 1
a. The likely diagnosis is meningococcal meningitis.
b. The petechial rash is a hallmark of disseminated intravascular coagulation (DIC) and septicemia, indicating a severe systemic response to the *Neisseria meningitidis* infection.
c. (1) A lumbar puncture [cerebrospinal fluid (CSF) analysis] is used to confirm the diagnosis of meningococcal meningitis; (2) Blood culture to confirm meningococcemia.

Ans. 2
a. X-ray of abdomen shows air around the right kidney.
b. Emphysematous pyelonephritis
c. USG of abdomen, CT of Kidneys, Ureters, and Bladder (KUB), and urine culture sensitivity (C/S)
d. Parenteral antibiotics for extended spectrum beta-lactamase-producing *Escherichia coli* (ESBL *E. coli*) (Meropenem), percutaneous drainage and if no improvement nephrectomy

Ans. 3
a. Granulomatous amebic encephalitis (GAE)
b. GAE caused by certain species belonging to the genus *Acanthamoeba*, *Balamuthia*, or *Naegleria* presents as a subacute or chronic illness. Amebic encephalitis caused by *Acanthamoeba* is seen more often in immunosuppressed individuals.
c. The treatment of *Acanthamoeba* GAE often involves a combination of drugs, such as miltefosine, pentamidine, sulfadiazine, and flucytosine. Additionally, an antifungal drug called voriconazole may be used in some cases.

Ans. 4
a. Conjunctival suffusion
b. Leptospirosis

Ans. 5
a. Eschar
b. Scrub typhus
c. Doxycycline and azithromycin
d. Multiorgan dysfunction syndrome (MODS), renal failure, hepatitis, meningoencephalitis, and shock

Ans. 6
a. Sister Mary Joseph's node
b. USG or CT abdomen and Fine needle aspiration cytology (FNAC) of the lesion

Ans. 7
a. Right apical opacity due to pleuroparenchymal changes with a cavity and small right basal effusion

Infectious Diseases

b. Old pulmonary tuberculosis (TB) with possible reactivation
c. Past history of TB and contact history of TB
d. Sputum for acid-fast bacillus (AFB), sputum for GeneXpert, sputum for TB culture, and ABST

Ans. 8

a. Black
b. Red
c. Red
d. Yellow
e. Blue

Ans. 9

a. Congenital rubella syndrome
b. Cataract, hearing impairments, and heart defects
c. Macular drusens, pigmentary changes like age-related macular degeneration (ARMD) in midperiphery, salt and pepper retinopathy
d. In acute infection serum IgM up to 6 weeks and IgG in chronic up to 1 year; MMR vaccine

Ans. 10

a. Pulmonary embolism
b. CT pulmonary angiography
c. Anticoagulants

Ans. 11

a. Drug-induced peripheral neuropathy
b. Most probably linezolid (Lzd)
c. Delamanid → pyrazinamide and ethionamide → para-aminosalicylic acid (PAS) → ethambutol → imipenem

Ans. 12

a. Acute pancreatitis
b. Elevated amylase and lipase levels, USG—bulky pancreas with peripancreatic fluid collection
c. Ranson's criteria and revised Atlanta criteria

Ans. 13

a. Anaphylaxis
b. Epinephrine
c. Glucagon

Ans. 14

a. Acute cerebrovascular accident (CVA)
b. Noncontrast head computed tomography (NCCT) head to rule out hemorrhagic CVA
c. Seizure, migraine, metabolic (hyper-/hypoglycemia)

Ans. 15

a. Poststreptococcal glomerulonephritis
b. Complete blood count (CBC), liver function test (LFT), kidney function test (KFT), urine routine, and antistreptolysin O (ASO) titer
c. Proteinuria, hematuria, and RBC cast

Ans. 16

a. Right lower lobe consolidation
b. CURB-65 (confusion, uremia, respiratory rate, blood pressure, age ≥65 years)
c. *Streptococcus pneumoniae*

Ans. 17

a. Four differentials are sarcoidosis, TB, lymphoma, and histoplasmosis
b. *Stage 0*—normal chest radiograph, *Stage I*—hilar or mediastinal nodal enlargement only, *Stage II*—nodal enlargement and parenchymal disease, *Stage III*—parenchymal disease only, and *Stage IV*—end-stage lung disease (pulmonary fibrosis)

Ans. 18

a. Miliary shadows seen on the chest X-ray
b. Miliary TB, silicosis, and histoplasmosis

Ans. 19

a. Ring-enhancing lesion seen
b. Two causes in immunocompetent are TB and neurocysticercosis and two causes in immunocompromised are TB and toxoplasmosis.

Ans. 20

a. CSF suggestive of (S/O) viral meningitis
b. 10 mg/kg of acyclovir intravenously every 8 h (30 mg/kg/day total dose) for 21 days

Ans. 21

a. TB meningitis
b. Antitubercular therapy (ATT) with corticosteroids

Ans. 22

a. Spontaneous bacterial peritonitis
b. Intravenous third-generation cephalosporin for 5 days with IV albumin

Ans. 23

a. *Mycobacterium tuberculosis* (MTB), *Nocardia*, and nontuberculous mycobacteria (NTM)
b. Bdq, levofloxacin (Lfx) or Mfx, Eto, E, Z, Hh, and Cfz for 4–6 months—intensive phase; Lfx or Mfx, Cfz, Z, and E for 5 months—continuation phase

Ans. 24

a. Pott's spine

Infectious Diseases

b. Surgical indications—lack of response to chemotherapy
  - Recurrent disease
  - Severe neurological weakness
  - Static or progressive neurodeficit despite a course of ATT
  - Deformity
  - Debilitating pain
  - Instability

Ans. 25

a. Emphysematous pyelonephritis—*E. coli*
b. (1) Nitrofurantoin—100 mg BD for 5–7 days; (2) fosfomycin—3 g single-dose sachet; (3) fluoroquinolones; and (4) β-lactams

Ans. 26

a. This is a chest X-ray posteroanterior (PA) view showing a well-defined heterogeneous opacity in the right upper lobe with bronchovascular markings. Other aspect of the lung field is normal and no other bony abnormality is detected.
b. Along with the given clinical history and the X-ray findings, this is a case of right upper lobe pneumonia with a *bulging fissure sign*.
c. The most likely causative organism with this particular radiological manifestation is *Klebsiella pneumoniae*.

Ans. 27

a. The tuberculin skin test (TST), first introduced in 1908, continues to be widely utilized for assessing TB infection globally, given its cost-effectiveness and applicability in resource-limited settings.
b. Administered with either five tuberculin units (5-TU) of standard purified protein derivative (PPD-S) or 2 TU of tuberculin PPD RT23, the tuberculin should be injected exclusively intradermally on the inner surface of the forearm. Correct administration should result in the formation of a discrete wheal (6–10 mm) and the test reaction should be read within 48–72 hours.
c.

Induration of 5 mm or more is considered positive among	Induration of 10 mm or more is considered positive among	An induration of 15 mm or more is considered positive among
- HIV-infected persons - Severely malnourished children - A recent contact of a person with TB disease - People with fibrotic changes on chest radiograph consistent with prior tuberculosis (TB)	- Recent immigrants (within 5 years) from high-prevalence countries - Injection drug users - Residents and employees of high-risk congregate settings (such as prisons, nursing homes, hospitals and health facilities, and homeless shelters)	Persons with no known risk factors for TB Reactions larger than 15 mm are unlikely to be due to previous BCG vaccination or exposure to environmental mycobacteria

Contd...

Contd...

Induration of 5 mm or more is considered positive among	Induration of 10 mm or more is considered positive among	An induration of 15 mm or more is considered positive among
• Organ transplant recipients and other immunosuppressed individuals who are on cytotoxic immune-suppress agents such as cyclophosphamide or methotrexate • People who are immunosuppressed for other reasons [such as taking the equivalent of >15 mg/day of prednisone for 1 month or longer taking tumor necrosis α (TNF-α) antagonists]	• Mycobacteriology laboratory personnel • Persons with clinical conditions that place them at high risk (such as diabetes, prolonged corticosteroid therapy, leukemia, end-stage renal disease, chronic malabsorption syndromes, and low body weight) • Children below 5 years of age, or children and adolescents exposed to adults in high-risk categories	

d. Factors affecting TST results include infection with non-TB mycobacteria. Previous BCG vaccination (may yield false-positive results for many years after vaccination). Low risk of TB exposure (given the low specificity of TST, positive reactions in low-risk individuals may be false-positives). Errors in TST administration or interpretation of reaction.
e. Conditions influencing cutaneous anergy or TST reactions include:
   • Weakened immune system or immune-suppressive medication causing cutaneous anergy
   • Recent TB infection (within 12 weeks of exposure) or very old TB infection (many years)
   • Children below 5 years of age with younger children having a higher probability
   • Recent live-virus vaccination (measles and smallpox) or viral illnesses (measles and chickenpox)
   • Overwhelming TB disease (miliary TB and TB meningitis)
   • Errors in TST administration (subcutaneous injection, insufficient dose) or interpretation of reaction

Ans. 28

a. Right upper zone consolidation
b. Pulmonary TB
c. Sputum AFB smear, cartridge-based nucleic acid amplification test (CBNAAT)
d. Isoniazid (5 mg/kg)
   • Rifampicin (10 mg/kg)
   • Ethambutol (15 mg/kg)
   • Pyrazinamide (25 mg/kg)

Ans. 29

a. Miliary pattern
b. *Differential diagnosis of miliary pattern:*
   • Miliary TB
   • Tropical pulmonary eosinophilia (TPE)
   • Sarcoidosis

- Carcinoma lung with lymphangitis carcinomatosis
- Metastatic carcinoma
- Viral pneumonia
- The spread of pyogenic infection from a remote site
- Pulmonary hemosiderosis
- Nocardiosis
- Coccidioidomycosis
- Blastomycosis
- Histoplasmosis

c. The diagnosis of miliary TB may be considered based on the following criteria: (1) A clinical presentation aligning with a TB diagnosis including persistent pyrexia with an evening rise in temperature, significant weight loss, anorexia, tachycardia, and night sweats lasting over 6 weeks, responsive to anti-TB treatment; (2) Identification of the classical miliary pattern on chest radiograph; (3) Presence of microbiological, cytopathological, histopathological, or molecular evidence supporting a TB diagnosis.

d. Complications are:
- Tubercular meningitis (TBM)
- Multiorgan dysfunction syndrome
- Acute respiratory distress syndrome (ARDS)
- Air leak syndromes (pneumothorax and pneumomediastinum)
- Tubercular pericardial effusion and pericarditis
- Tubercular meningitis with focal neurological deficits
- Systemic amyloidosis
- Immune complex glomerulonephritis
- Bone marrow suppression and DIC

e. Yes, it is required if disseminated TB or manifest with TBM or patient presented with low general condition.
Intravenous dexamethasone 0.4 mg/kg/24 hours in 3-4 divided doses with a slow switch to oral therapy and taper.

Ans. 30

a. Bedaquiline is a bactericidal drug which belongs to a new class of antibiotics (diarylquinolines). Although the drug is active against many different bacteria.
b. 400 mg OD for 14 days followed by 200 mg OD on thrice a week.
c. Side effects are:
- QT prolongation in ECG
- Increased transaminases in LFT
- Severe hepatotoxicity
- Pancreatitis
- Myopathy
- Myocardial injury

d. 188 pills, 4 × 14 (number of pills × number of days) for 14 days = 56 pills; For next 22 weeks (6 × 22 = 132), total no of pills—56 + 132 = 188 pills per jar

Ans. 31

a. Rapid-format immunochromatographic card test for *Wuchereria bancrofti*, enzyme-linked immunosorbent assay (ELISA), polymerase chain reaction (PCR), and detection of microfilaria in blood
b. Hydrocele, acute adenolymphangitis, and chronic lymphatic disease (e.g., elephantiasis)
c. Diethylcarbamazine and albendazole
d. Mass drug administration (MDA) employs albendazole in combination with either DEC or ivermectin, or a combination of all three. MDA entails providing an annual dose of these medications to the entire population at risk. While the medicines exhibit limited effectiveness against adult parasites, they efficiently decrease the microfilariae density in the bloodstream and impede the transmission of parasites to mosquitoes.

Ans. 32

a. The amastigote form of *Leishmania*, which has clear two parts—kinetoplast and basal body
b. Sandflies of the genus *Phlebotomus*
c. Post kala-azar dermal leishmaniasis (PKDL), cutaneous leishmaniasis, and mucocutaneous leishmaniasis
d. Absence of splenomegaly
e. Injection amphotericin B total 40 mg/kg in 10 divided doses on day 1–5, and then weekly.

Ans. 33

a. Gnathostomiasis
b. Larva migrans
c. Cyclops
d. Oral albendazole and steroid
e. Eosinophilic myeloencephalitis and even can cause CVA.

Ans. 34

a. Percent of patient encounter/patient prescribed with antibiotics × 100
 = 53,502/148,730 × 100
 = 35.9%
b. • *Access:* Amoxicillin, doxycycline, cefalexin, metronidazole, doxycycline, ampicillin, cloxacillin, clindamycin, and cotrimoxazole
 • *Watch:* Levofloxacin, ciprofloxacin, cefixime, and azithromycin
 • *Reserve:* Nil
c. DDD/1,000 inhabitants/day = Total units of daily dose (DD) × 1,000/365 × Total number of inhabitant
 = 3,884 × 1,000/365 × 28,000
 = 0.38/1,000 inhabitants/day
d. • DDD is a unit of measurement of "therapeutic intensity" and does not necessarily correspond to actually prescribed.
 • Individual dosage regimen will differ based on patient groups, age, and weight; hence, they differ from PDD.

- PDD relates to the diagnosis on which the dosage is based. So, DDD is not an exact picture of actual usage of antibiotics.
e. - Computerized physician order entry
- Strict implementation of antimicrobial stewardship program

Ans. 35

a. Disseminated cryptococcosis, disseminated histoplasmosis, molluscum contagiosum, and talaromycosis
b. Serum cryptococcal antigen (CrAg)
c. CSF CrAg, CSF for Indian ink, and CSF for fungal culture
d. The recommended induction regimen for treating individuals with cryptococcal meningitis involves a solitary high dose (10 mg/kg) of liposomal amphotericin B, coupled with a 14-day course of flucytosine (100 mg/kg/day, divided into four daily doses), and fluconazole (1,200 mg daily for adults; 12 mg/kg/day for children and adolescents, with a maximum of 800 mg daily).
   - Fluconazole (800 mg daily for adults, 6–12 mg/kg/day for children and adolescents, up to a maximum of 800 mg daily) is advised for the consolidation phase, extending for 8 weeks subsequent to the induction phase.
   - Fluconazole (200 mg daily for adults, 6 mg/kg/day for adolescents and children) is prescribed for the maintenance phase until immune reconstitution (CD4 >200 cells/mm^3) and effective suppression of viral loads on antiretroviral therapy (ART).

Ans. 36

a. Cryptosporidiosis (*Cryptosporidium parvum* and *Cryptosporidium hominis* cause the majority of human disease)
b. Differential diagnoses are:
   - Cystoisosporiasis
   - Cyclosporiasis
c. *Risk factor:* The nutritional supplements may have contained steroids
d. *Treatment:* Tablet nitazoxanide 500–1,000 mg PO BD for 14 days
   (In immunocompetent/HIV-negative nitazoxanide 500 mg BD for 3 days and immunocompromised/HIV-positive nitazoxanide 500–1,000 mg BD for 14 days)
e. *Extraintestinal manifestations:*
   - Primary sclerosing cholangitis
   - Biliary tract disease
   - Pancreatitis
   - Respiratory cryptosporidiosis—dyspnea and bilateral pulmonary infiltrates

Ans. 37

a. Infective endocarditis (vegetation in tricuspid valve) with probably septic emboli to lung
b. Bilateral nodular densities (CXR) and subpleural wedge-shaped opacities (HRCT)
c. Blood culture and echocardiography

d. Injection vancomycin 15 mg/kg IV q12h
   i. +
   Injection gentamicin 1 mg/kg IV q8h
   ii. or
   Injection ceftriaxone 2 g q24h
   HIV and hepatitis B
e. *Staphylococcus aureus*

Ans. 38

a. Tuberculosis preventive treatment (TPT)
b. Need to rule out active TB before TPT
c. Yes. All household contact (HHC) <5 years should receive TPT
d. Tuberculin skin test or interferon-γ release assay (IGRA)
e. 6H (isoniazid daily for 6 months) or 3HP (weekly isoniazid and rifapentine for 3 months)
f. Isoniazid (5 mg/kg) daily for 6 months and pyridoxine (vitamin B_6) supplementation

Ans. 39

a. Adrenal TB and adrenal histoplasmosis
b. Urinary histoplasma antigen
c. Liposomal amphotericin B 3 mg/kg for 2 weeks followed by itraconazole 200 mg tid for 3 days, 200 mg bd for at least 12 months
d. Hydrocortisone and fludrocortisone

Ans. 40

a. Actinomycosis, nocardiosis, and botromycosis
b. Examination of the discharge, Gram stain, modified acid-fast stain, crushed granules to be inoculated for culture on sabouraud dextrose agar (SDA) and Löwenstein–Jensen (LJ) media, and HPE
c. HPE will show Splendore–Hoeppli phenomenon
d. Flucloxacillin/cefazolin

Ans. 41

a. Pregnant individuals contracting varicella face a heightened risk of severe complications, primarily pneumonia.
b. During the first or early second trimester, there is a minimal risk (0.4–2.0%) of the infant being born with congenital varicella syndrome. If a woman develops a varicella rash from 5 days before to 2 days after delivery, the newborn becomes susceptible to neonatal varicella.
c. For women susceptible to varicella [varicella immunoglobulin G (IgG) <100 mIU/mL] exposed within the initial 20 weeks of pregnancy, varicella-zoster immunoglobulin (VZIG) is recommended. In cases where susceptible women (varicella IgG <100 mIU/mL) encounter exposure after 20 weeks of pregnancy, either VZIG or acyclovir (800 mg four times a day from days 7–14 postexposure) is advised. Alternatively, oral valaciclovir at 1,000 mg three times a day can be considered.

Ans. 42

a. Globally, HPV-16 and HPV-18 collectively account for 71% of cervical cancer cases.
b. There are three licensed prophylactic HPV vaccines: (1) The 9-valent (9vHPV, Gardasil 9, Merck) available in India; (2) The Quadrivalent (4vHPV, Gardasil, Merck) also available in India; (3) The Bivalent (2vHPV, Cervarix, GlaxoSmithKline), which is also available in India.
c. For individuals initiating the series between ages 15 and 26, as well as for immunocompromised individuals, three doses of the HPV vaccine are recommended. The three-dose schedule involves vaccinations at 0, 1–2, and 6 months.
d. Immunocompromised persons, including those with HIV infection, aged 9 through 26 years, are recommended to receive three doses of the HPV vaccine.

Ans. 43

a. ICTC, HBsAg, HBV DNA, anti-HCV antibody, and LFT
b. WHO recommends that if HBV DNA >200,000 IU/mL, the tenofovir disoproxil fumarate (TDF) (300 mg) prophylaxis from 28th week of pregnancy until at least birth. If HBV-DNA report not available, then all pregnant women who are HBsAg reactive should receive TDF prophylaxis.
c. *Dose of vaccine and immunoglobulin:* The birth dose, amounting to 0.5 mL (10 µg), is administered intramuscularly in the anterolateral aspect of the mid-thigh within 12 hours of birth. This initial dose should be followed by the prompt administration of the three-dose hepatitis B-containing vaccine, which could be a monovalent hepatitis B vaccine, a tetravalent combination vaccine with DPT (DPT-Hep B), or a pentavalent vaccine (DPT + HepB + Hib).

For the prevention of mother-to-child transmission of hepatitis B virus (HBV), hepatitis B immunoglobulin (HBIG) should be administered at a dosage of 0.5 mL or 100 IU. The injection is given intramuscularly within 12–24 hours after birth and is administered in the anterolateral aspect of the mid-thigh, separate from the site where the hepatitis B vaccine has been administered.

Ans. 44

a. *Vaccination:*
   - 1 site ID on day 0 and 3 or
   - 1 site IM on day 0 and 3
b. Rabies immunoglobulin is not indicated
c. *Staphylococcus aureus, Bacteroides, Capnocytophaga* spp.
d. Amoxicillin-clavulanate

Ans. 45

a. *Helicobacter pylori* bacteria
b. Quadruple therapy—omeprazole 20 mg OD, bismuth 120 mg QID, tetracycline 500 mg QID, and metronidazole 400 mg TDS (now triple drug regimen is preferred)
c. Tetracycline—blocks V2 receptors and leads to diabetes insipidus.

SECTION 2

Immunology

QUESTIONS

Q1. A 42-year-old lady presented with petechial rashes over the legs and hands. She also complains of menorrhagia, fatigue, dizziness, shortness of breath, and limitation of physical activity. Physical examination showed pallor and mild jaundice. The spleen was enlarged. Petechiae and purpura were seen in legs. All serological, biochemical, and microbiological tests were normal. Her hemoglobin, red blood cell (RBC) count, and platelet were significantly low with neutrophilic leukocytosis. Peripheral blood smear report showed anisopoikilocytosis with the presence of microcytes, four nucleated RBC/100 white blood cell (WBCs), neutrophilic leukocytosis, and reduced platelet with no other atypical cells and hemoparasites.

a. What is the diagnosis? Discuss two differential diagnoses (D/D). *(3 marks)*
b. What further investigations would be performed? *(3 marks)*
c. Enumerate the treatment. *(4 marks)*

Q2. A 22-year-old female patient who is known hypothyroid on regular medication for last 2 years presented in outpatient department (OPD) with erythematous skin rash over face and back of neck for last 1 month with associated small joint pain with swelling of both lower limbs. Image of the skin rash is shown below.

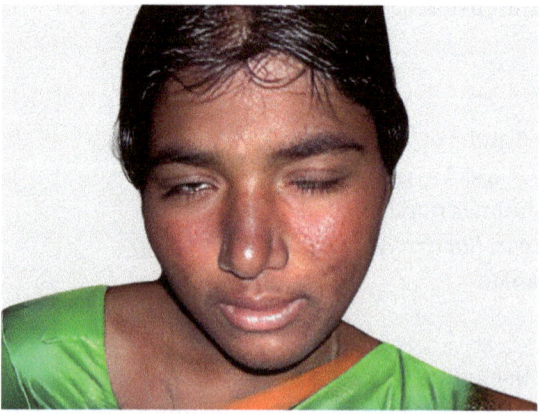

a. What is your diagnosis? *(1 mark)*
b. Mention different types of skin involvements in this disease. *(5 marks)*
c. What are the drugs you will prescribe to such a patient? *(4 marks)*

Q3.

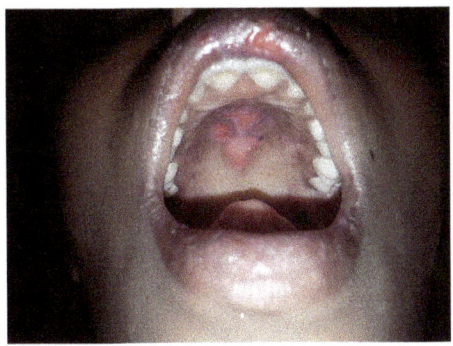

a. Describe the clinical sign seen. *(5 marks)*
b. What characteristic would distinguish a systemic lupus erythematosus (SLE) oral mucosal ulcer from other oral ulcers? *(5 marks)*

Q4.

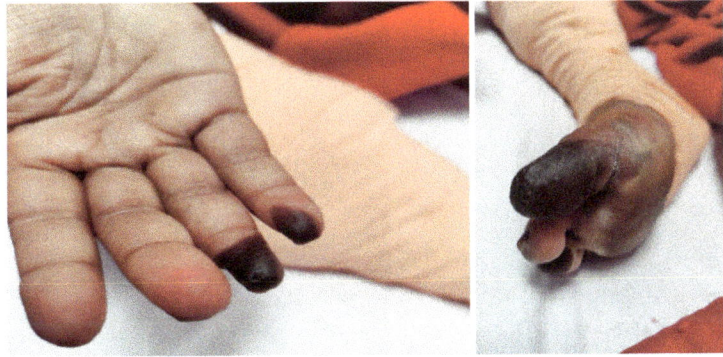

a. What is the clinical phenomenon seen above? *(3 marks)*
b. What is the difference between primary Raynaud's phenomenon and secondary Raynaud's phenomenon? *(3 marks)*
c. What procedures/tests would help in distinguishing primary Raynaud's from secondary Raynaud's? *(4 marks)*

Q5.

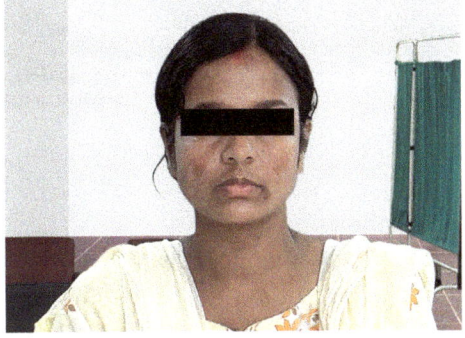

a. Describe the rash seen? (3 marks)
b. What are the differential diagnoses to be considered? (4 marks)
c. What is the screening test you would like to order for this patient? (3 marks)

Q6.

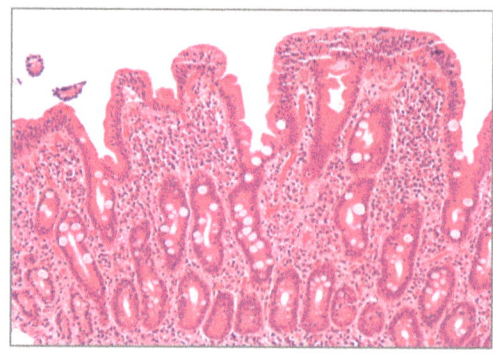
Image 1

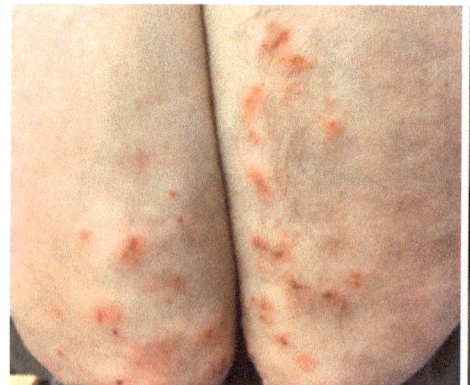
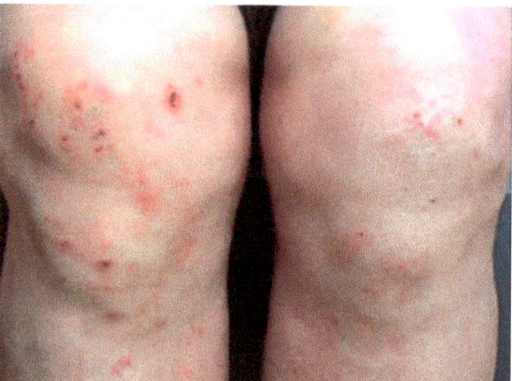
Image 2

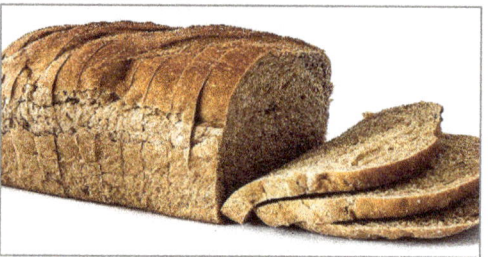
Image 3

a. Identify the disease. (3 marks)
b. Identify the associated skin condition. (2 marks)
c. Define the characteristic histological finding in Image 1. (2 marks)
d. Name the antibody involved in the pathogenesis of the disease. (3 marks)

Q7. A 27-year-old female presented with a history of systemic lupus erythematosus (SLE) of 2 years duration. She is stable on medication. She visited a physician with a following question. Kindly answer them.
a. I want to have a baby. Will pregnancy be safe? *(3 marks)*
b. Which drug is safe to be used in pregnancy for SLE? *(3 marks)*
c. Her urine examination done has shown protein 2 with red blood cells (RBCs). What further tests are required? *(4 marks)*

Q8. A 62-year-old male patient presented with new-onset abdominal pain, jaundice, and diabetes mellitus (DM). The image below depicts an abdominal computed tomography (CT) scan performed with the use of contrast.
a. What is the name of the sign and disease? *(1 mark)*
b. Close differential diagnosis (D/D) and what will be the finding then? *(2 marks)*
c. Other diagnostic clinical features? *(2 marks)*
d. How will you confirm? *(2 marks)*
e. What is the management? *(3 marks)*

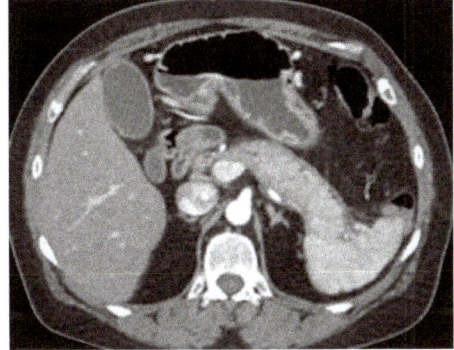

Q9. A 32-year-old man presented with recurrent bleeding from tongue when brushing teeth for several years. His mother has recurrent hemoptysis and brother has developed lung hemorrhage.

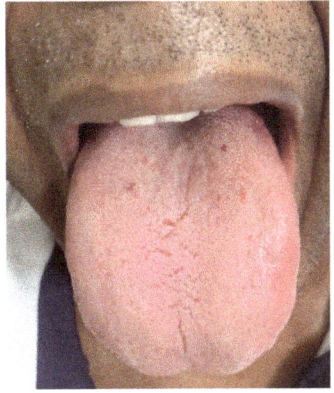

a. What is the abnormality seen in this picture? *(2 marks)*
b. What is the diagnosis? *(3 marks)*
c. What is the underlying pathology of this condition? *(3 marks)*
d. What is the inheritance? *(2 marks)*

Q10. A 30-year-old male presents with complaints of dysesthesia and weakness in the lower limbs since the last 2–3 days which has been progressive in nature rendering the patient unable to walk.

On examination, there is areflexia, hypotonia, and paraplegia. No sensory level is seen. No bowel/bladder involvement is seen.

Cerebrospinal fluid (CSF) studies show:
- Normal pressure and appearance
- Proteins: 90 mg/dL
- Glucose: 55 mg/dL
- Cell count: 3

a. Interpretation of the CSF studies and diagnosis. *(5 marks)*
b. Name the criteria used for the diagnosis of this condition. *(5 marks)*

Q11. A 40-year-old male presented with complaints of diarrhea, abdominal pain, and weight loss since past few days. On further enquiry, she had preceding history of arthritis and arthralgia. Endoscopy guided biopsy of small intestine showed following findings:

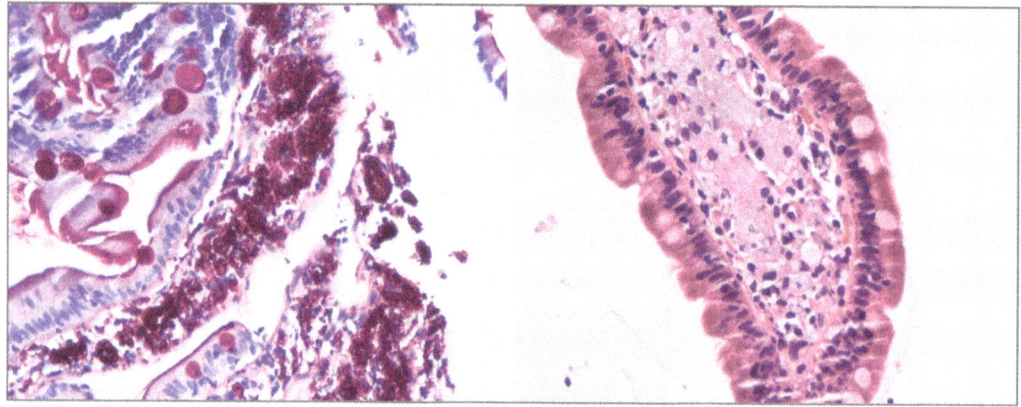

a. What is the most likely diagnosis and causative organism? *(5 marks)*
b. Name the extraintestinal features of celiac disease. *(5 marks)*

Q12. A 40-year-old female diagnosed with systemic lupus erythematosus (SLE) presented with oliguria, facial puffiness with elevated creatinine levels, and urine analysis showing proteinuria and presence of active sediments. Biopsy was done which is given below.

Immunology

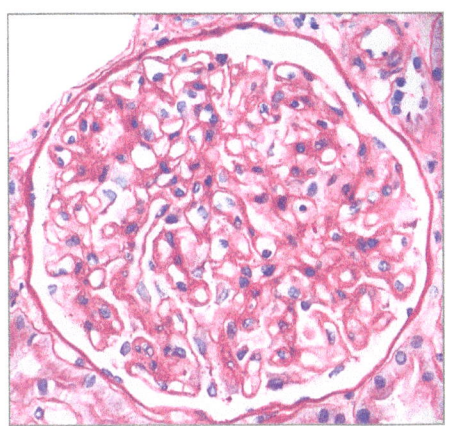

a. Name the condition. (3 marks)
b. Give its classification. (3 marks)
c. Name the various antibodies present in patients of SLE. (4 marks)

Q13.

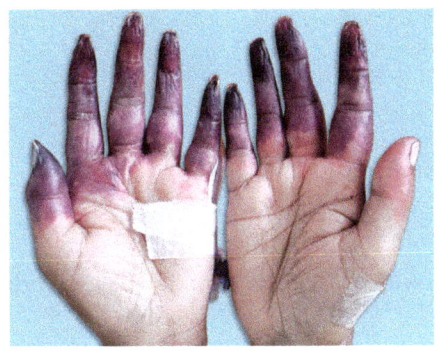

a. Give the differential diagnosis of the above conditions. (5 marks)
b. Enumerate clinical features of systemic sclerosis. (5 marks)

Q14.

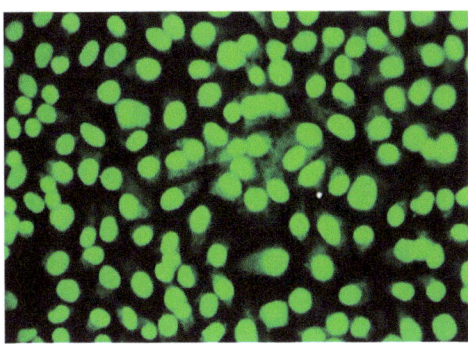

a. What is the test depicted in the picture? (2 marks)
   What pattern is present? (2 marks)
   What is the minimal dilution acceptable? (3 marks)
b. What test would the next logical step be? (3 marks)

Q15. A man presented with history of palpitations since last 1 year. He has undergone a weight loss of 10 kg in the last 6 months in spite of increase in appetite. Frequency of bowel habits has increase since last 6 months. He is also having tremor which is affecting his daily activities. Now within the last 3 months he complains of swelling in the anterior aspect of legs which is gradually progressive. On examination, HR—130/min, BP—122/60 mm Hg Intentional Tremor is present. On eye examination, proptosis is present.

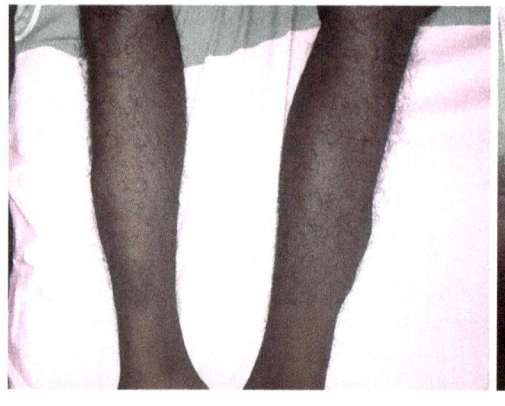
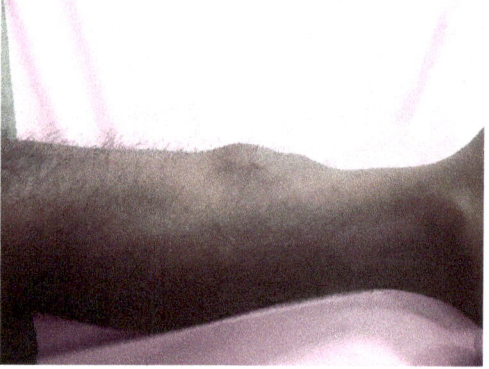

a. What is examination finding seen over lower limb? (4 marks)
b. What is your diagnosis? (3 marks)
c. What is device known as which is used to quantify the eye finding of proptosis? (3 marks)

Q16. A 55-year-old female presented with pain in multiple joints, involving the small joints of the fingers for the last 20 years. The pain was more in the morning and it was difficult to make a fist for her when she wakes up, but the pain decreases with activity. She consumed over-the-counter analgesics to deal with her pain for years and had developed deformity during the course of time as shown below.

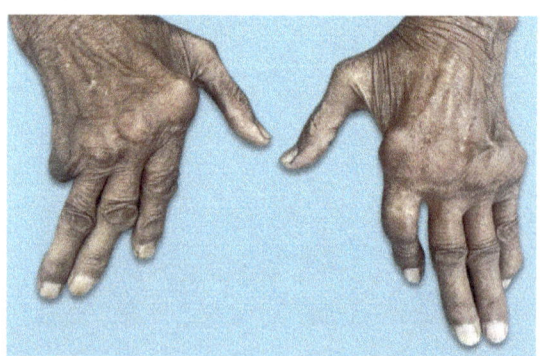

a. What is the diagnosis? (2 marks)
b. Name some bony deformities that are seen in this condition. (3 marks)
c. What are most common antibodies tested for in this condition for diagnosis? (2 marks)
d. Name the most common drugs used for managing the condition. (3 marks)

Q17. A 52-year-old man was referred to the clinic for evaluation of a pruritic rash and angioedema which started 7 hours after eating beef. His rash started on his extremities and later spread to become generalized pruritic hives. He reported tick bites in the past. He responded to the treatment.
a. What is the diagnosis? (4 marks)
b. How would you confirm the diagnosis? (3 marks)
c. How would you treat and advise? (3 marks)

ANSWERS

Ans. 1
a. Evans syndrome [autoimmune destruction of circulating blood cells in autoimmune hemolytic anemia (AIHA) and immune thrombocytopenic purpura (ITP)]. Differential diagnosis (D/D): Hemolytic uremic syndrome and disseminated intravascular coagulation
b. Direct Coombs test, antinuclear antibody (ANA), and viral antibodies
c. Corticosteroids with or without intravenous immunoglobulin (IVIG) and rituximab

Ans. 2
a. Systemic lupus erythematosus (SLE)
b. Malar rash, bullous lupus erythematosus (LE), psoriasiform lesion, annular lesion, discoid lupus erythematosus (DLE), scarring, or nonscarring alopecia
c. Hydroxychloroquine (HCQ), steroid, angiotensin receptor blocker (ARB), statin, cyclophosphamide (CYC), or mycophenolate mofetil (MMF)

Ans. 3
a. Oral mucosal ulcer on the roof of the palate. The characteristic SLE ulcer is at the junction of the hard and soft palate.
b. The SLE-associated oral ulcer is usually painless as compared to aphthous ulcers in the mouth or ulcers secondary to thermal or other trauma.

Ans. 4
a. Dry gangrene as a result of Raynaud's phenomenon in this particular patient. However, dry gangrene can also be a result of vascular insufficiency not related to Raynaud's phenomenon.
b. Primary Raynaud's phenomenon (also known as Raynaud's disease) is seen in young women with no underlying disease process. It is mandatory to do an antinuclear antibody (ANA) by indirect immunofluorescence (IIF) for this subset of patients and they must be screened with repeat ANA testing at regular intervals.
c. Nailfold capillaroscopic (NFC) changes would clearly indicate an underlying AICTD (autoimmune connective tissue disease as the cause for Raynaud's disease), whereas, in primary Raynaud's phenomenon, there will be no visible NFC changes.

Ans. 5
a. There is a visible hyperpigmentation in the malar region in the characteristic butterfly pattern with a sparing of the nasolabial folds. The rash is highly suggestive of systemic lupus erythematosus.
b. The most important differential diagnosis to be considered is dermatomyositis, especially if there is also associated muscular weakness; however, the rash in dermatomyositis would involve the nasolabial folds.
c. ANA by IIF (antinuclear antibody by indirect immunofluorescence)

Ans. 6

a. Celiac disease
b. Dermatitis herpetiformis
c. Histologic finding—loss of villi and lymphocytic infiltration
d. Anti-tissue transglutaminase/anti-endomysial antibodies

Ans. 7

a. Women with systemic lupus erythematosus (SLE) have more adverse pregnancy outcomes than control women. In a study of the nationwide inpatient sample that included 4,000 SLE pregnancies, lupus pregnancies had longer hospital lengths of stay, increased hypertension, higher rates of intrauterine growth restriction (IUGR), and C-section rate
b. Hydroxychloroquine, low-dose prednisolone, and low-dose azathioprine
c. Double-stranded deoxyribonucleic acid (dsDNA), compliment levels, and kidney biopsy to rule out lupus nephritis

Ans. 8

a. Computed tomography (CT) abdomen demonstrating a diffusely enlarged, hypoattenuating pancreas with a capsule-like rim—capsule sign (peripancreatic extension of inflammatory cell infiltration) and seen in type 1 autoimmune pancreatitis.
b. In poor response or high attenuation rim of compressed normal parenchyma by cancer, rule out for cancer.
c. Associated with other immunoglobulin G4 (IgG4)-related diseases—submandibular gland enlargement, renal lesion, and retroperitoneal fibrosis.
d. HISORt criteria—histology, imaging, serology (IgG4 levels), other organ involvement, response to steroid therapy, trial of steroid therapy.
e. 40 mg/day for 2–4 weeks followed by 5 mg/week tapering depending upon the signs and symptoms (s/s).

Ans. 9

a. Red spots in the base of the tongue
b. Hereditary hemorrhagic telangiectasia (HHT) or Osler–Weber–Rendu syndrome
c. An inherited disorder characterized by malformations of various blood vessels (vascular dysplasia). It results in external and internal bleeding and shunting of blood. The arteriovenous malformation of various blood vessels may occur in the lungs, brain, spinal cord, and liver.
d. Autosomal dominant

Ans. 10

a. Guillain–Barré syndrome (GBS)
b. BRIGHTON criteria for diagnosis of GBS

Ans. 11

a. Whipple disease—Tropheryma whipplei
b. Type 1 diabetes mellitus (DM)/autoimmune thyroid disease/dermatitis herpetiformis

Ans. 12

a. Lupus nephritis
b. Classification:
   - *Class I:* Minimal mesangial lupus nephritis
   - *Class II:* Mesangial proliferative lupus nephritis
   - *Class III:* Focal lupus nephritis
   - *Class IV:* Diffuse lupus nephritis
   - *Class V:* Membranous lupus nephritis
   - *Class VI:* Advanced sclerotic lupus nephritis
c. Antinuclear antibodies
   - Anti-dsDNA
   - Anti-C1q
   - Anti-Sm
   - Anti-RNP
   - Anti-Ro and Anti-La
   - Antihistone
   - Antiphospholipid

Ans. 13

a. Ischemic digital ulcers—differentials include:
   - Systemic sclerosis
   - Peripheral arterial disease
   - Diabetes mellitus
   - Vasculitis
   - Hypercoagulability
b. Skin involvement—Raynaud's phenomenon, bilateral (BL) symmetrical skin thickening, and calcinosis cutis
   - Interstitial lung disease and pulmonary arterial hypertension
   - Gastrointestinal tract (GIT) features—gastroesophageal reflux disease (GERD), gastroparesis
   - Scleroderma renal crisis

Ans. 14

a. ANA by IIF (antinuclear antibody by indirect immunofluorescence)
   - *Homogenous pattern:* Minimal acceptable dilution is 1:80 as per International Consensus on Antinuclear Antibody Patterns (ICAP). The reason is that at dilutions <1:80 (e.g., 1:40) much larger numbers of asymptomatic and normal healthy population would test as positive for the ANA by IIF.
   - ANA by IIF is the recommended screening test and is considered superior to ANA by enzyme-linked immunosorbent assay (ELISA) as it screens for a larger number of antigens.
   - www.ANApatterns.org is an excellent site to refer to and learn from.
b. ANA profile or CENA (combined extractable nuclear antigen)

Ans. 15

a. The examination findings seen over the lower limbs are firm, nontender, and noninflammatory nodular swellings. In view of the above clinical history provided, it is suggestive of *pretibial myxedema*.
b. In view of the given history (loss of weight, tremor, palpitations, increased frequency of bowel habits) with corroborative examination findings of tachycardia, proptosis, and pretibial myxedema, a diagnosis of *Graves' disease* is made.
c. The device used to quantify the eye findings is *Hertel's exophthalmometer*.

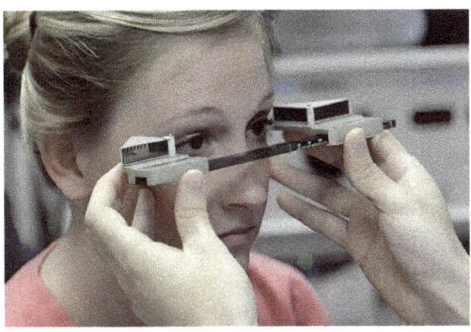

Ans. 16

a. Rheumatoid arthritis (RA)
b. Swan neck deformity, Boutonniere deformity, Hitchhiker's thumb, and Vaughan-Jackson deformity
c. RA factor and anti-cyclic citrullinated peptide (anti-CCP) antibody
d. Methotrexate, hydroxychloroquine, sulfasalazine, leflunomide, Janus kinase inhibitor (JAK) Inhibitors, tumor necrosis factor (TNF) inhibitors, rituximab, and steroids

Ans. 17

a. *Alpha-gal syndrome:* α-gal syndrome, also known as red or mammalian meat allergy, results from immunoglobulin E-mediated hypersensitivity responses to the carbohydrate galactose-α-1,3-galactose (α-gal).
b. The diagnosis is made through careful history-taking, identification of tick exposure, and positive α-gal serum-specific immunoglobulin E (sIgE) serology. Patients with α-gal sIgE of >2% of the total serum IgE is highly suggestive for diagnosis
c. Current management of α-gal syndrome involves avoidance of mammalian meats and tick bites and patients may use an antihistamine for very mild symptoms; intramuscular epinephrine is the treatment of choice for anaphylaxis.

SECTION 3

Rheumatology

QUESTIONS

Q1. A 35-year-old female presented with a fever of 102.2 for 1 week, arthralgia or arthritis lasting at least 2 weeks. She had the appearance of a pink or salmon-colored rash during fever spikes. She had an elevated white blood cell count (leukocytosis) and a negative antinuclear antibody (ANA) by immunofluorescence.
a. What diagnosis comes to your mind with the above presentation? *(3 marks)*
b. What further investigations would you carry out? *(4 marks)*
c. How would you manage? *(2 marks)*
d. Mention one recently approved drug in addition. *(1 mark)*

Q2. A 55-year-old female presented with swelling feet for 3 months. She had a long-standing history of rheumatoid arthritis (RA) diagnosed 20 years back. She tested positive 2+ for urine albumin to creatinine ratio (ACR).
a. What is the likely complication has she developed? Give full diagnosis. *(3 marks)*
b. How will you confirm the diagnosis? Mention the stain used. *(4 marks)*
c. Enumerate three drugs to control this disorder. *(3 marks)*

Q3. A enthusiastic PG teacher was teaching the residents importance of history-taking in rheumatology. He asked the following questions. Please answer them:
a. Enumerate three basic questions to be asked to a patient with joint pains. *(3 marks)*
b. Describe three conditions presenting with asymmetric joint pains of >3 weeks. *(3 marks)*
c. Enumerate three joints typically involved the ankylosing spondylitis. What is enthesitis? *(4 marks)*

Q4. A 24-year-old lady visited the general practitioner with history of joint pains and a rash. She was advised to get the ANA and rheumatoid factors (RFs) done:
a. Describe the methods of doing ANA. What titer is considered diagnostic of systemic lupus erythematosus (SLE) in a suspected case? *(2 marks)*
b. Name three conditions with a positive ANA apart from SLE. *(3 marks)*
c. Describe three conditions with a positive RF. *(3 marks)*
d. How do you confirm the diagnosis of RA with a biochemical test? Give its full form. *(2 marks)*

Q5. A 30-year-old lady presented with a long-standing diastolic murmur. Her hand examination is shown in the image below.

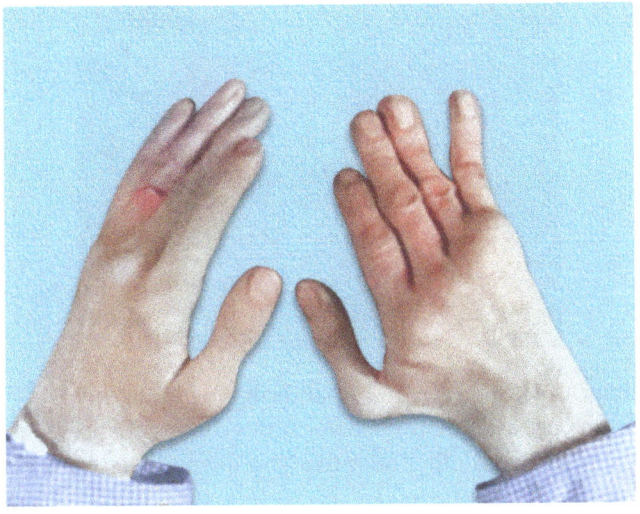

a. Identify the condition. (5 marks)
b. List two causes. (5 marks)

Q6. A 62-year-old woman comes to the hospital due to activity-related joint pain in the hands and periodic morning stiffness that lasts 10–15 minutes. The pain is moderately severe and has begun to limit her activities. The patient has attempted to treat the pain with paracetamol, which provided only partial relief. Past medical history is notable for hypertension (HTN) and diabetes mellitus. Physical examination shows firm nodules over the distal interphalangeal joints bilaterally as shown in the image below.

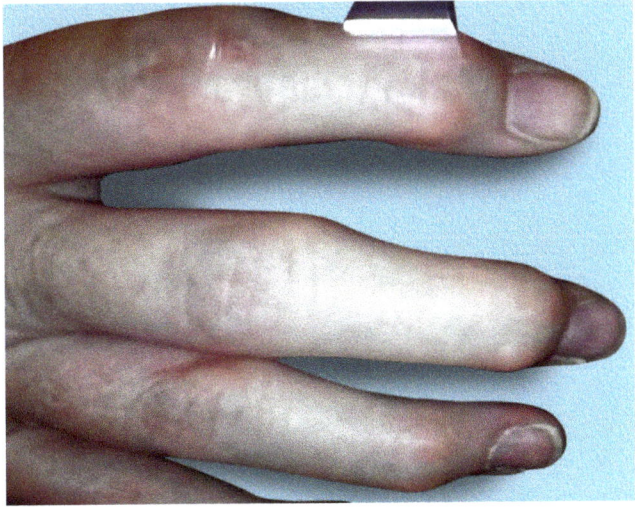

What is the diagnosis? (10 marks)

Q7.

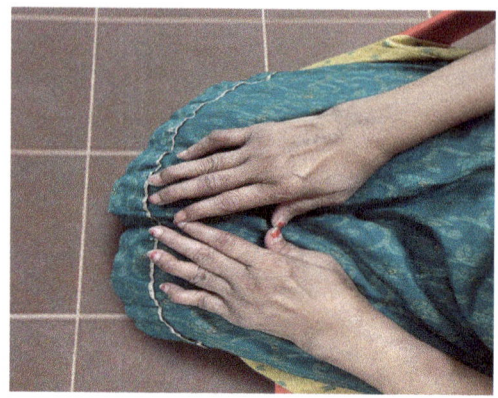

a. What kinds of deformities are seen in the hands in the photograph? (1 mark)
b. Which inflammatory arthritis are these deformities characteristically seen in? (2 marks)
c. What are the serological and other tests that you would like to specifically order for this patient? (1 mark)
d. What are the ACR-EULAR (American College of Rheumatology and the European League Against Rheumatism) 2010 criteria for classification of RA? (2 marks)
e. What is the nondeforming form of inflammatory arthritis seen in SLE known as? (1 mark)
f. What is the eponymous name for arthritis resulting due to neuropathy? (1 mark)

Q8.

The homunculus represents a 32-year-old male patient who has developed pain and swelling of the bilateral knee joints and left ankle joint over the last 3 months.

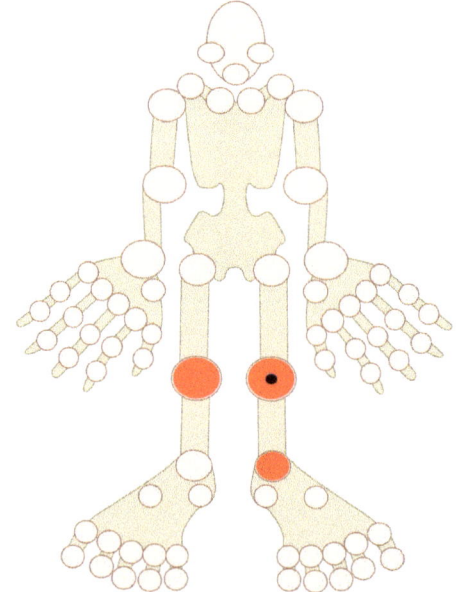

What is the pattern of arthritis? (10 marks)

Q9.

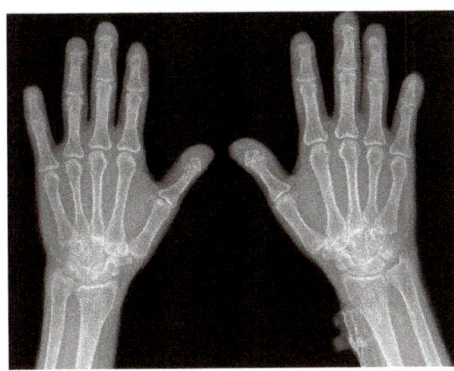

a. What are the features seen on the radiograph? (5 marks)
b. What is the differential diagnosis of acroosteolysis? (5 marks)

Q10.
A 45-year-old female comes to medicine outpatient department (OPD) with complaints of multiple joint pain (small > large) with morning stiffness lasting for >60 minutes for the last 2 years. On examination, following are seen:

a. What is RF and two conditions associated with positive RF? (3 marks)
b. What is Felty's syndrome? (2 marks)
c. Name some disease-modifying antirheumatic drugs (DMARDs) used in treatment. (2 marks)
d. How will you define remission in RA, mention any two criteria? (3 marks)

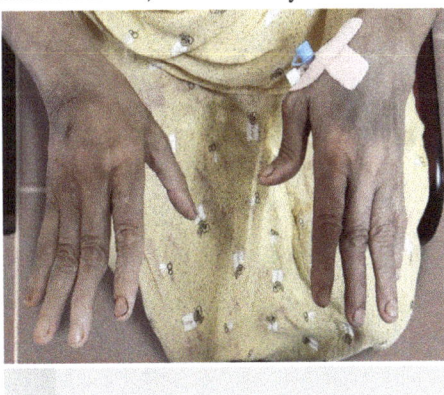

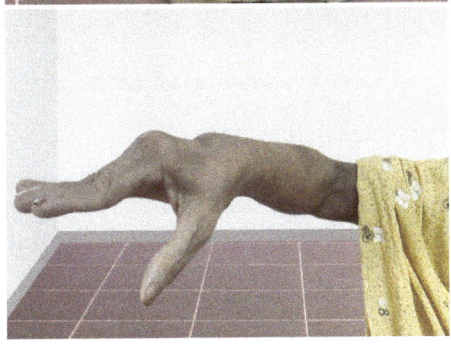

Q11.

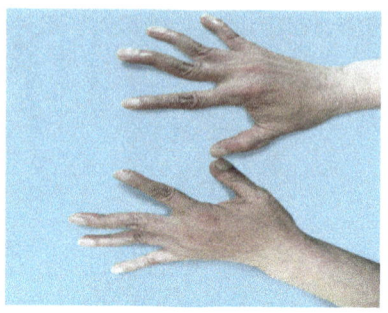

a. Identify the deformity. (5 marks)
b. EULAR criteria for RA. (5 marks)

Q12.

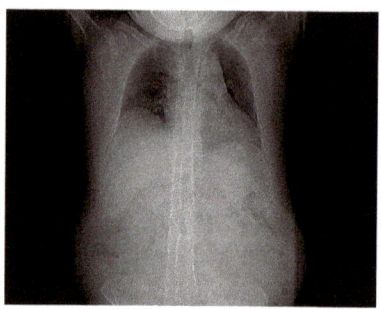

a. Identify the above X-ray and name the condition associated with it. (5 marks)
b. Name the extra-articular manifestations of above condition. (5 marks)

Q13.

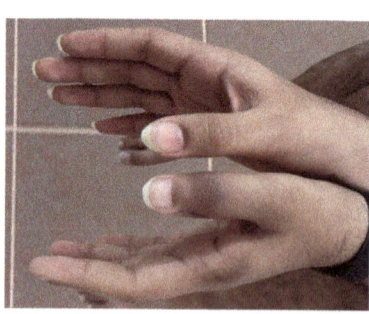

a. Identify the clinical sign depicted in the image. (2 marks)
b. Describe dactylitis. (2 marks)
c. In which conditions are you likely to see dactylitis in a patient? (2 marks)
d. What are the clinical patterns of arthritis seen in psoriatic arthritis as described by Moll and Wright? (2 marks)
e. What are the CASPAR (Classification criteria for Psoriatic Arthritis) criteria for classification of psoriatic arthritis? (2 marks)

Q14.

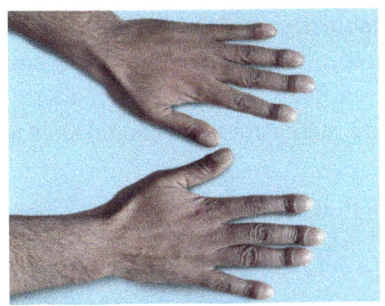

a. What is the clinical sign seen? (5 marks)
b. What is primary hypertrophic osteoarthropathy (PHO)? (5 marks)

Q15.

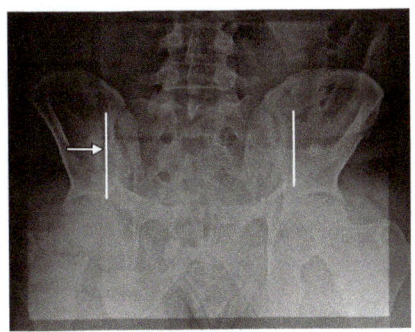

a. What is the pathological finding seen on the radiograph? (4 marks)
b. What are the grades of sacroiliitis (New York criteria)? (3 marks)
c. What is meant by active sacroiliitis on MRI as per ASAS (Assessment in Spondyloarthritis International Society) criteria? (3 marks)

Q16.

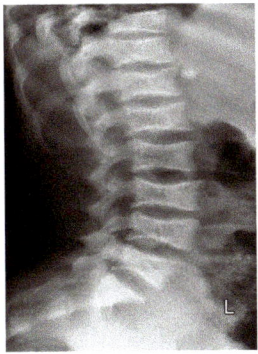

a. What abnormality does the X-ray lateral spine? (3 marks)
b. What are the differential diagnoses for this condition? (4 marks)
c. What specific investigations to be done for final diagnosis? (3 marks)

Rheumatology

Q17. A 48-year-old male presented with history of severe joint pain in bilateral knee and small joints of the foot with unable to walk due to severe pain. He is a known alcoholic for last 10 years. He has a history of cerebrovascular accident (CVA) [intracerebral hemorrhage (ICH)] with left sided hemiparesis 1 year back. No history of diabetes or HTN. There were multiple nodular lesions over the dorsum of the foot and bilateral knee was swollen and tender. Serum uric acid was 11.3 mg/dL.

Aspirate from knee joint and nodular swelling was taken. X-ray of bilateral foot was done.

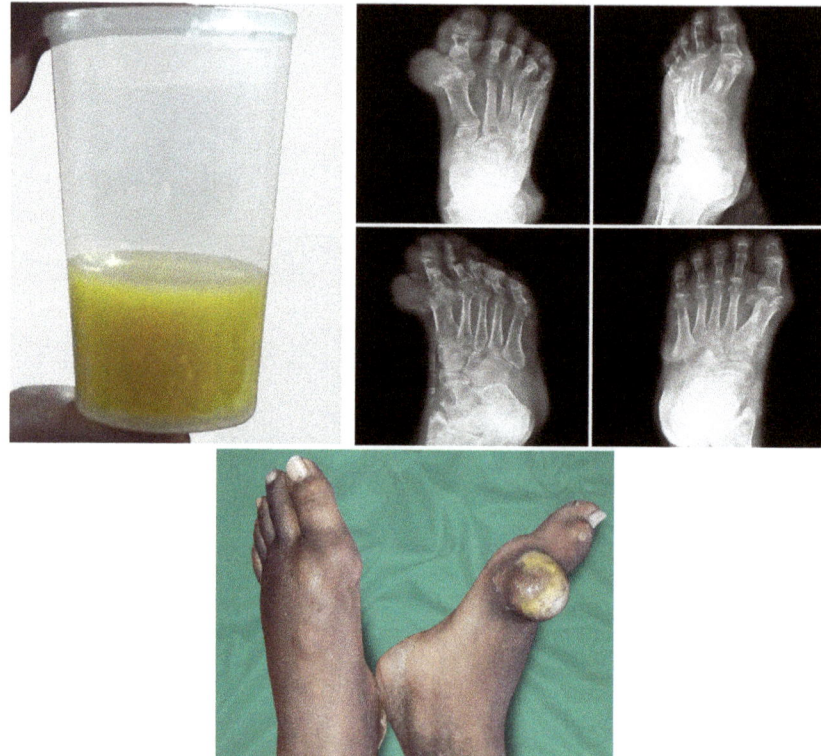

Microscopy from the aspirate shows the following:

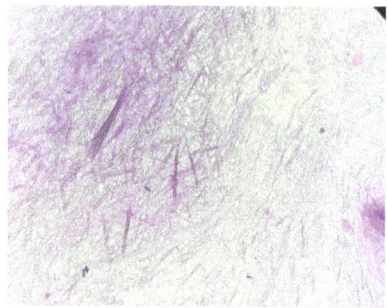

a. Read the X-ray findings. (4 marks)
b. What is your diagnosis? (3 marks)
c. What are the drugs used in the acute phase of the disease process? (3 marks)

Rheumatology

Q18. A 33-year-old female complains of (c/o) dry mouth and brittle eyes since 6 months and has now started having lower limb cramps and weakness since 1 month.
On evaluation, Hb—7.6 mg/dL, hypokalemia—2.9 mEq/L, ECG—U-waves, and urine pH—6.1

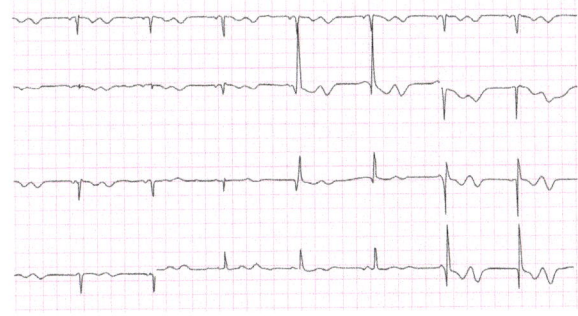
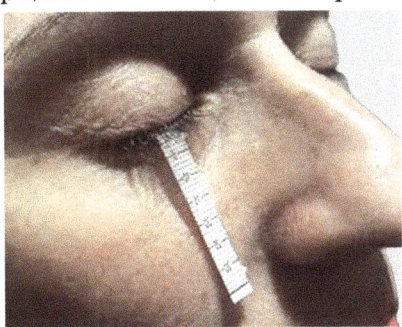

a. Identify the clinical image. *(4 marks)*
b. Diagnosis is: *(6 marks)*
- Type 1 (distal) renal tubular acidosis (RTA)
- Type 2 (proximal) RTA
- Type 3 RTA
- Type 4 RTA

Q19.

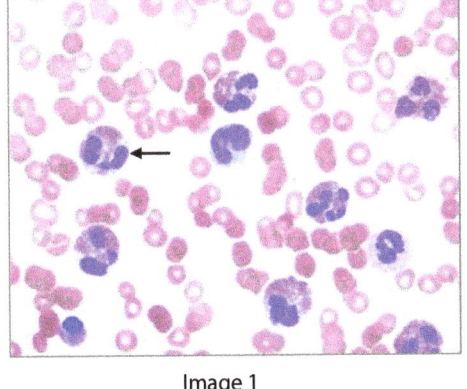

Image 1

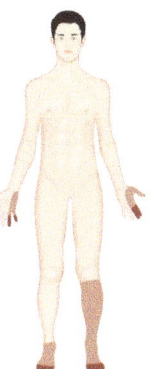

Image 2

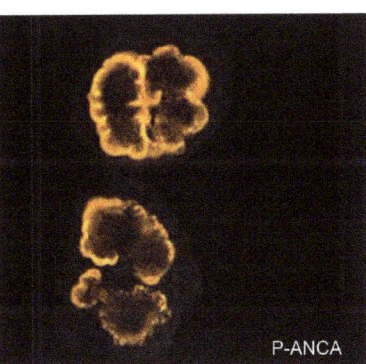

P-ANCA

Image 3

a. Identify the condition. *(2 marks)*
b. Identify the clinical entity in Image 1, 2, and 3. *(4 marks)*
c. State the classification of type of renal involvement in this condition. *(4 marks)*

Q20. A 60-year-old male presented with complaints of progressive muscle weakness involving the proximal lower limb. Laboratory examination revealed mild increase in serum creatine kinase (CK) levels. Muscle biopsy was performed which showed cytoplasmic inclusions staining positive with p62 immunostain.
a. What is the most likely diagnosis? *(5 marks)*
b. Enumerate the skin manifestations seen in dermatomyositis. *(5 marks)*

Q21. A 42-year-old woman presented with progressive shortness of breath on exertion. There is a history of episodic bluish discoloration of fingers on exposure of cold. On examination, fine bibasal inspiratory crepitations and thickening and hardening of the skin involving the fingers and face. Observations are as follows: heart rate 95 beats/min, respiratory rate 22 breaths/min, blood pressure 155/90 mm Hg, temperature 37.5°C, and oxygen saturation 94% on air. A high-resolution computed tomography (HRCT) is performed.

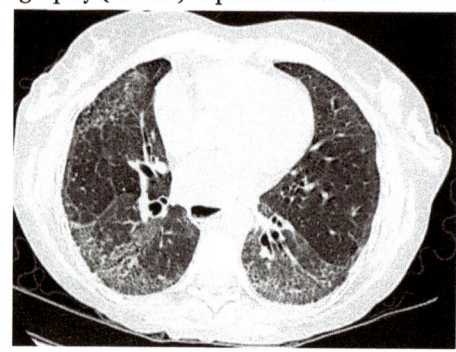

a. What is the most likely diagnosis? Mention other differential diagnosis of thickened tethered skin. *(2 marks)*
b. Mention antibodies present in this condition. *(2 marks)*
c. What antibody is associated with the high risk of interstitial lung disease (ILD)? *(2 marks)*
d. What is the CREST (calcinosis, Raynaud phenomenon, esophageal dysmotility, sclerodactyly, and telangiectasia) syndrome? *(2 marks)*

Q22. A 70-year-old presented with dyspnea on exertion and following features:

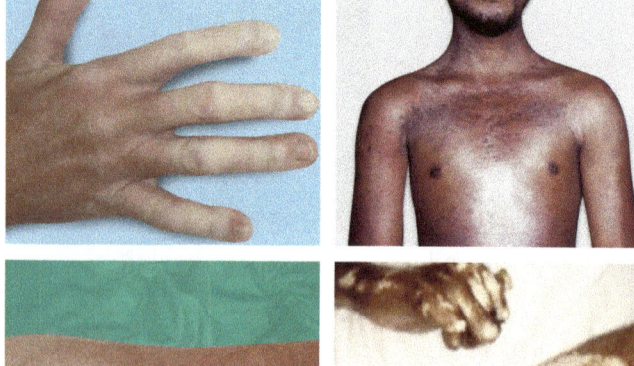
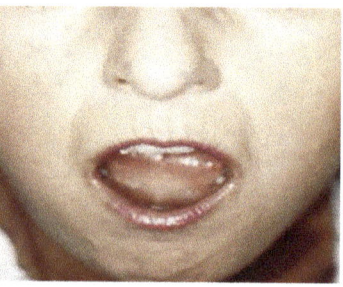

a. What is diagnosis? *(3 marks)*
b. What are specific antibodies? *(4 marks)*
c. What are pulmonary complications? *(3 marks)*

Rheumatology

Q23. A 44-year-old woman who has had Sjögren's syndrome for 4 years presents with diffuse muscle weakness. She uses carboxymethylcellulose eye drops. Physical examination findings and laboratory test results are shown in table below. A computed tomographic scan of the abdomen is shown in image below.

Component	Finding
Body mass index	19
Blood pressure, mm Hg	98/60
Pulse, beats per minute	98
Respiratory rate, breaths per minute	20
Edema	Absent
Sodium, mEq/L	134
Potassium, mEq/L	2.3
Chloride, mEq/L	114
Bicarbonate, mEq/L	12
Serum creatinine, mg/dL	0.8
Anion gap, mEq/L	8
Arterial blood gas:	
• pH	7.27
• PCO_2, mm Hg	27
Urinalysis:	
• pH	6.7
• Protein	Trace
• Glucose	Negative
• Red blood cells per high-power field	3–10

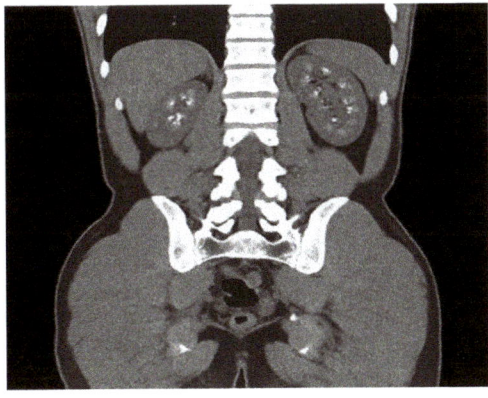

a. What is the diagnosis? *(3 marks)*
b. What is the CT finding? *(3 marks)*
c. What are the other causes of this disease? *(4 marks)*

ANSWERS

Ans. 1

a. Adult-onset Still's disease (AOSD)
b. Elevated inflammatory markers, namely the C-reactive protein (CRP) and erythrocyte sedimentation rate (ESR). Serum ferritin, which is frequently disproportionally elevated in AOSD. Liver function tests (LFTs) may be deranged.
c. Nonsteroidal anti-inflammatory drugs (NSAIDs) for symptomatic relief, corticosteroids, and methotrexate.
d. In 2020, the US Food and Drug Administration (USFDA) approved canakinumab to treat patients with active Still's disease including AOSD.

Ans. 2

a. She has developed AA type amyloidosis secondary to RA
b. Biopsy and histopathological examination from any of the sites, such as subcutaneous fat, spleen, adrenal gland, liver, labial salivary gland, and sites in the alimentary canal ranging from the tongue and gingiva to the rectum. The stain used is Congo Red. Deposits of amyloid bind Congo Red and exhibit apple-green birefringence when viewed by polarization light microscopy.
c. *Biologics:* Anti-tumor necrosis factor (anti-TNF), anti-interleukin-6 (anti-IL-6), rituximab, abatacept, tofacitinib, and antifibril drug—eprodisate.

Ans. 3

a. Duration, pattern of joint involvement, and symmetry
b. Reactive arthritis, rheumatic fever and arthritis, and psoriatic arthritis
c. Sacroiliac (SI) joint, hips, and vertebra. "Enthesitis is inflammation of the "enthesis," which is where a tendon or ligament attaches to bone.

Ans. 4

a. Enzyme-linked immunosorbent assay (ELISA), immunofluorescence. A positive ANA titer (>1:80) with the associated clinical signs (e.g., skin disease and polyarthritis) and laboratory findings (e.g., proteinuria and thrombocytopenia) is diagnostic for SLE.
b. Polymyositis/dermatomyositis, juvenile idiopathic arthritis, juvenile idiopathic arthritis with uveitis, Sjögren's syndrome, and RA
c. Rheumatoid arthritis, primary Sjögren's syndrome, and mixed connective tissue disease
d. Anti-cyclic citrullinated peptide (anti-CCP) antibody testing is particularly useful in the diagnosis of rheumatoid arthritis with high specificity.

Ans. 5

a. Jaccoud's arthropathy is a benign chronic arthropathy without functional impairment and needs to be differentiated from fixed and noncorrectable deformities of RA.
b. Rheumatic heart disease, systemic lupus erythematous, etc.

Ans. 6

Heberden's nodes in osteoarthritis

Ans. 7

a. Swan neck deformity, Z deformity of the thumb, ulnar subluxation, and ulnar deviation at the MCPs.
b. Rheumatoid arthritis
c. Rheumatoid factor, anticyclic citrullinated polypeptide (ACCP), CRP quantitative, complete blood counts, LFTs, renal function tests (RFTs), virological markers [hepatitis B surface antigen (HBsAg), anti-hepatitis C virus (anti-HCV), and human immunodeficiency virus (HIV)], radiographs [X-ray both hands and wrists posteroanterior (PA) view, X-ray both knees anteroposterior (AP) and lateral, chest X-ray (CXR)—PA view].
d. There are four domains of the criteria and a patient is classified as RA if the cumulative score is 6/10 or more. The maximum possible is 10/10. Patient may fulfill the criteria prospectively or retrospectively.

Joint distribution (0–5):	
1 large joint	0
2–10 large joints	1
1–3 small joints (large joint not counted)	2
4–10 small joints (large joint not counted)	3
>10 joints (at least 1 large joint)	5
Serology (0–3):	
Negative RF and anticitrullinated protein auto-antibody (ACPA)	0
Low titer positive RF or ACPA	1
High titer positive RF or ACPA	3
Symptom duration (0–1):	
<6 weeks	0
>6 weeks	1
Acute phase reactants (0–1):	
Normal C-reactive protein (CRP) and erythrocyte sedimentation rate (ESR)	0
Raised CRP or ESR	1

e. Jaccoud's arthropathy
f. Charcot's arthritis

Ans. 8

The pattern is suggestive of inflammatory oligoarthritis.

Term	Explanation
Single joint involvement	Monoarthritis
Four or less joints involved	Oligoarthritis
More than four joints involved	Polyarthritis

Contd...

Contd...

Term	Explanation
Axial skeleton	Cranium, vertebral column, sternoclavicular joints, and sacroiliac joints
Symmetrical arthritis	Involvement of the same joints on both sides of the skeleton
Additive arthritis	As new joints are involved, arthritis in the previously involved joints persists
Migratory or fleeting arthritis	As new joints are involved, arthritis in the previously involved joints resolves

Ans. 9

a. The following features are seen:
   - Acrosteolysis of the distal phalanges
   - Features suggestive of erosive arthritis involving the bilateral wrist joints. There is decreased intercarpal joint space with periarticular sclerosis and erosions.
b. Systemic sclerosis and scleroderma, psoriatic arthritis, idiopathic inflammatory myositis, mixed connective tissue disease (MCTD), hyperparathyroidism, post-traumatic, drugs—phenytoin/ergot poisoning, and primary PHO

Ans. 10

a. Rheumatoid factors are antibodies directed against Fc portion of immunoglobulin G. Positive association in—Rheumatoid arthritis, Sjögren's syndrome, mixed essential cryoglobulinemia, and primary biliary cholangitis.
b. Clinical triad of neutropenia, splenomegaly, and RA
c. Methotrexate, sulfasalazine, hydroxychloroquine, and leflunomide
d. At any time point, the patient on treatment must satisfy all of the following:
   - Tender joint count ≤1
   - Swollen joint count ≤1
   - C-reactive protein ≤1 mg/dL
   - Patient global assessment ≤1 (on a 0–10 scale)

Ans. 11

a. Swan neck deformity
b.

2020 ACR-EULAR classification—rheumatoid arthritis

Joint involvement:	
1 large joint	0
2–10 large joints	1
1–3 small joints, +/- large joints	3
>10 joints (at least 1 small joint)	5
Serology (need at least 1):	
Negative RF, negative anticyclic citrullinated peptide antibody (anti-CCP Ab)	0
Low positive RF or low positive anti-CCP Ab	2
High positive RF or high positive anti-CCP Ab	3

Contd...

Contd...

Acute phase reactants (need at least 1):	
Normal CRP and normal ESR	0
Abnormal CRP or abnormal ESR	1
Duration of symptoms:	
<6 weeks	0
≥6 weeks	1

For patients with at least one joint with definite clinical synovitis, not better explained by another disease
Rule out:
- Psoriatic arthritis
- Viral polyarthritis
- Gout
- Calcium pyrophosphate deposition (CPPD)
- SLE

≥6/10 definite RA

Source: Studenic P, Aletaha D, de Wit M, et al. Ann Rheum Dis. 2023;82:74-80.

Ans. 12

a. Bamboo spine—ankylosing spondylitis
b. Acute anterior uveitis, inflammatory bowel disease (IBD), psoriasis, ischemic heart disease (IHD), and heart block

Ans. 13

a. Dactylitis of the thumb
b. A uniform swelling and inflammation along with a cylindrical appearance of the entire digit is considered as dactylitis, also known as sausage digit.
c. - *Inflammatory conditions:* (1) Psoriatic arthritis and enthesitis, (2) gouty arthritis, and (3) RA
   - *Infectious conditions:* (1) Lyme disease (2) syphilis, and (3) tuberculosis
   - *Miscellaneous:* (1) Sarcoidosis and (2) sickle cell disease
d. - Distal arthritis
   - Asymmetric oligoarthritis
   - Symmetric polyarthritis
   - Arthritis mutilans
   - Spondyloarthritis
e. These criteria can only be applied to patients who have evidence of musculoskeletal disease in the form of peripheral arthritis, enthesitis, or axial spondyloarthritis)
   Three points are required:
   - Skin psoriasis:
   - Present at the time of examination—2 points
   - Historically present—1 point
   - Family history of psoriasis—1 point

- Nail lesions in the form onycholysis and pitting—1 point
- Dactylitis—1 point
- Negative RF—1 point
- Juxta-articular bone formation distinct from osteophytes on radiograph—1 point

Ans. 14

a. Grade 5 clubbing

Grade 1	Fluctuation of the nail bed is increased.
Grade 2	Increase in the angle between the nail bed and the proximal nail fold
Grade 3	Increase in convexity of the nail
Grade 4	Parrot beaking and drumstick appearance
Grade 5	In addition to grade 4 features, appearance of shiny and glossy appearance of nail and adjacent skin with longitudinal striations.

b. These patients come to medical attention due to grade 5 clubbing; they generally do not have any underlying lung disease. There is subperiosteal new bone formation especially at the end of long bones. They may also have features of synovitis and due to the rarity of the disease; there are no clear treatment guidelines. It is also known as pachydermoosteolysis when there is skin involvement of the face and scalp in the form of excessive wrinkling due to hypertrophy of the underlying glands and subcutaneous tissue.

Ans. 15

a. Bilateral sacroiliitis is seen. There is periarticular sclerosis is seen on both the iliac and sacral aspects of the SI joints bilaterally. There are a few erosions seen especially on the iliac aspect of the right SI joint.

b.
- *Grade 0:* Normal
- *Grade I:* Suspicious changes (some blurring of the joint margins)
- *Grade II:* Minimum abnormality (small localized areas with erosion or sclerosis, with no alteration in the joint width)
- *Grade III:* Unequivocal abnormality (erosions, widening, narrowing, sclerosis, or partial ankyloses).
- *Grade IV:* Severe abnormality (ankylosis)

c. MRI can characterize sacroiliitis as active inflammation, whereas conventional radiograph and CT scan are only able to demonstrate and document chronic changes.

Required MRI features:
- Bone marrow edema (BME)/osteitis on T2-weighted sequence sensitive for free water (STIR or T2FS) or bone marrow contrast enhancement on T1FS post GAD.
- Inflammation must be present in a typical anatomical area (subchondral bone).
- MRI appearance must be highly suggestive of spondyloarthropathy.

Corroborative but not mandatory/required MRI features:
- The isolated presence of lesions such as synovitis, enthesitis, and capsulitis without BME will not qualify as active sacroiliitis.
- The isolated presence of lesions, such as fat metaplasia, sclerosis, erosions, and ankylosis without BME will not qualify as active sacroiliitis.

Ans. 16

a. X-ray lateral spine depicts concave shape of upper and lower bodies of vertebrae known as *fish mouth vertebrae*.
b. Differential diagnoses are osteoporosis, osteomalacia, renal osteodystrophy, osteogenesis imperfecta, sickle cell disease, thalassemia major, hereditary spherocytosis, and homocystinuria
c. *Investigations for evaluating a case of fish mouth vertebrae:* Serum calcium, phosphorus, vitamin D3, urea, and creatinine
   - Ultrasonography kidney, ureter and bladder (USG KUB) (if RFT deranged) dual X-ray absorptiometry (DEXA) scan (for osteoporosis)
   - High performance liquid chromatography (HPLC) [to rule out (r/o) hereditary hemolytic anemia]
   - Serum homocysteine and methionine levels (only if other causes are ruled out and a strong suspect for homocystinuria present)

Ans. 17

a. The X-ray of the foot shows a large nodular swelling in right metatarsophalangeal (MTP) joint and a small nodular swelling over left MTP joint and with the clinical history in the background it is signs of (s/o) *gouty tophi*.
b. Our clinical diagnosis is *acute gouty arthritis with tophi* which is evident by history of alcoholism, tophi seen clinically and on X-ray and microscopic evidence of needle-shaped crystals with hyperuricemia.
c. *Drugs used in m/m of acute attacks:* Colchicine and NSAIDs. In cases of renal impairment, steroids are useful.

Ans. 18

a. Clinical image is of Sjögren's disease.
b. Associated with distal (type 1) RTA which is characterized by hypokalemia and acidosis.

Ans. 19

a. Eosinophilic granulomatosis with polyangiitis (Churg-Strauss syndrome)
b. Image 1—eosinophilia, Image 2—mononeuritis multiplex, and Image 3—p-ANCA (perinuclear anti-neutrophil cytoplasmic antibody) positive
c. Renal involvement—crescentic glomerulonephritis

Ans. 20

a. Inclusion body myositis (IBM)
b. Heliotrope rash (erythematous discoloration of eyelids with periorbital edema)
   - Gottron sign (erythematous rash over the extensor surfaces of joints, such as the knuckles, elbows, knees, and ankles)
   - Gottron papules (raised erythematous rash over knuckles)
   - V-sign (rash on the sun-exposed anterior neck and chest)
   - Shawl sign over the back of the neck and shoulders, nail bed telangiectasias, and subcutaneous calcium deposits

Ans. 21

a. Systemic sclerosis (scleroderma). Other differential diagnosis of thickened tethered skin are mixed connective tissue disease (a distinct disorder with features of scleroderma, SLE, RA, and myositis) and graft-versus-host disease
b. Antibodies present in this condition are:
   - Antinuclear antibody
   - Anti-RNA polymerase III, Scl-70 (anti-topoisomerase) with diffuse subset of scleroderma
   - Anticentromere with limited subset of scleroderma
c. Anti-Scl-70 positivity in this disease is useful in predicting those at high risk for.
d. The combination of calcinosis cutis, Raynaud's phenomenon, esophageal dysmotility, sclerodactyly, and telangiectasia is termed CREST syndrome.

Ans. 22

a. Systemic sclerosis
b. Anti-centromere (limited)/Scl-70/RNA polymerase III
c. Pulmonary HTN/ILD/pulmonary hemorrhage

Ans. 23

a. This is a classic case of distal RTA.
b. Distal RTA is associated with calcium phosphate nephrolithiasis and nephrocalcinosis.
c. **Distal RTA (type 1)**
   What is it?
   - Failure to acidify urine in distal tubular
   - Consequent impaired NH_4^+ secretion
   - Cannot lower pH <5.5

   Causes:
   - *Primary (isolated):*
     - Autosomal dominant-AE1/Band-3/SLC4A1 (Cl^-/HCO_3^- XC)
     - Autosomal recessive-Apical H^+-ATPase (sensorineural deafness)

   Secondary:
   - *Autoimmune disease:*
     - Sjögren's syndrome
     - Rheumatoid arthritis
     - SLE
   - Dysproteinemias
   - *Drugs:*
     - Amphotericin
     - Toluene toxicity
     - Ifosfamide
     - Lithium
   - *Hypercalciuric conditions (nephrocalcinosis):*
     - Hyperparathyroidism

- Idiopathic hypercalciuria
- Sarcoid
- Medullary sponge kidney

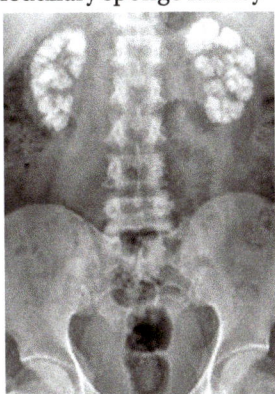
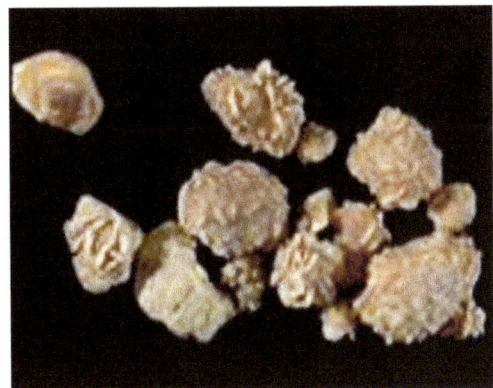

- *Clinical phenotype:*
  - Hypercalciuria (acidosis "leaches" bones)
  - Hypocitraturia
  - Nephrocalcinosis
  - $CaPO_4$ stones (alkaline urine)
  - Propensity to urinary tract infection (UTI)
  - No Fanconi syndrome
  - HCO_3 variable (may be <10)
- *Diagnosis:*
  - Urine pH always >5.5
- *Take note caveats:*
  - Urea-splitting organism (exclude)
  - Acute kidney injury (AKI), low urine Na, prolonged ↓K
  - Presence of nephrocalcinosis
  - Urine anion gap (UAG) *positive* (take note measure NH_4^+)
- *If doubt:*
  - Acidification test (NH_4Cl)
  - Furosemide and fludrocortisone (F'n'F test)
- *Treatment:*
  - Treat underlying cause
  - Withdrawal of toxins
  - Combination of Na and K alkali salts.

SECTION 4

Endocrinology

QUESTIONS

Q1. A 64-year-old lady presented with chronic fatigue, muscle weakness, weight loss, vomiting, abdominal pain, and hyperpigmented skin, particularly in sun-exposed areas, axillae, palmar creases, and mucous membranes. Her laboratory tests are given.

Thyroid-stimulating hormone (TSH): 14.5 mU/L

Free thyroxine (FT4): 0.49 ng/dL

Luteinizing hormone (LH): 14 mUI/mL

Follicle-stimulating hormone (FSH): 19.1 mUI/mL

Adrenocorticotropic hormone (ACTH): 4,292 pg/mL

a. What is the diagnosis? (4 marks)
b. List two associations. (2 marks)
c. How should it be treated? (4 marks)

Q2. A postgraduate medical resident was asked during the rounds to demonstrate all the methods of assessing the size of the spleen.

a. Enumerate the three methods of splenic palpation. (4 marks)
b. Enumerate the two methods of percussion for the spleen. (4 marks)
c. List four causes of massive splenomegaly. (2 marks)

Q3. A 48-year-old male visited the clinic, reporting a gradual onset of swelling and deformities in his hands. He had a 36-year history of (H/O) type 1 diabetes mellitus (T1DM) and had been undergoing hemodialysis for the past 5 years due to end-stage renal failure induced by diabetic nephropathy. Upon examination, the patient displayed swollen and deformed digits in the absence of acute inflammation or signs of infection.

Investigations are as follows:
- Urea: 52.5 mg/dL
- Creatinine: 5.38 mg/dL
- Corrected calcium: 13.6 mg/dL
- Phosphate: 6.2 mg/dL

- *Parathyroid hormone (PTH):* 1,263.30 pg/mL.

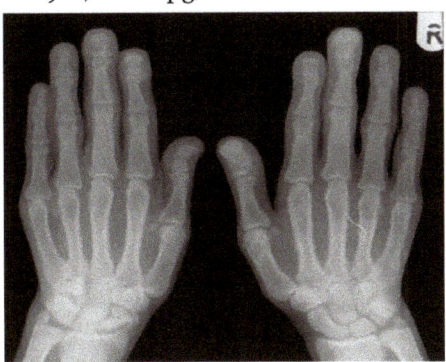

He underwent an X-ray of the hands.

a. Name the condition. (2 marks)
b. X-ray of the hand shows. (3 marks)
c. Type of calcification seen in this condition. (2 marks)
d. Most appropriate approach to manage the condition. (3 marks)

Q 4. A 35-year-old woman visits an outpatient department (OPD) with complaints of irregular and infrequent menstrual cycles. She is also upset that she has gained 11 kg over the past few months. Her face appears as shown in the image below. On an examination her blood pressure (BP) is 148/98 mm Hg and she has multiple purple striae over her abdomen and weakness in the proximal muscle group in the four limbs.

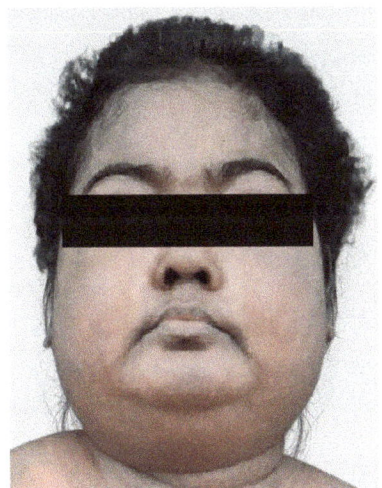

a. What sign is shown in this picture and what is its diagnosis? (2 marks)
b. Write the etiology. (2 marks)
c. Name the investigations that you should advise this patient for screening. (3 marks)
d. Write a cause of pseudo-Cushing syndrome. (3 marks)

Endocrinology

Q 5. A 34-year-old female presented with low-grade fever, neck pain, sweating, and heat intolerance of 4 weeks duration. Her investigation revealed a low TSH and elevated T3 and T4. Her investigation done is given below.

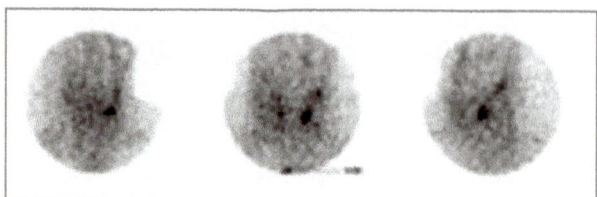

a. What investigation has been done and what does it suggest? (2 marks)
b. What is the diagnosis? (2 marks)
c. What is the difference between thyrotoxicosis and hyperthyroidism (3 marks)
d. Enumerate three causes of thyrotoxicosis without hyperthyroidism (3 marks)

Q 6.

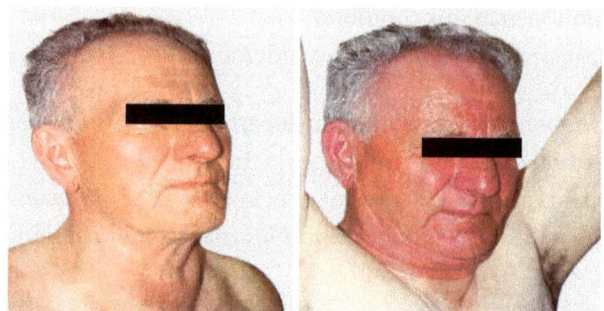

a. What is the sign depicted in the image? (5 marks)
b. Enlist some common causes of the sign. (5 marks)

Q 7.

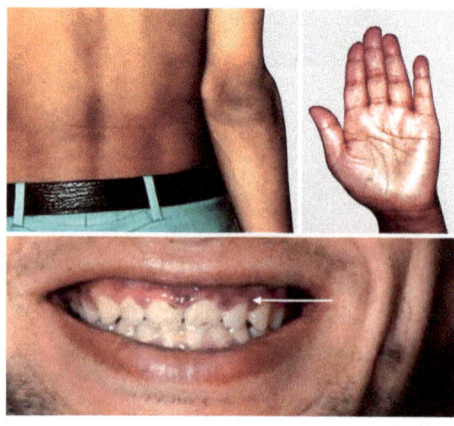

a. Which endocrinological abnormality presents with the following disease? (5 marks)
b. Which hormone is elevated in the following disease? (5 marks)

Q8. A 72-year-old patient who is a chronic smoker gives the H/O type 2 diabetes mellitus (T2DM) for the last 8 years. For the 6 months, he noticed a gradually progressive decline in his near vision which suddenly increased in the last 1 week. His diabetes is not well controlled even with insulin and he does not have any other comorbid illness.
a. What are the two most common likely causes for his visual loss? (2 marks)
b. Name three risk factors for his sudden visual impairment. (3 marks)
c. What other complications are likely to be present? (2 marks)
d. Name one treatment modality for each of the likely causes of the visual loss. (2 marks)
e. What is the World Health Organization (WHO) definition of blindness? (1 mark)

Q9. A 68-year-old male presents with symptoms of fatigue, bone pain, and arthralgias. His medical history is notable for chronic kidney disease (CKD), a left nephrectomy due to renal cell carcinoma, hypertension, and degenerative joint disease. With a height of 173 cm, a weight of 65 kg, BP at 133/77 mm Hg, and a heart rate of 62 beats per minute, he exhibits diffuse arthralgias and mild pitting edema in the lower extremities. Laboratory results indicate a serum creatinine of 2.3 mg/dL, serum calcium of 8.2 mg/dL, phosphorus of 5.8 mg/dL, PTH at 298 pg/mL, and hemoglobin at 10.2 g/dL. The only medication he is currently taking is the extended-release formulation of diltiazem at 360 mg.
a. What is your next recommendation? (5 marks)
b. What are the target PTH levels in nondialysis and dialysis populations? (5 marks)

Q10. Sarah comes to the clinic with a 2-month H/O increased heart rate, weight loss, and anxiety. She reports difficulty sleeping and occasional hand tremors. She also mentions an increased appetite but notes that despite eating more, she has lost about 10 pounds over the last month. Sarah denies any recent illness, fever, or changes in her diet. She reports a family H/O autoimmune disorders, including thyroid disorders.
a. What is the provisional diagnosis? (4 marks)
b. What investigations will you send for workup? (3 marks)
c. What is the drug of choice in pregnancy? (3 marks)

Q11. Magnetic resonance imaging (MRI) findings of female presenting with headaches, visual disturbances, amenorrhea, infertility, and decreased libido.

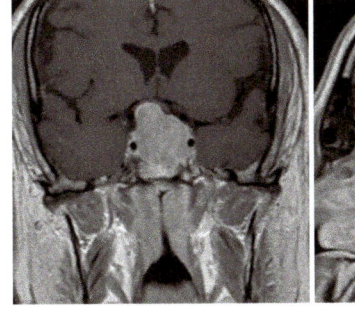
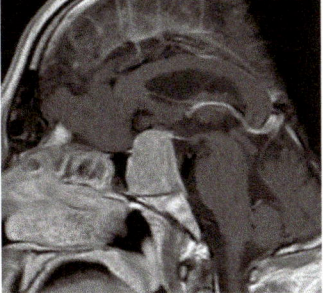

a. Discuss the most likely radiological diagnosis. (5 marks)
b. Enumerate the treatment options of the given condition. (5 marks)

Q12. A 40-year-old female presented with heat intolerance, palpitations, weight loss, and oligomenorrhea. On examination she was having tachycardia, the lid retraction sign was positive and skin changes on the lateral aspect of shins. The laboratory findings showed low TSH levels and total thyroid hormones are raised.

a. Identify the condition. *(5 marks)*
b. Name the other eye signs seen in the above condition. *(5 marks)*

Q13. A 29-year-old male presented with episodic palpitations, headache, and profuse sweating. He was found to be hypertensive, to evaluate further, 24 hours of urinary catecholines were done which was raised with elevated plasma metanephrine levels.

a. Discuss its diagnosis. *(5 marks)*
b. Discuss the imaging techniques used for the diagnosis. *(5 marks)*

Q14. A 34-year-old female came to Sriram Chandra Bhanj Medical College and Hospital (SCBMCH) casualty with an H/O altered sensorium since last 8 hours with two episodes of generalized tonic–clonic seizure (GTCS) in the last 4 hours. She gave H/O similar such episodes (two times) in the past within the last 1 year for which she was treated in other hospital symptomatically and discharged. Her BP was 88/56 mm Hg.

On observing the routine reports she had serum Na$^+$ of 112 mEq/L.

She has one living issue which was vaginally delivered 2 years back, but on removing the placenta the cord was detached and the placenta was retained. The retained placenta was associated with an atonic uterus and severe bleeding for which the patient was taken to OT and the placenta was removed surgically. She received three units of BT.

After birth she was able to feed her child with breast milk for 1 week after which her milk production decreased gradually and then stopped.

On general examination there was no pubic and axillary hair and her menses has stopped since last 8 months.

Her hormonal profile was suggestive of (S/O) decrease TSH, FT3, FT4, LH, and FSH.

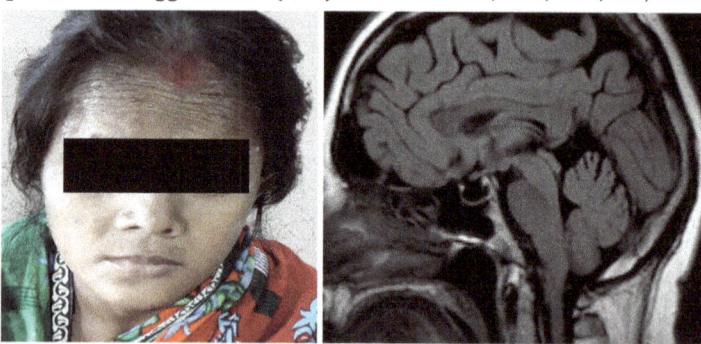

a. What is the diagnosis? *(4 marks)*
b. What are the embryological origins of the parts of the above mentioned gland? *(3 marks)*
c. What is the sequence of fall in hormonal levels in this case? *(3 marks)*

Q15. Mrs Fatma, a 52-year-old female presented with acute onset nasal regurgitation of food and nasal intonation of the voice of 1-month duration. She had an H/O weight loss (approximately 6 kg), palpitation, and sweating for the last 6 months.

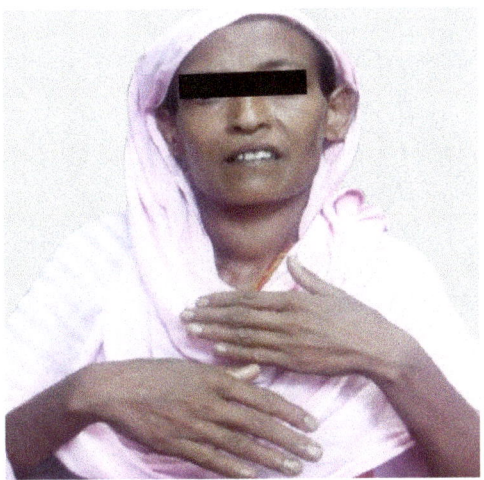

Her thyroid profile was:

T3: 534.6 ng/dL

T4: 19.5 µg/dL

TSH: 0.005 mIU/L

a. What is your provisional diagnosis? (4 marks)
b. What is your investigation plan? (4 marks)
c. How do you manage the subject? (2 marks)

Q 16. A 12-year-old boy presented to endocrinology OPD with a neck swelling that moves with deglutition. His T3, T4, and TSH are within normal range.

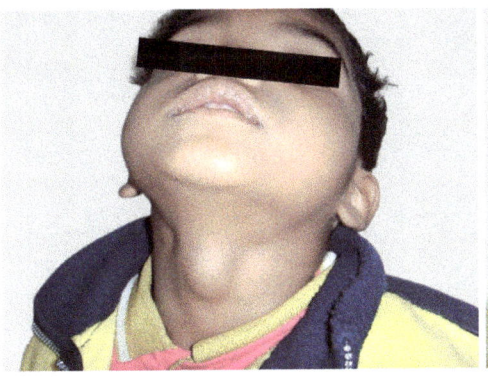 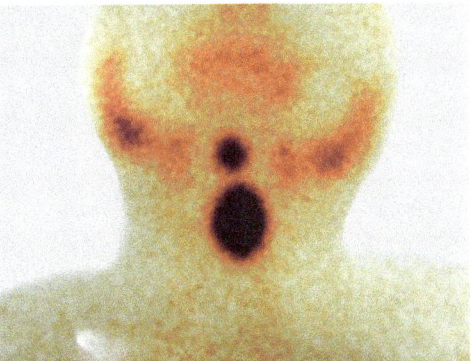

a. What are the differential diagnosis (D/D)? (2 marks)
b. What is your diagnosis? (3 marks)
c. How you will manage the case? (5 marks)

Q17. A 60-year-old male subject is presented with an H/O headache and visual difficulty in form of injuring his body on the sides when walking.

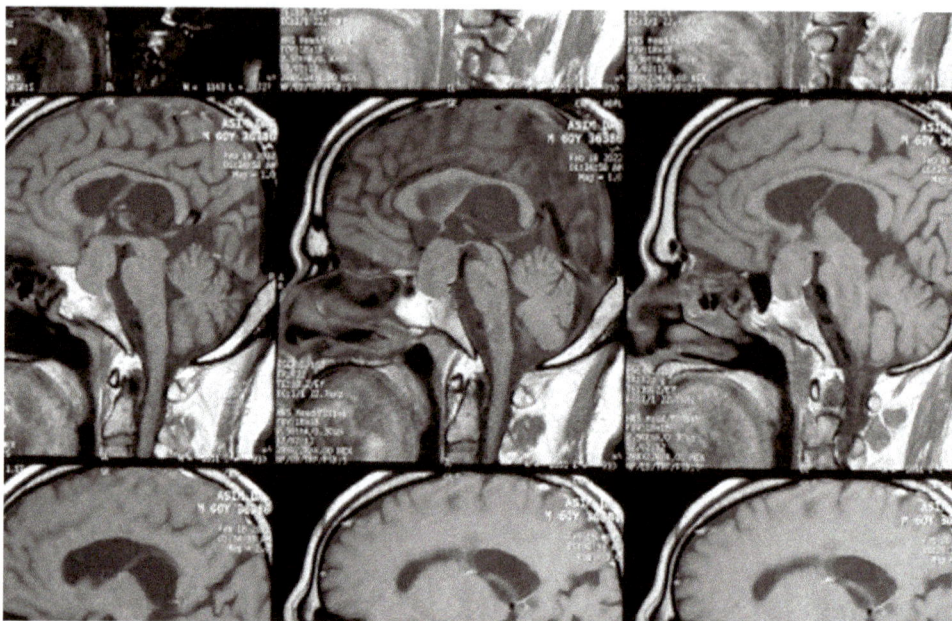

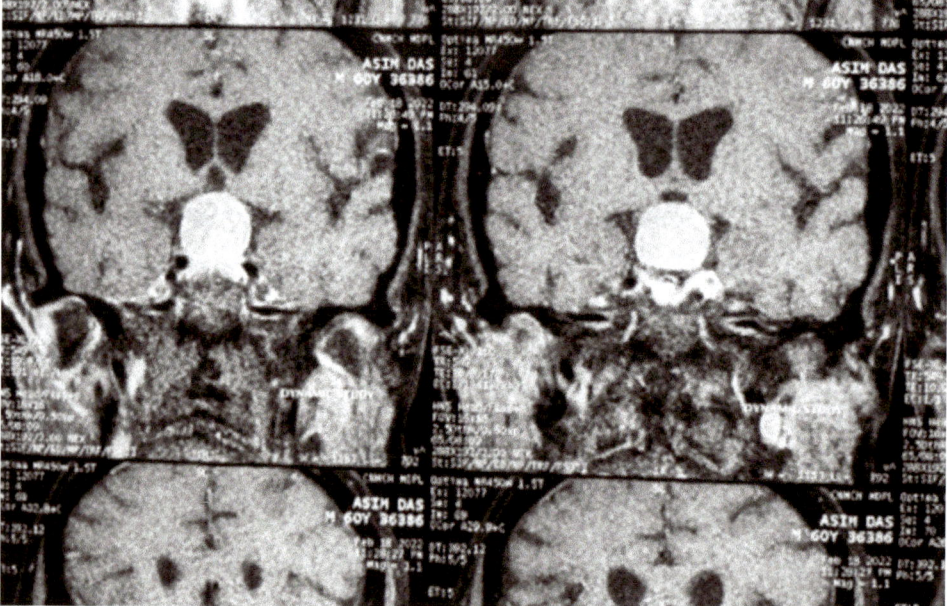

a. Describe the MRI findings. (3 marks)
b. Discuss the investigation plan. (3 marks)
c. Briefly discuss the treatment plan. (4 marks)

Endocrinology 67

Q18. A 29-year-old male subject attended an endocrinology clinic for infertility. On further questioning, he has preserved libido with difficulty in releasing objects from the handgrip.

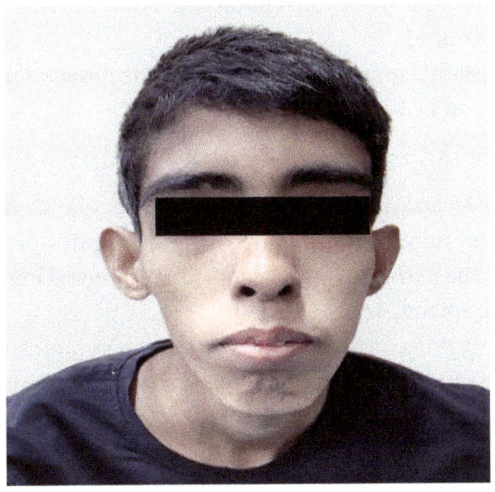

a. Describe the face. (2 marks)
b. What is your diagnosis? (2 marks)
c. Describe the neurological and EMG findings. (6 marks)

ANSWERS

Ans. 1

a. Autoimmune polyendocrine syndrome characterized by adrenal insufficiency and thyroid disease (Schmidt syndrome).
b. Coeliac disease, myasthenia gravis, and idiopathic thrombocytopenic (ITP).
c. Glucocorticoids followed by thyroid replacement.

Ans. 2

a.
- *Supine palpation technique:* Instruct the patient to lie in the supine position. The examiner, using the right-hand fingertips, gently applies pressure just below the left costal margin. Ask the patient to take a deep and prolonged breath, facilitating palpation for the descending spleen.
- *Middleton's hooking procedure:* Position the patient supine and approach from the left side, placing fingers under the left costal margin. Instruct the patient to inhale while the examiner attempts to detect the spleen's tip.
- *Right lateral decubitus and supine:* Have the patient lie in the right lateral decubitus position.
- The examiner's left hand is passed anterior to posterior around the left lower thorax, gently lifting the lowermost left rib cage.
- Apply gentle pressure beneath the left costal margin with the right-hand fingertips, palpating the spleen during deep inspiration.

b.
- *Traube's space percussion:* Position the patient supine with the left arm slightly abducted for full Traube's space assessment. Percuss the medial to lateral margins of the triangle during normal respiration. Normally, a resonant or tympanitic sound is expected; dullness on percussion indicates potential splenomegaly.
- *Castell's technique:* Instruct the patient to lie supine. Percuss the lowest left intercostal space in the anterior axillary line during full inspiration. Normally resonant, a dull sound suggests possible splenomegaly.
- *Nixon's maneuver:* Have the patient lies in the right lateral decubitus position. Initiate percussion midway along the left costal margin, moving perpendicular to it. If dullness extends >8 cm above the left costal margin, it suggests a potential splenomegaly.

c. Chronic myeloid leukemia, Hodgkin's lymphoma, kala azar, hairy cell leukemia, and chronic malaria.

Ans. 3

a. Tertiary hyperparathyroidism is characterized by elevated levels of calcium and PTH in individuals with end-stage renal failure.
b. Generalized osteopenia, erosion of terminal phalangeal tufts (acroosteolysis), and subperiosteal bone resorption, particularly in the radial aspects of the second and third middle phalanges, are observed. Additionally, hand X-rays reveal soft tissue calcification.
c. The presence of metastatic calcification is identified.
d. Elective parathyroidectomy remains the preferred treatment for tertiary hyperparathyroidism in patients.

Ans. 4

a. Moon face, Cushing's syndrome, or Cushing disease.
b. ACTH-dependent Cushing's syndrome—Cushing's disease, ectopic ACTH syndrome, ectopic corticotropin-releasing hormone (CRH) syndrome.
   - *ACTH-independent Cushing's syndrome:* Adrenal adenoma, adrenal carcinoma micronodular hyperplasia, and macronodular hyperplasia.
c. The following four investigations are used to establish an initial diagnosis of endogenous Cushing's syndrome as per the clinical guidelines of the endocrine society.
   - A 24-hour urinary free cortisol (increased 3 × above normal).
   - Midnight salivary cortisol (>5 nmol/L)
   - Overnight dexamethasone suppression (plasma cortisol >50 nmol/L at 8–9 AM after 1 mg dexamethasone at 11 PM)
   - Standard 2-day (low dose) dexamethasone suppression test (plasma cortisol >50 nmol/L after 0.5 mg dexamethasone sixth hourly for 48 hours).
d. It may occur secondary to the following conditions:
   - Severe major depressive disorder
   - Polycystic ovarian syndrome
   - Insulin-resistant obesity
   - Obstructive sleep apnea
   - Chronic alcoholism
   - End-stage renal disease

Ans. 5

a. Thyroid scintigraphy (radio-active Iodine Uptake)
b. Shows markedly reduced radioiodine uptake and markedly decreased glandular activity
c. Hyperthyroidism is distinguished by an augmented synthesis and release of thyroid hormones from the thyroid gland, while thyrotoxicosis denotes the clinical syndrome of having an excess of circulating thyroid hormones, regardless of the origin.
d. Subacute thyroiditis, ingestion of thyroid hormone or recent excess iodine exposure.

Ans. 6

a. Pemberton sign
b. Intrathoracic goiter and lung cancer

Ans. 7

a. Addison disease.
b. Excess ACTH on the melanocytes to produce melanin.

Ans. 8

a. Cataract and diabetic retinopathy
b. Age, duration, and severity of diabetes and smoking
c. Diabetic neuropathy and diabetic nephropathy
d. Cataract surgery with posterior chamber intraocular lens (PCIOL), antivascular endothelial growth factor therapy (anti-VEGF)/laser photocoagulation
e. Visual acuity <3/60 in the better eye

Ans. 9

a. Insufficiency of 1,25-dihydroxyvitamin D is prevalent in individuals with CKD. Commencing vitamin D therapy is recommended for addressing secondary hyperparathyroidism in CKD patients, with the goal of attaining specified target levels of PTH.
b. For individuals with CKD stages G3a-G5 not undergoing dialysis, the ideal PTH level remains uncertain. Nevertheless, it is advised to assess levels of intact PTH that show a gradual increase or consistently exceed the upper normal limit for the assay. This evaluation should consider modifiable factors such as hyperphosphatemia, hypocalcemia, and vitamin D deficiency. In the case of CKD G5D dialysis, it is recommended to maintain the intact parathyroid hormone (iPTH) level within approximately two to nine times the upper normal limit for the assay.

Ans. 10

a. Thyrotoxicosis
b. Thyroid function test (TFT), anti-thyroid peroxidase (anti-TPO), and anti-thyroglobulin (anti-Tg).
c. Propylthiouracil

Ans. 11

a. Pituitary adenoma (prolactin secreting)
b. The treatment options of the given condition are as follows:
   - *Medical therapy:* Dopamine agonists (bromocriptine and cabergoline)
   - *Surgical therapy:* Transsphenoidal surgery
   - Radiation therapy

Ans. 12

a. *Hyperthyroidism:* Grave's disease
b. *Von Graefe sign:*
   - Rosenbach's sign
   - Stellwag sign
   - Joffroy sign
   - Moebius sign

Ans. 13

a. Pheochromocytoma
b. T2-weighted MRI abdomen with gadolinium contrast
   - Computed tomography (CT) of the abdomen
   - Metaiodobenzylguanidine (MIBG) scintigraphy
   - 18F DOPA PET (18F-dihydroxyphenylalanine positron emission tomography)
   - 68 Ga–DOTATATE PET

Ans. 14

a. The patient presented with recurrent seizures for last 1 year (due to recurrent hyponatremia) with hypotension with H/O severe blood loss [requiring three units of packed red

blood cells (PRBCs)] during childbirth with inability to breastfeed her child with absent pubic and axillary hairs and hormonal profile showing secondary hypothyroidism and hypogonadotropic hypogonadism all suggesting toward pituitary failure secondary to postpartum hemorrhage (PPH). Adrenocorticotropic hormone has negative action on antidiuretic hormone (ADH), so in hypopituitarism hyponatremia occurs due to increase in ADH. Hypoglycemia can also be a manifestation due to decrease in growth hormone (GH). Hypotension can be explained by decrease in ACTH. Magnetic resonance imaging brain shows absent pituitary bright spot on T1-weighted sequence, so all are suggestive of diagnosis of *Sheehan syndrome*.
b. Anterior pituitary/adenohypophysis: *Rathke's pouch*, posterior pituitary/neurohypophysis—*neural ectoderm*
c. *Sequence of decrease in level of hormones:* GH > gonadotropins > TSH > ACTH

Ans. 15

a. Acute bulbar palsy is an uncommon manifestation of Graves' disease (GD). While GD is typically diagnosed based on clinical findings, confirming tests include thyroid profile, radioactive uptake studies (using iodine or technetium), and TRAB (TSH receptor antibody) assays.
b. Treatment options for Graves' disease include anti-thyroid drugs (ATDs), radioactive iodine therapy (iodine 131), or surgery.
c. Symptomatic relief is provided for acute bulbar palsy, alongside managing hyperthyroidism through the use of anti-thyroid drugs.

Ans. 16

a. Differentials are:
   - Ectopic thyroid
   - Hypoglossal cyst
b. Ectopic thyroid, as confirmed by increased uptake of Tc^{99}
c. *Management:* Radioablation by I^{131}

Ans. 17

a. Large pituitary macroadenoma.
b. Biochemical assessment of pituitary function.
c. Surgical intervention in case there is a pressure on the optic chiasma or features of raised intracranial pressure (ICP), hormone replacement if it is a nonfunctioning adenoma causing hypopituitarism, and treatment with cabergoline, if it is a case of prolactinoma (in this patient, prolactin level was >1,200 πg/L.

Ans. 18

a. Face appeared hatchet shaped with bilateral ptosis along with visible atrophy of masseter and temporalis muscles.
b. Myotonic dystrophy.
c. Electromyography (EMG) of distal extremity muscles revealed myotonic discharges with a waxing and waning frequency and a characteristic "engine revving" sound.

SECTION 5

Diabetology

QUESTIONS

Q1. A 65-year-old male presented with a tingling numbness typically starting in the feet and gradually ascending in glove and stocking way. The symptoms were worse at night. He complained of sexual dysfunction and had a postural hypotension on examination.
a. What is the specific neurological diagnosis? *(3 marks)*
b. What is the characteristic feature in neurological examination? *(4 marks)*
c. List three causes. *(3 marks)*

Q2. A 58-year-old diabetic male was evaluated in the outpatient for a routine check-up. He has a strong familial hypercholesterolemia (FH) of coronary artery disease (CAD). His blood pressure (BP) was 136/90 mm Hg. His body mass index (BMI) is 28 kg/m². His glycated hemoglobin (HbA1c) was 8.2%. His serum creatinine is 1.2 mg% [estimated glomerular filtration rate (eGFR) 50 mL/min/1.73 m²)] and his albumin-to-creatinine ratio (ACR) is 240 mg/g. He is on metformin 1 g twice a day.
a. Write is full diagnosis with staging. *(4 marks)*
b. Enumerate three additional medications/strategies to prevent the progression of the disease. *(4 marks)*
c. Discuss two findings expected on fundoscopic examination. *(2 marks)*

Q3. A 15-year-old girl comes to the emergency department complaining of fever, vomiting, and abdominal pain for the last 2 days. The patient's temperature is 38.9°C (102°F), the pulse is 115/min, respirations are 25/min, and BP is 95/60 mm Hg. Physical examination shows a thin, uncomfortable girl with legs flexed to her chest. She is breathing deeply. Laboratory studies show the following:

Laboratory value	Result
Hemoglobin	12 g/dL
Leukocyte count	16,000/mm³
Platelet count	400,000/mm³
Sodium	130 mEq/L

Contd…

Contd...

Laboratory value	Result
Potassium	5.0 mEq/L
Chloride	100 mEq/L
pH	7.23
Bicarbonate	14 mEq/L
Blood urea nitrogen	15 mg/dL
Creatinine	1.0 mg/dL
Glucose	500 mg/dL

a. Which type of diabetes mellitus (DM) does the patient have? What is the diagnosis of the associated condition? *(2 marks)*
b. Write pathophysiology. *(3 marks)*
c. Name the autoantibodies seen in this type of DM. *(2 marks)*
d. Outline the treatment of the associated condition. *(3 marks)*

Q4. Mr X is a 32-year-old male who was diagnosed with type 1 diabetes mellitus (T1DM) at the age of 12 years. He has been managing his condition with multiple daily insulin injections and regular blood glucose monitoring. Recently, he has been experiencing weight gain, increased hunger, and high BP. During the examination, it is noted the BMI has increased from 23 to 30 over the past year. His BP is consistently elevated, and his fasting blood glucose levels are often above the target range.

a. What is this condition referred to as? *(2 marks)*
b. How do you define it? *(2 marks)*
c. What is the pathogenetic mechanism? *(3 marks)*
d. What are the management strategies? *(3 marks)*

Q5. A 62-year-old woman presents with generalized body swelling, decreased stamina, and fatigue. She has had type 2 diabetes mellitus (T2DM) for 24 years, hypertension, and hyperlipidemia. She has a history of migraine headaches. She has pale skin and pitting edema up to the thigh. On auscultation, breath sounds are mildly decreased in the bases bilaterally. Other physical examination findings and laboratory test results are shown below.

Component	Finding
Height, cm	170
Weight, kg	82
Blood pressure, mm Hg	98/62
Heart rate, BPM	102
Serum creatinine, mg/dL	1.2
Serum albumin, g/dL	2.0
Total cholesterol, mg/dL	260

Contd...

Contd… Component	Finding
Low-density lipoprotein cholesterol, mg/dL	180
High-density lipoprotein cholesterol, mg/dL	30
Triglycerides, mg/dL	198
Hemoglobin, g/dL	9.6
Hemoglobin A1c, %	9.2

She is taking neutral protamine Hagedorn (NPH) insulin, simvastatin 40 mg daily, aspirin 81 mg daily, metoprolol 100 mg twice daily, and naproxen 500 mg SOS basis. A renal biopsy was performed.
a. What is the first probable diagnosis on renal biopsy? *(3 marks)*
b. What renal biopsy finding would be most likely? *(3 marks)*
c. Patients with DM and chronic kidney disease (CKD) should be treated with a comprehensive strategy to reduce risks of kidney disease progression and cardiovascular disease. Mention the first-line drugs. *(4 marks)*

Q6. A 55-year-old male, with rheumatoid arthritis (RA) on hydroxychloroquine and uncontrolled T2DM was referred for a yearly eye checkup.

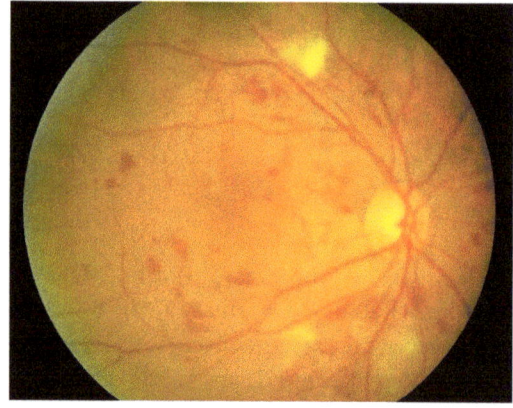

a. What is the retinal abnormality? *(5 marks)*
b. How will you treat it and mention the name of the lipid-lowering agent that has a specific role in the reduction of disease progression? *(5 marks)*

Q7. Maria is brought to the emergency department by her family due to the sudden onset of severe abdominal pain, persistent vomiting, and difficulty breathing. She has a known history of T1DM for the past 15 years. Her family reports that she has been feeling unwell for the past 2 days, with increased thirst and frequent urination. Maria has not been compliant with her insulin regimen.
a. What is the provisional diagnosis? *(2 marks)*
b. What will be the expected arterial blood gas (ABG) changes? *(4 marks)*
c. What is the line of management? *(4 marks)*

Q8

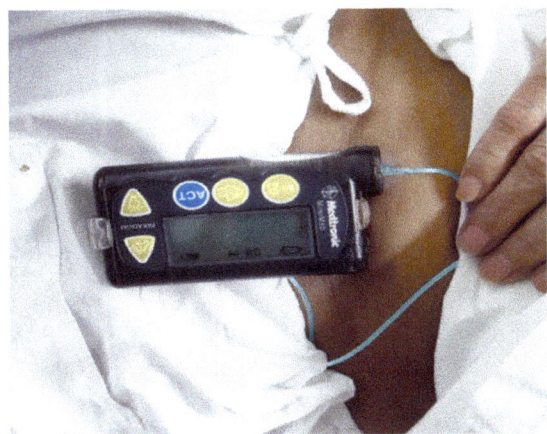

a. Identify the device and give any two indications. (5 marks)
b. What is the Dawn phenomenon and Somogyi effect? (5 marks)

Q9. The following instrument is given.

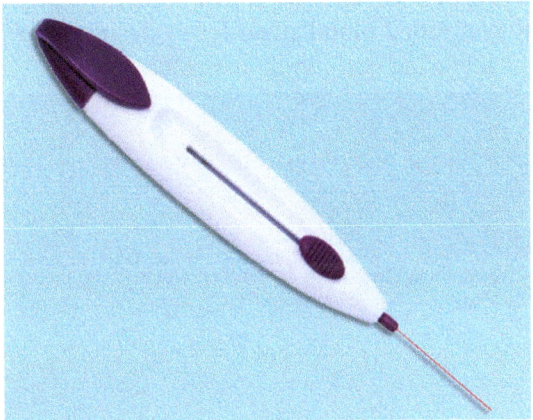

a. Name the test and the complication for which it is used. (5 marks)
b. Enumerate the acute and chronic complications of DM. (5 marks)

Q10.
A 50-year-old female, [known case of T2DM (8 years)], on oral hypoglycemic agents (OHA), discontinued for last month, presented with headache right (RT) side with nasal discharge, convulsion, and altered sensorium. Random blood sugar (RBS) >500, HbA1c 22.4, urine ketone body (KB) present, total leukocyte count (TLC) 26.400, N80, L15, E5, urea 86, creatinine 3.6, and ABG showed a picture of Metabolic acidosis. She developed swelling of the face and RT eye, and bloody nasal discharge during the hospital stay. Coronavirus disease of 2019 (COVID) real-time reverse transcriptase-polymerase chain reaction (RT PCR) and rapid antigen test (RAT) negative. Computerized tomography of the paranasal sinus (CT PNS) is as shown below.

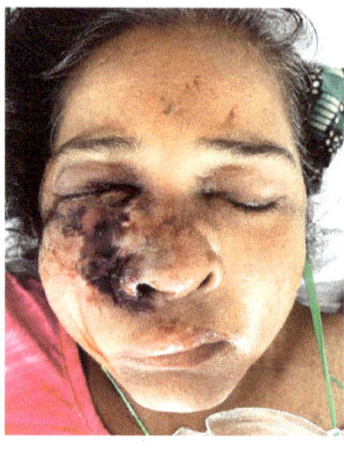 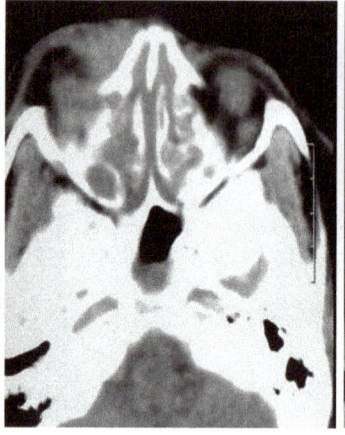 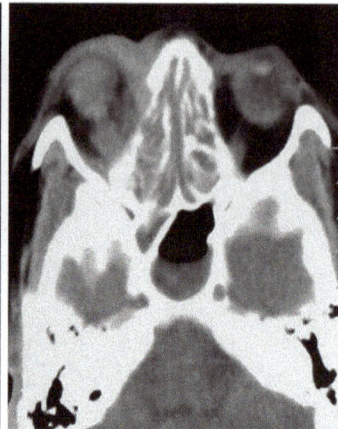

a. What is the probable diagnosis? (3 marks)
b. What is the most common organism involved? (3 marks)
c. What are the risk factors? (2 marks)
d. Modalities of treatment. (2 marks)

Q11. A 45-year-old, with a case of T2DM for 8 years with diabetic neuropathy and diabetic retinopathy had poorly controlled blood sugar levels despite four oral antidiabetics. His examination revealed the following skin condition in his neck.

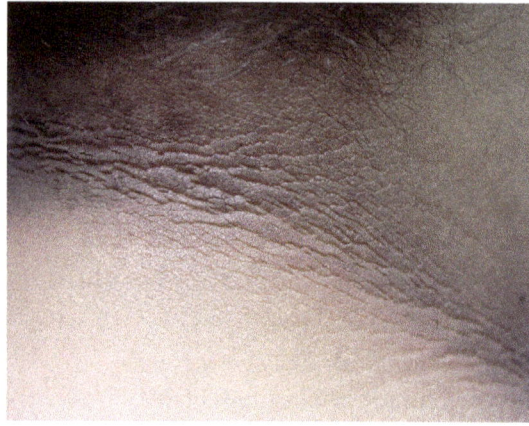

a. Identify the skin condition. (1 mark)
b. Identify the other areas where this condition may be found. (1 mark)
c. What is the significance of this condition in DM? (2 marks)
d. Enumerate other diseases associated with this skin disorder. (3 marks)
e. Enumerate the other cutaneous manifestations of DM. (3 marks)

Q12. 55-year-old, a case of T2DM for 10 years presented with progressive blurring of vision of both eyes. He also had an infected diabetic foot. His fundoscopy examination revealed this.

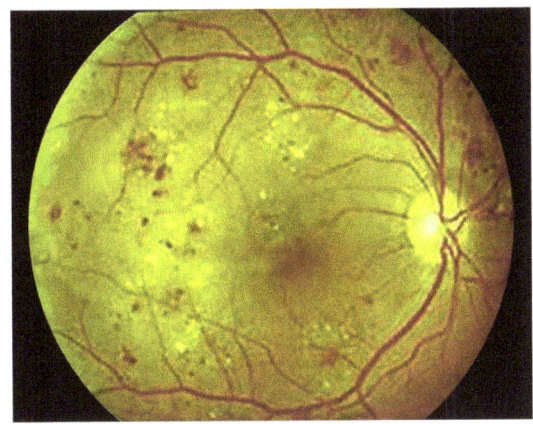

a. Mention the stages of diabetic retinopathy. (3 marks)
b. Identify the stage of diabetic retinopathy in this figure. (1 mark)
c. Enumerate the fundus features of diabetic retinopathy. (3 marks)
d. Enumerate microvascular and macrovascular complications DM. (3 marks)

Q13. 62-year-old, a case of T2DM for 8 years on oral antidiabetics was staying alone at home. He developed acute enteritis after which he had reduced intake and stopped his antidiabetics. His intake deteriorated over the next few days and he developed altered sensorium and drowsiness. He was brought to the hospital in a comatose state with hypotension, tachycardia, and features of dehydration. He was comatose responding to the painful stimuli. His urgent blood sugar done was 680 mg/dL. His ketone bodies in urine were negative and serum osmolality was 345 mOsm/kg. An urgent ABG done is given below.

	ABG
pH	7.34
HCO_3	22
CO_2	48
O_2	86
Na	148
K	4.5
Cl	118
Ca	1.1
Glucose	664

a. Identify the disorder of hyperglycemia. (1 mark)
b. Mention the primary pathogenic mechanism or abnormality. (1 mark)
c. Enumerate the precipitating factors for this condition. (2 marks)
d. Mention the diagnostic features of this condition. (3 marks)
e. Outline the management of this condition. (3 marks)

Q14. 38-year-old, a case of T1DM for 18 years has been on insulin therapy for several years. He is presently on a long-acting insulin preparation (36 units at 10 PM) and 12 units before each meal. He developed this cutaneous disorder in his anterior abdominal wall.

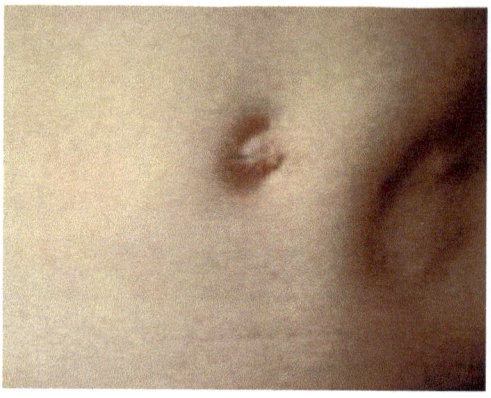

a. Identify the skin condition. (1 mark)
b. Name a few long-acting and short-acting insulin preparations. (3 marks)
c. Name the absolute indications of insulin therapy. (3 marks)
d. What are the side effects of insulin therapy? (3 marks)

Q15. A 45-year-old, chronic alcohol consumer with a history of alcohol-related pancreatitis presented to the hospital with pain abdomen, nausea, and vomiting. His blood sugars were 330 mg/dL with ketone bodies negative and a normal ABG. His X-ray abdomen is given below. After stabilization, he persisted in having high blood sugars. He was added on oral antidiabetics and insulin, and he had a predictable glycemic control with frequent hypoglycemia and hyperglycemia episodes.

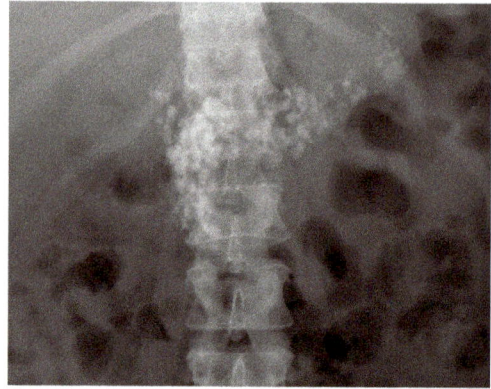

a. Identify the T1DM. (1 mark)
b. Identify the condition shown in the X-ray abdomen. (1 mark)
c. Enumerate the systemic conditions that can lead to DM of this type. (3 marks)
d. Enumerate drugs that can cause DM. (2 marks)
e. Name the various classes of oral antidiabetic drugs. (3 marks)

Q16. A 50-year-old male presented with fever and lower abdominal pain for three days. He has had DM for 30 years with poor glycemic control. His last HbA1c was 11. He has had a history of ureteric stones. After admission, a urine catheter was inserted. A picture of the urine sample is given below.

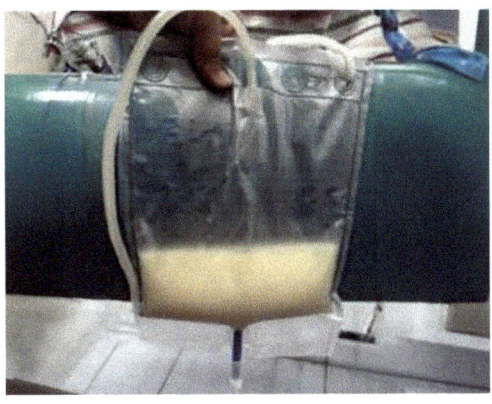

a. What causes the appearance of the urine? (2 marks)
b. Enumerate two risk factors for pyuria in this patient. (4 marks)
c. Mention one complication that can occur in this patient. (4 marks)

Q17.

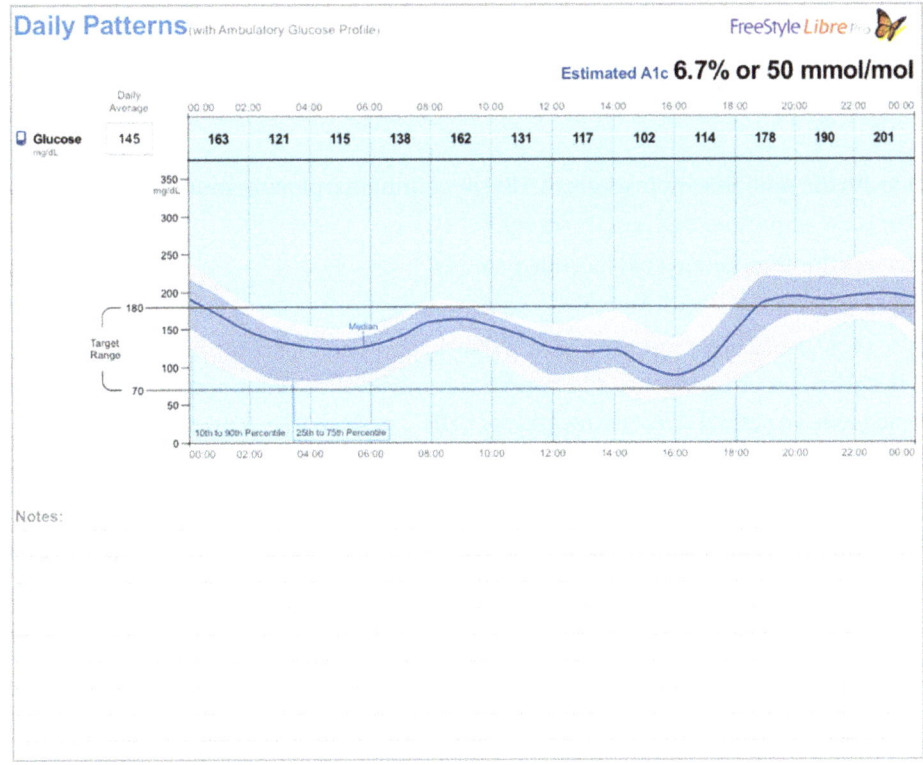

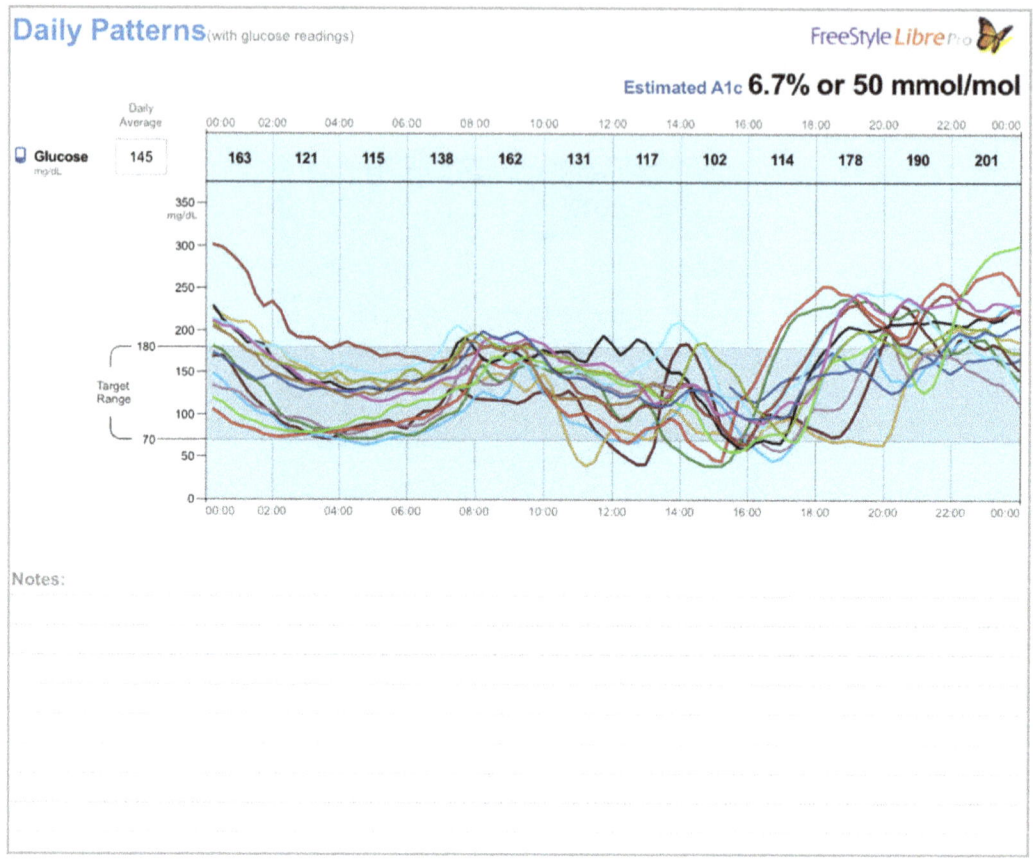

a. What are the probable indications of ABG or continuous glucose monitoring? (3 marks)
b. What is the importance of time-in-range (TIR)? (4 marks)
c. What are the components of glycemic pentad? (3 marks)

Q18. A 14-year-old boy presented with polyuria and polydipsia for 6-month duration. No visual disturbances or headache, and growth is normal. After water deprivation tests, he was concluded to have central diabetes insipidus (CDI).

Magnetic resonance imaging (MRI) of the pituitary showed a thickened pituitary stalk and an absent posterior pituitary bright spot.

a. How do you classify DM insipidus? (3 marks)
b. Do you consider further investigation for the boy? (4 marks)
c. How do you treat CDI? (3 marks)

Q19.

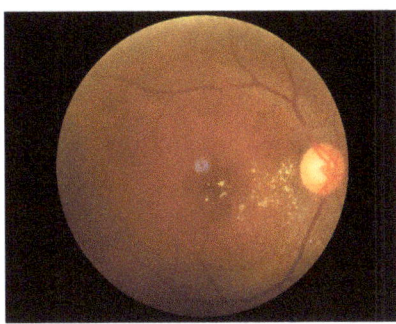

a. What is the provisional diagnosis? (2 marks)
b. What is the cause of this? (2 marks)
c. What is other common differential diagnosis? (2 marks)
d. What is the management? (4 marks)

Q20.
A 76-year-old female patient with poorly controlled DM presented to the emergency department with progressive bilateral lower limb weakness and high-grade fever for 1 week with evidence of acute urinary retention. Her inflammatory markers were significantly elevated, and the MRI spine image is shown below.

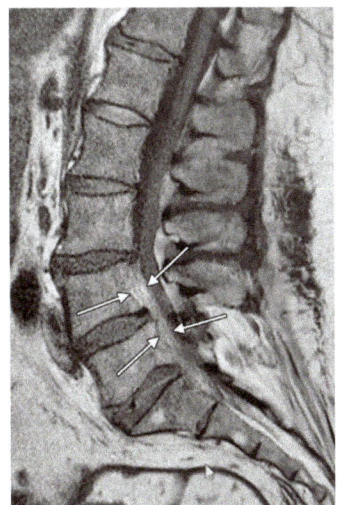

a. Describe MRI spine findings. (2 marks)
b. What is the underlying diagnosis? (3 marks)
c. What are the most appropriate treatment options to prevent long-term complications? (3 marks)
d. State two long-term complications associated with delaying the treatments. (2 marks)

ANSWERS

Ans. 1

a. Small fiber neuropathy with dysautonomia.
b. Normal light touch, vibratory sensation, and proprioception is normal. Reflexes are preserved.
c. DM mellitus, amyloidosis, and Sjögren's disease.

Ans. 2

a. Uncontrolled DM with CKD (diabetic kidney disease) stage G3aA2.
b. Sodium–glucose transport protein 2 (SGLT2) inhibitors, angiotensin II receptor blockers (ARBs)/angiotensin-converting enzyme (ACE) inhibitors, glucagon-like peptide-1 (GLP1) receptor agonist, strategies lifestyle modifications, 0.8 g/kg protein diabetic diet, and moderate intensity statins.
c. Blot hemorrhages, microaneurysms, hard exudates, and neovascularization

Ans. 3

a. T1DM and diabetic ketoacidosis (DKA)
b. Autoimmune destruction of β-cells results in insulin deficiency.
c. Anti-glutamic acid decarboxylase (anti-GAD), anti-islet cell autoantibodies (anti-ICA), anti-ZnT8 antibodies (anti-ZnT8A)
d. Give intravenous (IV) fluids and Insulin

Ans. 4

a. This condition is referred to as "double DM."
b. "Double DM" refers to a condition where individuals who have T1DM also develop features of insulin resistance, which is typically associated with T2DM. It is characterized by the coexistence of autoimmune destruction of insulin-producing cells in the pancreas (as seen in T1DM) and reduced responsiveness of body tissues to the action of insulin (as seen in T2DM).
c. Beta cell depletion in T1DM, resulting in insulin deficiency, can lead to a compensatory increase in insulin production by the pancreas, potentially contributing to insulin resistance. Genetic predisposition, obesity and adipose tissue dysfunction, sedentary lifestyle, and inflammatory factors.
d. Insulin therapy along with metformin, lifestyle measures, weight management, and education.

Ans. 5

a. Diabetic nephropathy
b. Mesangial matrix expansion and cell proliferation, thickening of the glomerular basement membrane, mesangial nodular sclerosis, fusion of podocyte foot processes on electron microscopy, and hyaline arteriosclerosis.

c.

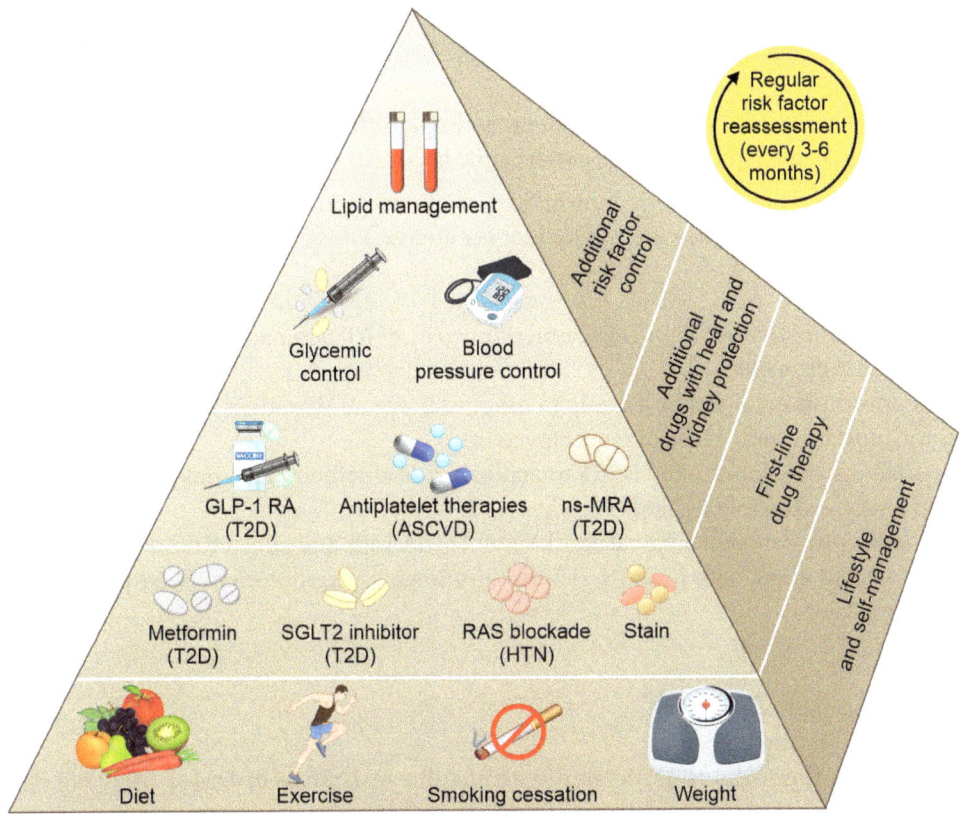

Diabetes with CKD

(ASCVD: atherosclerotic cardiovascular disease; HTN: hypertension; ns-MRA: nonsteroidal mineralocorticoid receptor antagonist; RAS: renin–angiotensin system)
Source: KDIGO Diabetes Work Group. Kidney Int. 2022 Nov;102(5S):S1-S127. 36272764.

Ans. 6

a. Nonproliferative diabetic retinopathy showing retinal hemorrhages and yellow lipid exudates.
b. Lowering triglyceride with fenofibrate (accord eye study) has been shown to reduce some beneficial effects.

Ans. 7

a. DKA
b. ABG—metabolic acidosis
c. IV fluids, IV insulin, and electrolyte management

Ans. 8

a. Insulin pump, brittle DM, and T1DM
b. The Dawn phenomenon is an observed increase in blood sugar levels that takes place in the early morning, often between 2 and 8 AM

The Somogyi phenomenon states that early morning hyperglycemia occurs due to a rebound effect from late-night hypoglycemia.

Ans. 9

a. Microfilament tests-to-test for peripheral neuropathy (diabetic foot).
b. *Acute complications:* DKA and hyperglycemic hyperosmolar state (HSS).

Chronic complications: Diabetic neuropathy, diabetic retinopathy, diabetic nephropathy, cardiovascular diseases, and cerebrovascular accidents.

Ans. 10

a. This is a case of T2DM with DKA, mucormycosis of RT paranasal sinus with intracranial and orbital extension.
b. Mucormycosis is caused by a group of fungus known as Mucorales out of which *Rhizopus* is the most common cause of mucormycosis.
c. Risk factors are uncontrolled DM, ketoacidosis, iron overload states, deferoxamine therapy, and prolonged steroid intake.
d. *Modalities of treatment:* Surgical debridement of necrotic and infected tissue is the mainstay of treatment along with broad-spectrum antifungals (amphotericin B, caspofungin, and voriconazole)

Ans. 11

a. Acanthosis nigricans
b. Axillae, groin, and body folds
c. Acanthosis nigricans is associated with insulin resistance in DM is associated with hyperinsulinemia and metabolic syndrome.
d. Polycystic ovarian syndrome, Down's syndrome, congenital lipodystrophy, malignancies especially adenocarcinoma, drugs such as steroids, oral contraceptive (OC) pills, nicotinic acid; metabolic syndrome, and obesity.
e. Diabetic dermopathy, necrobiosis lipoidica, bacterial infections, fungal infections, skin xerosis, metabolic prurigo, scleredema and skin thickening, scleredema diabeticorum, bullosis diabeticorum, ichthyosiform changes, acquired perforating dermatosis, eruptive xanthomas, benign fibromas, fibroepithelial polyps, pigmented purpuric dermatoses, and palmar erythema granuloma annulare.

Ans. 12

a. Stages of diabetic retinopathy:
   - *Stage 1:* Mild nonproliferative diabetic retinopathy.
   - *Stage 2:* Moderate nonproliferative diabetic retinopathy.
   - *Stage 3:* Severe nonproliferative diabetic retinopathy.
   - *Stage 4:* Proliferative diabetic retinopathy.
b. Proliferative diabetic retinopathy
c. Microaneurysms, hard exudates, macular edema, neovascularization, intraretinal hemorrhages, venous beadings, intraretinal microvascular anomalies, and vitreous hemorrhage

Diabetology

d. Microvascular—retinopathy, nephropathy, and neuropathy.

Macrovascular—ischemic heart disease, peripheral vascular disease, and cerebrovascular disease.

Ans. 13

a. Hyperosmolar nonketotic hyperglycemic state
b. Prolonged relative insulin deficiency associated with prolonged hyperglycemia causing osmotic symptoms and gradual dehydration.
c. Infection, sepsis, drug default, stress, skipping insulin, trauma, pancreatitis, myocardial infarction, and stroke.
d. Hyperglycemia (about 500–1,200), serum osmolality >320 mOsm/kg, pH >7.3, minimal or no ketosis, severe volume depletion, and altered sensorium or coma.
e. Fluid replacement (IV and oral) (use of isotonic or hypotonic normal saline depending on the levels of dehydration and sodium levels), insulin bolus followed by infusion (to correct hyperglycemia), correction of dyselectrolytemia, correction of potassium levels, and the treatment of underlying cause like infection.

Ans. 14

a. Lipodystrophy (insulin-related).
b. Long-acting preparations—glargine and detemir
   Short-acting preparations—regular insulin, lispro, aspart, and glulisine.
c. T1DM, T2DM with failure of oral antidiabetic drugs (OADs), T2DM with major surgery, illness, sepsis; hyperglycemic states such as DKA and nonketotic coma, pregnancy—labor and delivery, myocardial infarction, and allergy to OADs.
d. Hypoglycemia, weight gain, lipoatrophy and lipodystrophy, formation of insulin antibodies, allergy, edema, and insulin resistance.

Ans. 15

a. Secondary DM
b. Multiple calcifications in the pancreas.
c. Conditions causing pancreatic beta cell destruction (e.g., hemochromatosis, chronic pancreatitis, cystic fibrosis, and pancreatic cancers), endocrine conditions (acromegaly, Cushing's, and hyperthyroidism), infections [such as *Cytomegalovirus* (CMV), Coxsackievirus, and rubella)], and drugs (like steroids).
d. Steroids, phenytoin, thyroxine, thiazides, and interferon.
e. Sulfonylureas (glipizide, glyburide, gliclazide, and glimepiride), meglitinides (repaglinide and nateglinide), biguanides (metformin), thiazolidinediones (rosiglitazone and pioglitazone), α-glucosidase inhibitors (acarbose, miglitol, and voglibose), dipeptidyl peptidase 4 (DPP-4) inhibitors (sitagliptin, saxagliptin, vildagliptin, linagliptin, and alogliptin), and SGLT2 inhibitors (dapagliflozin and canagliflozin).

Ans. 16

a. Pyuria

b. Poor glycemic control, ureteric stones causing obstruction
c. Pyonephrosis and renal failure

Ans. 17

a. Continuous glucose monitoring (CGM) or ambulatory glucose profile is indicated for diagnosis of nocturnal hypoglycemia or to diagnose suspected glycemic variability.
It is very useful in situations where HbA1c appears to be falsely elevated or very low, clearly indicating a mismatch between fasting/postmeal blood glucose and the HbA1c
b. The TIR indicates the amount of time during which glucose readings are within the target range of 70–180 mg/dL (or 63–140 mg/dL for pregnancy). It is a new metric for glucose control.
c. Pentad consists of fasting, postmeal, HbA1c, glycemic variability, and quality of life.

Ans. 18

a. DI can be classified as central and nephrogenic. But close differential diagnosis (D/D) is primary polydipsia.
b. The absence of bright spot is seen in all cases of CDI, thus not specific for etiological diagnosis. The patient is at risk of panhypopituitarism, so a complete workup for pituitary function is needed. A thickened pituitary stalk implies the risk of infiltrating disorders, such as germ cell tumor, Langerhans cell histiocytosis, or hypophysitis. Follow-up MRI and tumor markers from cerebrospinal fluid (CSF) [human chorionic gonadotropin (hCG) and alfa-fetoprotein] are to be done.
c. Desmopressin is available as a pill or nasal spray in India. Duration of action is variable, so dose titration is needed in each child.

Ans. 19

a. Hard exudates
b. DM and nonproliferative diabetic retinopathy
c. Hypertension
d. Adequate glycemic control, BP control, and periodic check-up

Ans. 20

a. Heterogeneous signal material demonstrated in the anterior aspect of the epidural space at the L4 to S1 levels
b. L4 to S1 epidural abscess
c. Laminectomy and evacuation of ventral epidural abscess.
Long-term (4–12 weeks) IV/oral antibiotics preferably—meropenem, ceftazidime, ceftriaxone, metronidazole, and vancomycin
d. Permanent bilateral lower limb paralysis.
Fecal/urinary incontinence

SECTION 6

Hematology

QUESTIONS

Q1. A 10-year-old boy with pallor since 6 months of age, requiring regular blood transfusions.

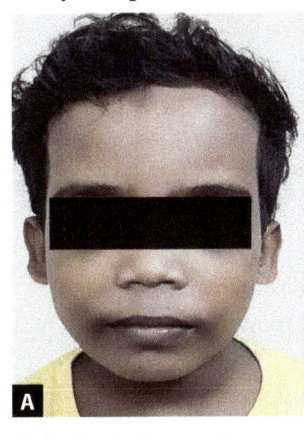
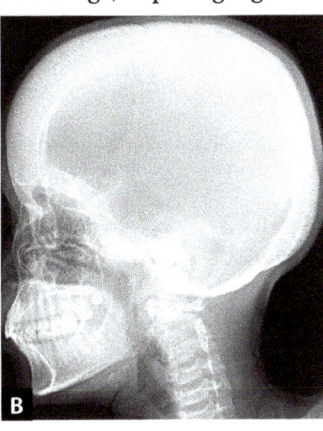

a. Name the classic facies in Image A. (3 marks)
b. Name the appearance in Image B. (3 marks)
c. Enumerate the mechanism for the above two Images A and B. (2 marks)
d. What is the diagnosis? (2 marks)

Q2. A 4-year-old girl with pallor since 4 months of age, requiring regular blood transfusion. Peripheral blood smear (PBS) image shown below.

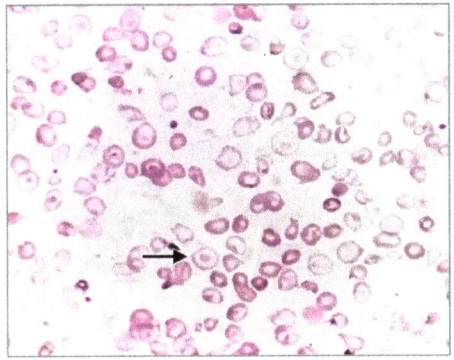

a. Identify the marked cells. *(2 marks)*
b. Name four conditions where these cells are seen. *(4 marks)*
c. What is the probable diagnosis? *(2 marks)*
d. How to confirm the diagnosis? *(2 marks)*

Q3. A 21-year-old male with hepatic vein thrombosis. Urine at different times of the day is shown below.

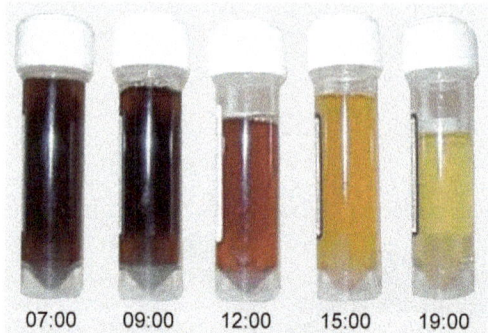

Source: Suyama D. Paroxysmal nocturnal hemoglobinuria: Recommendations for diagnostic testing. BC Med J. 2016;58(6):306-09.

a. What is the diagnosis? *(2 marks)*
b. What is the characteristic triad of the disease? *(3 marks)*
c. Name the genetic mutation and pattern of inheritance of this disease. *(2 + 2 marks)*
d. Name one complement inhibitor drug used to treat this condition. *(1 mark)*

Q4. An 8-year-old boy with a short stature with an image of a hand is shown below.

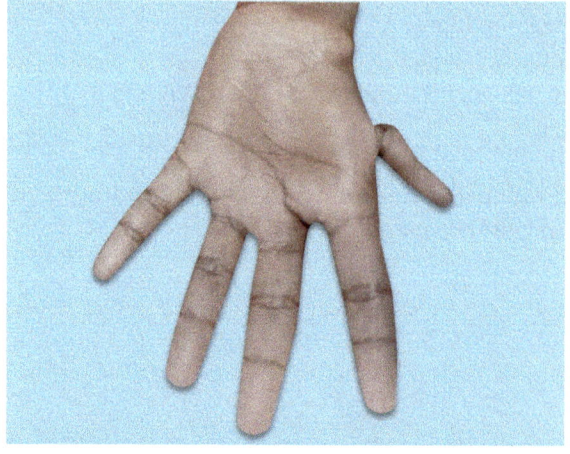

a. Identify the thumb abnormality. *(2 marks)*
b. It is found most commonly in which hematological condition? *(3 marks)*
c. What is the mode of inheritance of this disease? *(3 marks)*
d. Name two malignancies people with this disease are prone to develop. *(2 marks)*

Q5. A 10-year-old girl had an episode of the upper respiratory tract infection, and after 7 days developed extensive nonblanching red skin lesions all over the body and gum bleeding with no lymphadenopathy or organomegaly.

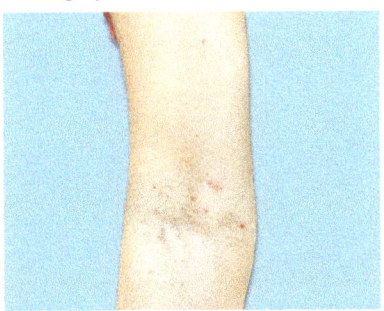

a. Identify the skin lesion. (2 marks)
b. What is the probable diagnosis? (3 marks)
c. Name two agents used as frontline therapy to treat this disease. (2 marks)
d. Name three infections causing this disease. (3 marks)

Q6. A 12-year-old boy with a history of (H/O) recurrent bony pains relieved by blood transfusion.

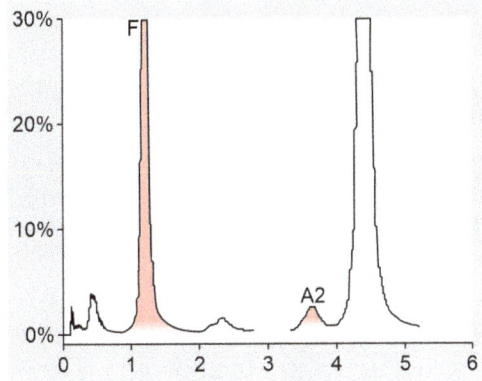

(Ao: 1.2%, A2: 2.1%, F: 21%, S window: 74%)

a. Identify the graph plot. (1 mark)
b. Discuss the diagnosis of the condition. (2 marks)
c. Name four complications of this disease. (4 marks)
d. Name three newer drugs used in this condition. (3 marks)

Q7. A 76-year-old female presented to the outpatient department (OPD) with H/O fatigue, tiredness, and backache for 6 months. The resident, after evaluation and scanning his bunch of reports made a diagnosis of monoclonal gammopathy of undetermined significance (MGUS).

a. What are the diagnostic criteria of MGUS? (3 marks)
b. Enumerate three adverse risk factors for progression. (4 marks)
c. Name three conditions that they are at high risk to get developed. (3 marks)

Q8. A 64-year-old male with anemia and recurrent urinary tract infection for the last 1 year.

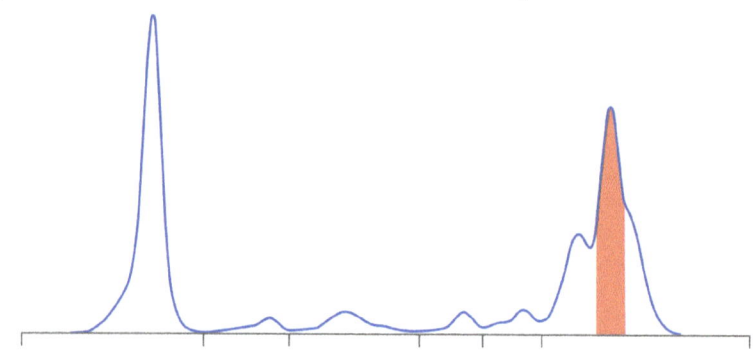

Fractions	%	Reference (%)	g/dL	Reference (g/dL)
Albumin	30.7	55.8–66.1	3.79	3.57–5.42
Alpha 1	2.5	2.9–4.9	0.26	0.19–0.40
Alpha 2	5.5	7.1–11.8	0.57	0.45–0.96
β-1	2.8	4.7–7.2	0.29	0.30–0.59
β-2	3.8	3.2–6.5	0.39	0.20–0.53
γ	48.7	11.1–18.8	5.03	0.71–1.54

a. Name the investigation. (2 marks)
b. What is the peak marked in black called? (2 marks)
c. What is the diagnosis in this case? (2 marks)
d. Name two other conditions where such a spike can be found. (4 marks)

Q9. A 5-year-old boy with recurrent pain and swelling since 6 months of age after minor trauma.

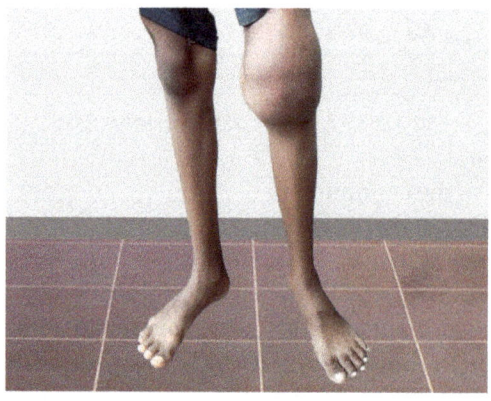

a. What is the probable diagnosis? (3 marks)
b. Name two tests to confirm the diagnosis. (2 + 2 marks)
c. What is the mode of inheritance of this disease? (3 marks)

Q10. A 17-year-old male presented with severe pallor and bleeding gums. PBS (photomicrograph) is shown below.

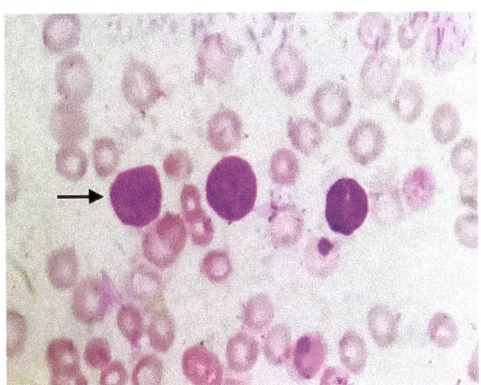

a. What is the diagnosis? (3 marks)
b. What is the characteristic chromosomal anomaly found in this disease? (3 marks)
c. Name one life-threatening complication encountered in such a situation. (2 marks)
d. Name two drugs used to treat this condition. (2 marks)

Q11. A 60-year-old man presents to the OPD with low back pain for the last 6 months and was complaining of easy fatigability on doing moderate-level work.
On examination (O/E), pallor present (PR) = 90/min, blood pressure (BP) = 144/80 mm Hg.
Routine examination revealed: Hemoglobin (Hb) = 9 g/dL, TLC = 9,000/mm^3, TPC = 2.34 lacs/mm^3, Na$^+$ = 136 mEq/L, K$^+$ = 4.2 mEq/L, calcium = 10 mg/dL, urea = 35 mg/dL, and creatinine = 1.3 mg/dL
Peripheral smear: No atypical cells bone marrow (BM) aspiration report shows:
- The percentage of the above cells was 15%
- *Serum M protein:* 50 g/L
- *Magnetic resonance imaging (MRI) of the lumbar spine (LS) spine was normal*
- *Serum-free light chain (AL) ratio:* 70 mg/L

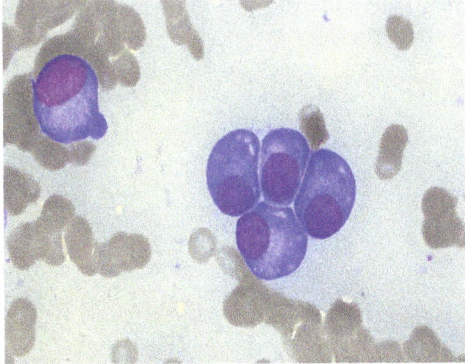

a. What is the clinical diagnosis? (5 marks)
b. Name the score used for the prognosis of the disease. (5 marks)

Q12.

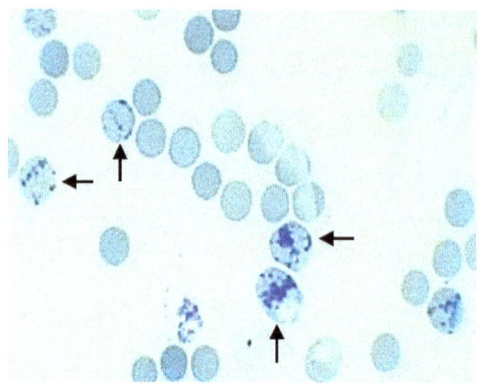

a. Name the cell depicted here. (5 marks)
b. Name the stain used to view the cells. (5 marks)

Q13.

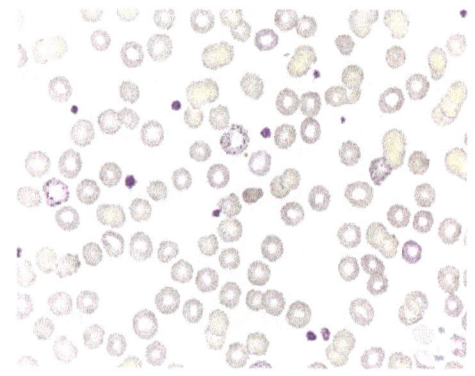

a. What is depicted in the given image? (5 marks)
b. Name the poisoning associated with given condition. (5 marks)

Q14.

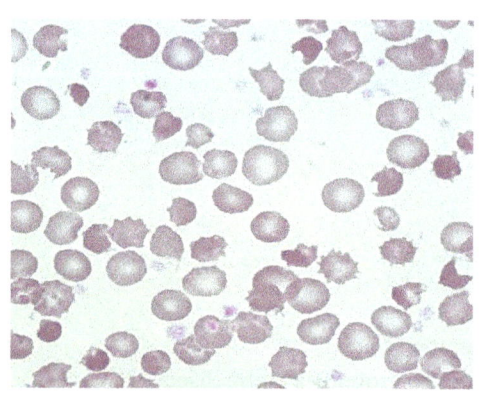

a. Name the cell shown in the image. (5 marks)
b. Name the conditions associated with the given image. (5 marks)

Q15.

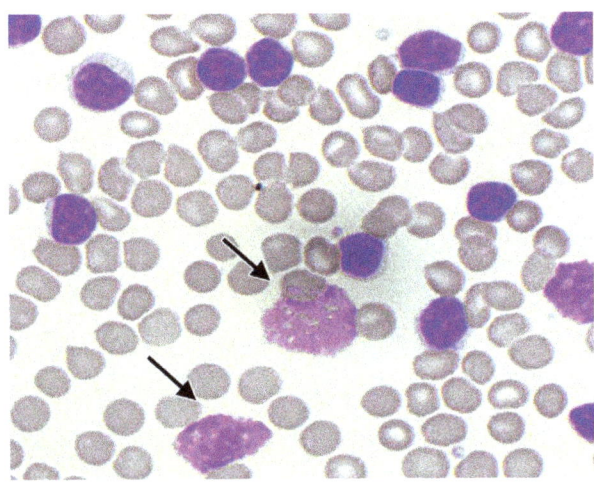

a. What is the type of cell shown in the image? (5 marks)
b. In which malignancy is this cell found? (5 marks)

Q16. PBS of a child with weight loss, anorexia, and diarrhea shows this.

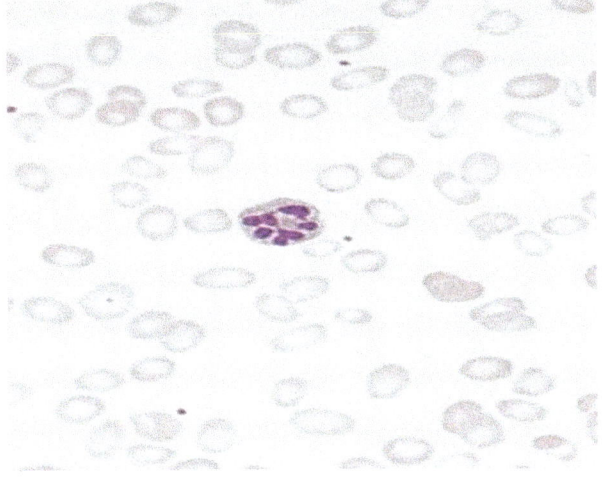

a. What is in the smear? (2 marks)
b. Mention two other findings in the smear. (2 marks)
c. What could be the cause? (2 marks)
d. Mention two other clinical features. (2 marks)
e. How will you reach a diagnosis? (2 marks)

Q17.

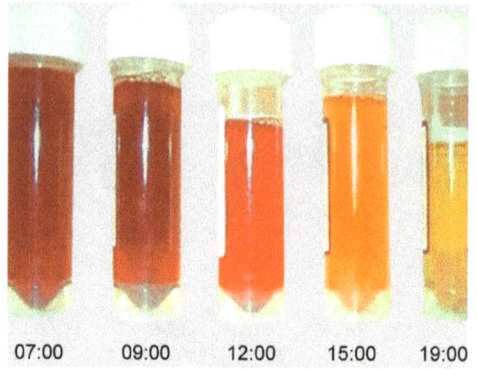

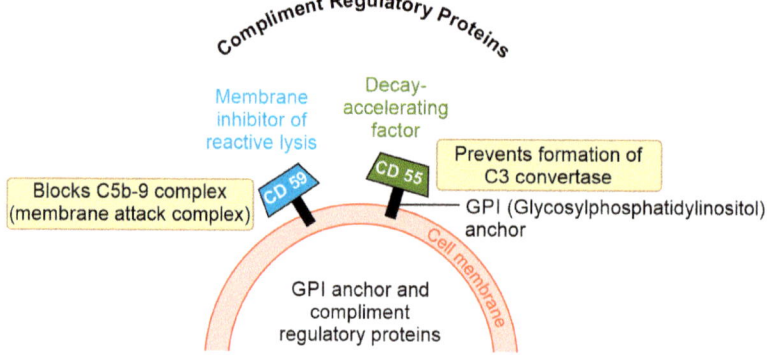

a. Identify the condition and the type of hemolysis involved. (2 marks)
b. Name the mutation involved in the condition. (2 marks)
c. Name the triad of symptoms involved in the condition. (2 marks)
d. Name the gold standard investigation and treatment of the condition. (4 marks)

Q18.
A 30-year-old mother of four children has had menorrhagia for several months. This is her PBS.

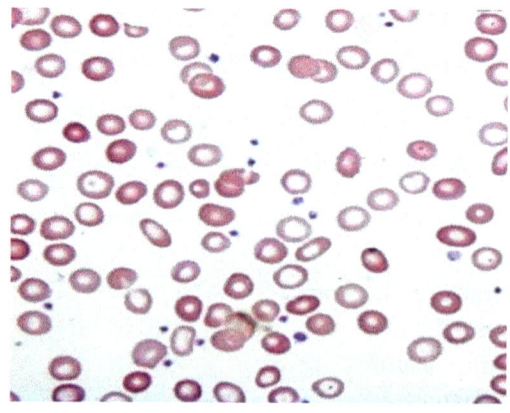

a. What does this peripheral smear show? (2 marks)
b. Name some causes. (3 marks)
c. What is Plummer–Vinson syndrome? (2 marks)
d. What are the stages of iron deficiency anemia? (3 marks)

Q19.

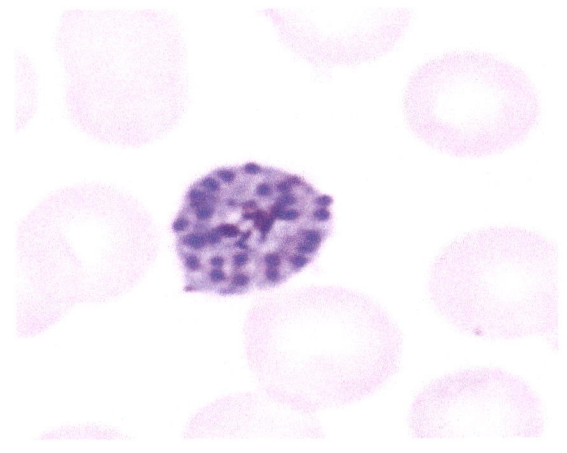

a. Identify the given slide. (5 marks)
b. Enumerate clinical features of the same. (5 marks)

Q20.

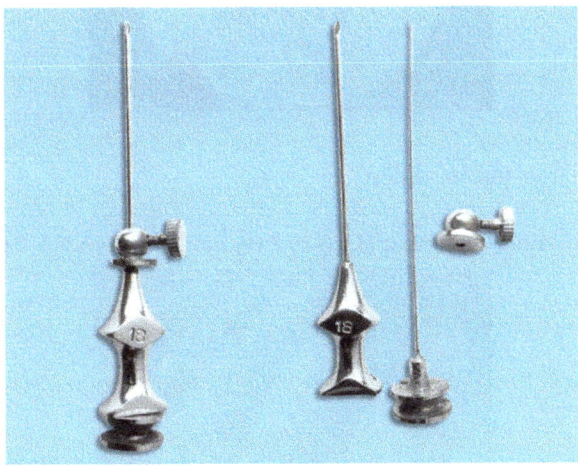

a. Identify the instrument. (½ mark)
b. Name the parts of this needle. (1½ marks)
c. Name two preferred sites in an adult for the procedure done by this needle.
   (½ + ½ = 1 mark)
d. Name two more needles that can be used for the procedure as indicated above.
   (1 + 1 = 2 marks)

Q21.

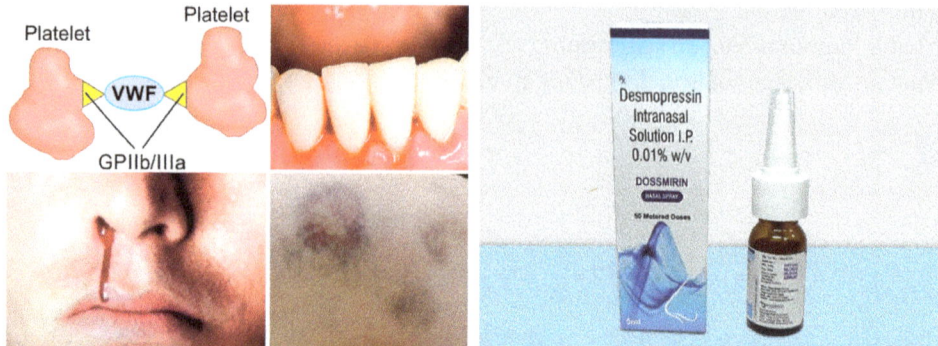

a. Identify the condition. (2 marks)
b. What is the result of the ristocetin test related to this condition? (3 marks)
c. Discuss the treatment of the condition. (5 marks)

Q22. A 55-year-old smoker was found to have this problem during a routine check-up.

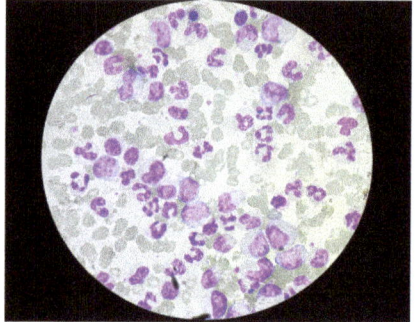

a. Describe the PBS. (5 marks)
b. Name the drug to treat the condition. (5 marks)

Q23. A 50-year-old female with complaints of easy fatigability and O/E pallor present.

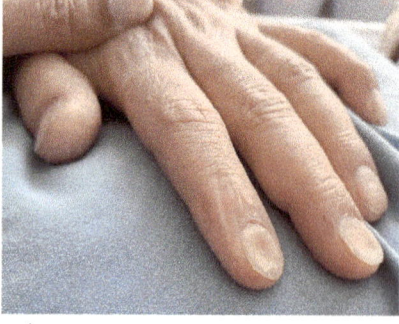

a. Identify the finding seen in the image. (3 marks)
b. What is the condition associated with it? (3 marks)
c. Findings expected in a peripheral smear of the patient. (4 marks)

ANSWERS

Ans. 1

a. Chipmunk facies (seen in chronic hemolytic anemias, e.g., beta-thalassemia major)
b. Hair on-end appearance or crew-cut skull
c. Excessive bone marrow hyperplasia
d. Congenital hemolytic anemias (transfusion-dependent thalassemia—beta-thalassemia major)

Ans. 2

a. Target cells
b. Postsplenectomy, iron deficiency anemia, hemoglobin C (HbC) disease, and liver disease.
c. Congenital hemolytic anemias (transfusion-dependent thalassemia—beta-thalassemia major), PBS showing anisopoikilocytosis, microcytic hypochromic red blood cells (RBCs), target cells, and teardrop cells.
d. *Cation exchange:* High-performance liquid chromatography (CE-HPLC) of Hb.

Ans. 3

a. Paroxysmal nocturnal hemoglobinuria (PNH)
b. Intravascular hemolysis, thrombosis, and cytopenias
c. (i) *PIGA* gene and (ii) acquired genetic disorder
d. Eculizumab (anti-C5 monoclonal antibody)

Ans. 4

a. Hypoplastic thumb
b. Fanconi anemia
c. *Autosomal recessive:* The most common, can show autosomal dominant, and X-linked inheritance.
d. Squamous cell carcinoma (cutaneous/head and neck) and acute leukemia (acute myeloid leukemia).

Ans. 5

a. Petechiae
b. Immune thrombocytopenia/immune thrombocytopenic purpura (ITP)
c. Intravenous immunoglobulin (IVIG) and corticosteroids
d. Human immunodeficiency virus (HIV), hepatitis C virus (HCV), and *Helicobacter pylori* (*H. pylori*)

Ans. 6

a. Hb high-performance liquid chromatography (Hb-HPLC)
b. Sickle cell anemia (HbSS)
c. Vaso-occlusive crisis, hemolytic crisis, sequestration crisis, and aplastic crisis
d. Crizanlizumab, voxelotor, and L-glutamine

Ans. 7

a. MGUS is a clinically asymptomatic premalignant clonal plasma cell or lymphoplasmacytic proliferative disorder. It is defined by the presence of a serum monoclonal protein (M protein) at a concentration <3 g/dL, a bone marrow with <10% monoclonal plasma cells, and the absence of end-organ damage (lytic bone lesions, anemia, hypercalcemia, renal insufficiency, and hyperviscosity) related to the proliferative process.
b. The risk stratification system promoted by the IMWG combines three adverse risk factors to predict the risk of progression of MGUS (non-IgM and IgM) to multiple myeloma (MM) or a related malignancy. They are:
   - Serum M-protein level ≥1.5 g/dL (≥15 g/L)
   - Non-IgG MGUS [i.e., immunoglobulin A (IgA), immunoglobulin M (IgM), and immunoglobulin D (IgD) MGUS]
   - Abnormal serum free light chain (FLC) ratio (i.e., ratio of the kappa to lambda free ALs <0.26 or >1.65)
c. Increased risk of fractures, infections, and thromboembolic disease.

Ans. 8

a. Serum protein electrophoresis
b. Monoclonal peak (M band)
c. Multiple myeloma
d. Systemic AL amyloidosis and Waldenström's macroglobulinemia

Ans. 9

a. Hemophilia
b. (i) Prothrombin time (PT) and activated partial thromboplastin time (aPTT) and (ii) Factor VIII and IX assay
c. X-linked recessive

Ans. 10

a. Acute promyelocytic leukemia (PBS showing abnormal promyelocytes with an arrow showing "Angel wing" or "buttock cell" appearance)
b. t(15;17)
c. Disseminated intravascular coagulation
d. All trans-retinoic acid and arsenic trioxide

Ans. 11

a. The clinical diagnosis in the above question is nothing but multiple myeloma. So going as per the new diagnostic criteria "SLIM CRAB" are defined as myeloma defining events (MDE). So, the presence of bone marrow plasma cells >10% (in our case 15%) with any one of the MDE (in our case Hb—9 g/dL (<10 g/dL) is suggestive of multiple myeloma.

Myeloma-defining events (SLIM + CRAB)

S: Bone marrow plasma cells >60%

LI: Involved : Uninvolved SFLC ratio ≥100 (involved LC must be >100 mg/L)

M: ≥2 focal lesions on MRI (>5 mm in size)

C: Hypercalcemia (>2.75 mml/L or >0.25 above ULN)

R: Renal insufficiency (serum Cr >177 umol/L or CrCl <40 mL/min)

A: Anemia: Hb <100 g/L

B: ≥1 lytic lesion on X-ray/CT/PET-CT (>5 mm in size)

(CT: computed tomography; Hb: hemoglobin; LC: locus coeruleus; MRI: magnetic resonance imaging; PET: positron emission tomography; SFLC: serum free light chains; ULN: upper limit of normal)

b. The score used for disease prognostication is the Revised International Staging System (R-ISS) score.

Ans. 12
a. Reticulocytes
b. New methyl blue

Ans. 13
a. Basophilic stippling
b. Lead poisoning

Ans. 14
a. Acanthocyte
b. Liver disease and abetalipoproteinemia

Ans. 15
a. Smudge cell
b. Chronic lymphocytic leukemia (CLL)

Ans. 16
a. Hypersegmented neutrophil (>5 nuclear lobes)
b. Few macrocytes, Howell–Jolly bodies, elliptocytes, and some hypochromic RBCs
c. Vitamin B_{12} deficiency.
d. Cognitive impairment and psychotic disturbances.
e. PBS, test for pernicious anemia (serum gastrin level, antibodies to IF or partial cells), serum methylmalonic acid level.

Ans. 17
a. Paroxysmal nocturnal hemoglobinuria and intravascular hemolysis
b. *PIGA* gene mutation
c. Triad—hemolysis, pancytopenia, and venous thromboses
d. Flow cytometry, treatment—eculizumab (anti-CD5 monoclonal antibody)

Ans. 18

a. Severely hypochromic and microcytic picture
b. Iron deficiency anemia, thalassemia, lead poisoning, and sideroblastic anemia
c. Iron deficiency anemia, postcricoid dysphagia, and upper esophageal webs
d. (i) Stage 1—iron stores depletion; (ii) Stage 2—iron-deficient erythropoiesis; and (iii) Stage 3—iron deficiency anemia

Ans. 19

a. Schizont of *Plasmodium vivax*
b. Initially, patients have fever, chills, sweating, headache, weakness, and other symptoms mimicking a "viral syndrome." Later, severe disease may develop, with an abnormal level of consciousness, severe anemia, renal failure, and multisystem failure.

Ans. 20

a. Salah bone marrow aspiration (BMA) needle
b. Trocar
   - Cannula
   - Adjustable side guard
c. The posterior superior iliac spine is the most preferred sternum.
d. (i) Klima BMA needle
   (ii) Jamshidi disposable BMA needle

Ans. 21

a. Von Willebrand disease
b. The ristocetin test is negative
c. Treatment is desmopressin

Ans. 22

a. CML
b. *Treatment:* Tyrosine kinase inhibitors [imatinib and 2 g tyrosine kinase inhibitor (TKI); such as dasatinib, nilotinib, and bosutinib)

Ans. 23

a. Koilonychia
b. Seen in iron deficiency anemia
c. Findings expected on a peripheral smear of this patient are hypochromia, microcytosis, anisocytosis, and poikilocytosis.

SECTION 7

Oncology

QUESTIONS

Q1. A 55-year-old male presented in an emergency with an acute onset of breathlessness. He was a smoker with a 30-pack-year history. Examination revealed clubbing. His X-ray chest is shown below.

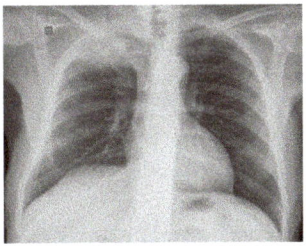

a. Name the condition. (2 marks)
b. Enumerate the components. (4 marks)
c. How will you confirm the diagnosis and which histopathology (HP) is commonly associated with it? (2 marks)
d. Name the full name of the scientist who first described it. (2 marks)

Q2. A 62-year-old male presented with fatigue, weakness, fever, weight loss, and/or abdominal discomfort for 6 months. On examination, he had pallor2+ and an enlarged hepatosplenomegaly. He gave a history of pneumonia 6 months back. Laboratory tests were suggestive of pancytopenia. His peripheral cell is shown below.

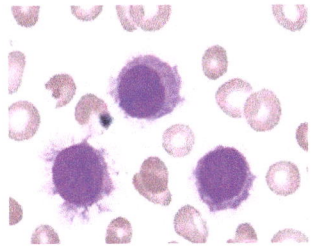

a. Describe the peripheral smear. (2 marks)
b. What is the diagnosis? Which category does it belong to? (3 marks)
c. Suggest further test and treatment. (5 marks)

Oncology

Q3. A 58-year-old woman presented with headache, dizziness, and blurred vision for 2 months. Examination of the abdomen revealed mild-moderate splenomegaly.

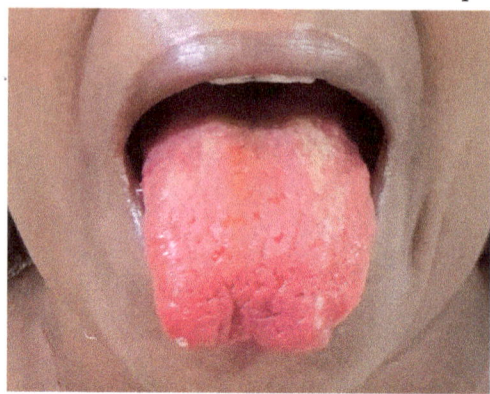

a. What characteristic appearance is shown in the picture? *(2 marks)*
b. What is the diagnosis? *(2 marks)*
c. What are the complications of this condition? *(2 marks)*
d. How do you diagnose this condition? *(4 marks)*

Q4. *Scenario*: You are evaluating a patient with fatigue, pale skin, and bleeding gums. Laboratory results show pancytopenia. Physical examination reveals hepatosplenomegaly.
a. What is the most likely diagnosis? *(3 marks)*
b. Describe the pathophysiology of pancytopenia in this condition. *(4 marks)*
c. Name one genetic mutation associated with this disorder. *(3 marks)*

Q5. A 34-year-old female with pallor and massive splenomegaly for the last 1-year peripheral blood smear is shown below.

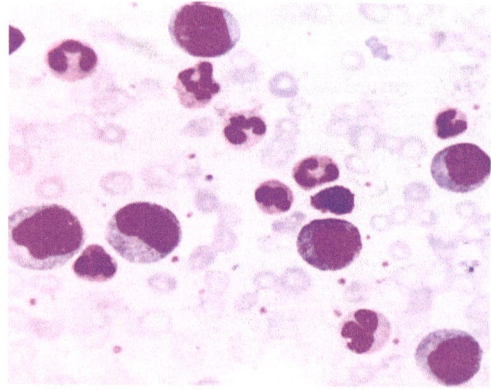

a. Identify the disease. *(3 marks)*
b. Name the chromosomal abnormality found in this condition. *(3 marks)*
c. Name the scientists who discovered the above chromosomal abnormality. *(2 marks)*
d. What is the drug of choice for this condition? *(2 marks)*

Q6.

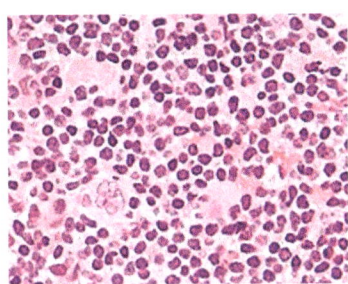

a. Identify the above cell. (5 marks)
b. In which condition this cell is found? (5 marks)

Q7. A 63-year-old female with complaints of back pain, fatigability, and oliguria.
Creatinine: 3.3 mg/dL
Calcium: 11.6 mg/dL
Complete blood count (CBC): 7.5/5,600/230,000

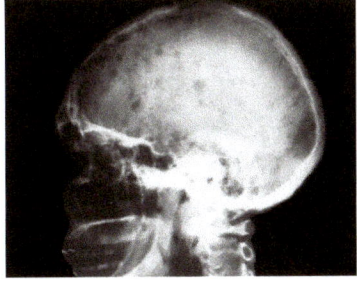

a. Identify the findings seen in the above image. (5 marks)
b. Staging of the above condition. (5 marks)

Q8. A 35-year-old patient presented with acute promyelocytic leukemia (APML). He was treated with ATRA + ATO. 5 days later, he developed dyspnea, pericardial plus pleural effusion, and weight gain with the saturation of peripheral oxygen (SpO_2) 85%.

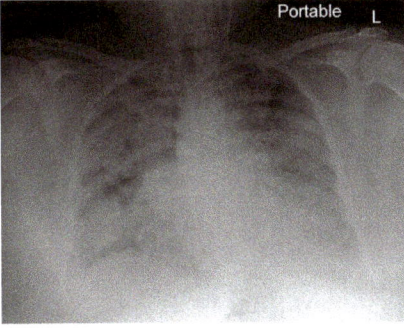

a. What is the diagnosis for the above condition? (5 marks)
b. What will be the treatment for the above condition? (5 marks)

Q9. A patient presents with lymphadenopathy. Peripheral smear findings are shown below.

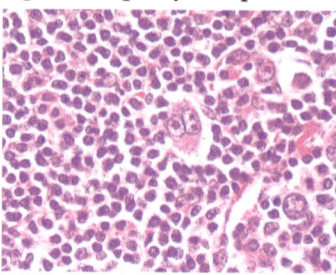

a. Identify the finding seen on the peripheral smear and the condition in which it is seen?
(5 marks)
b. Name the staging system used for the condition and causes of generalized lymphadenopathy.
(5 marks)

Q10. A patient with a known case of bronchogenic carcinomas has the following findings:

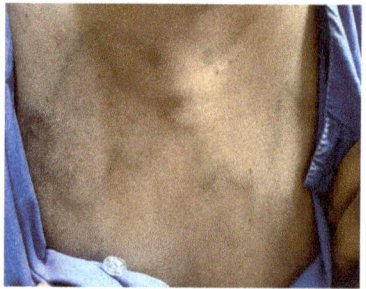

a. Identify the condition. (5 marks)
b. Give the histological classification if lung cancers. (5 marks)

Q11. A 20-year-old female has a history of fever with night sweats for the last 3 months. On examination, she had multiple swellings over the postcervicals region which were rubbery in consistency and matted. Biopsy was taken from the swelling and the histopathological examination (HPE) is demonstrated below.

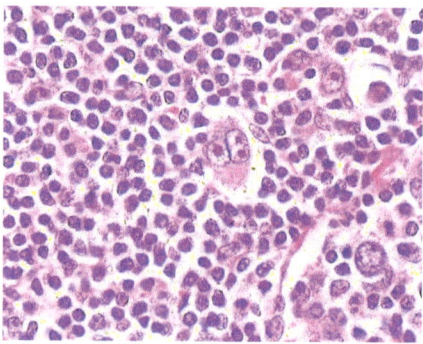

a. What are the pathological cells in the HPE? (3 marks)

b. What is your diagnosis? *(2 marks)*
c. What are the markers to look for? *(3 marks)*
d. What is the classification system known as? *(2 marks)*

Q12. A 55-year-old male presented to the casualty with generalized fatigability, difficulty in getting up from a sitting position, and lifting his arms above his head for the last 2 months. He is also complaining of difficulty in swallowing the food. But he is saying his symptoms are more during the morning after getting up from bed and improve as the day passes. He is recently complaining of a dry cough for the last 1 month without any fever or night sweats although he has significant weight loss. He is a known smoker for the last 20 years.

A chest X-ray was done which showed:

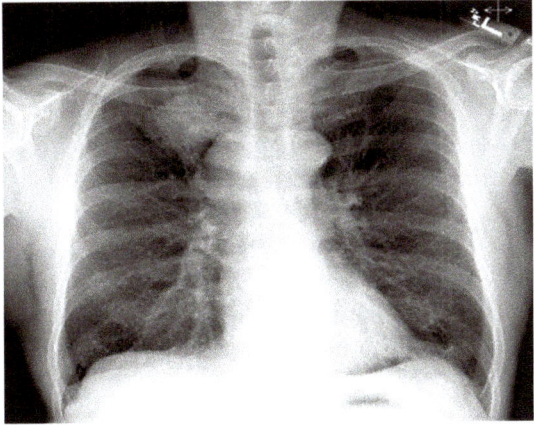

Immediately a bronchoscopy-guided biopsy was ordered and the specimen was sent for HPE. Histopathological examination revealed:

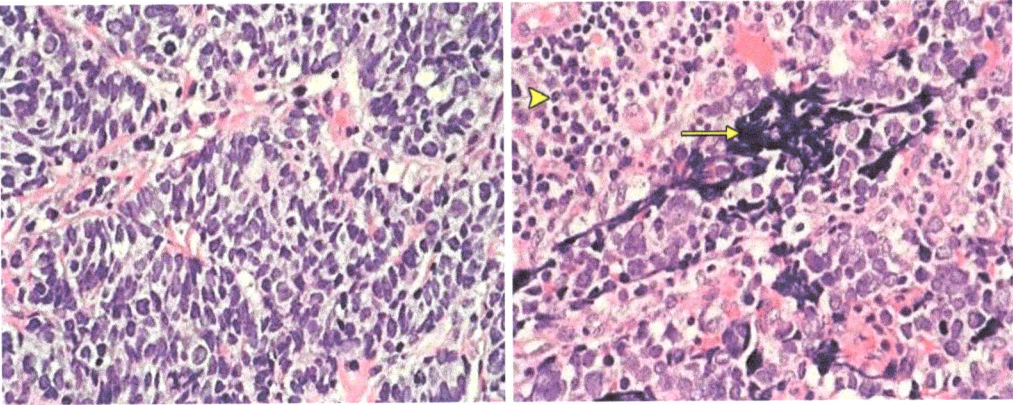

a. What is the clinical diagnosis? *(3 marks)*
b. What is the classical site affected in this person with the aforementioned neurological disease process? *(3 marks)*
c. Describe the HP slide from the biopsy obtained. *(4 marks)*

Q13.

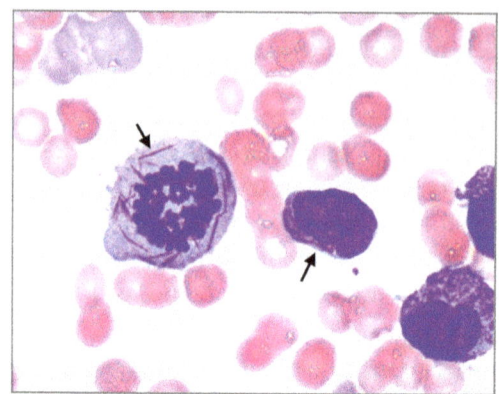

a. What is the name of the labeled structure? (2 marks)
b. What is the diagnosis? (2 marks)
c. What do you expect to see in a complete hemogram? (2 marks)
d. Discuss the various management options. (4 marks)

Q14.
A 65-year-old male presented with a fever of 101°F for 3 weeks with no evidence of infection, unintentional weight loss for the last 6 months, drenching night sweats, extreme fatigue, and early satiety. On examination, he had anemia, generalized lymphadenopathy moderate, nontender and firm splenomegaly, and hepatomegaly. His blood smear was as below.

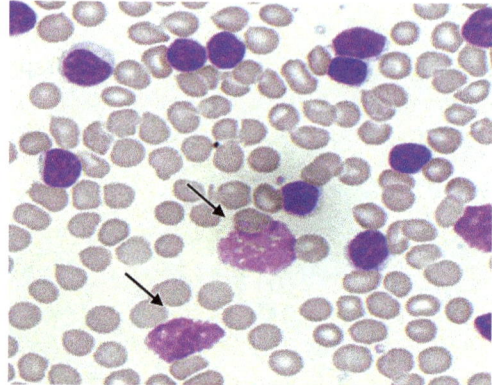

a. What is the probable diagnosis? (1 mark)
b. What are the arrow-marked cells called? (1 mark)
c. How are these cells formed? (1 mark)
d. What is its significance in the prognosis of the disease? (1 mark)
e. This condition is common in children. True or False? (1 mark)

Q15. A 72-year-old lady came with recurrent multiple falls with a long lie. She has a history of reduced memory and functional decline over the last 6 months.
- *Serum calcium:* 3.22 mmol/L [relative risk (RR) 2.15–2.65 mmol/L]
- *Corrected calcium:* 3.40 mmol/L (RR: 2.15–2.65 mmol/L)
- *Plasma parathyroid hormone (PTH) (intact):* <0.3 pmol/L (2.0 015–8.5 pmol/L)
- *25 hydroxyl vitamin D:* 70 nmol/L (>50 nmol/L)
- *Creatine kinase (CK):* 1,855 → 594 U/L (0–170 U/L)
- *Urea:* 9.8 mmol/L (3–10 mmol/L)
- *Creatinine:* 114 umol/L (40–90 umol/L)
- *Estimated glomerular filtration rate (eGFR) (mL/min):* 39 (>60/1.73 m^2)

Computed tomography of the chest, abdomen, and pelvis (CTCAP)-enlarged lymph nodes demonstrated at both and below the diaphragm as described above includes marked retroperitoneal involvement with partial encasement of the left kidney and the bilateral ovarian veins extending inferiorly into the pelvis.

a. Name two acute complications. *(2 marks)*
b. What do you expect in urine testing? *(2 marks)*
c. Name two immediate treatments that can be used to manage each complication in an acute setting. *(4 marks)*
d. What is the underlying diagnosis? *(2 marks)*

ANSWERS

Ans. 1

a. Pancoast syndrome
b. Superior sulcus tumor along with ipsilateral shoulder and arm pain, paresthesias, paresis, and atrophy of the thenar muscles of the hand and Horner's syndrome (ptosis, miosis, and anhidrosis).
c. Bronchoscopy and biopsy/CT-guided biopsy. Squamous cell/adenocarcinoma.
d. Professor Henry Pancoast in 1932.

Ans. 2

a. The peripheral smear is suggestive of abnormal lymphocytes—"The Hairy cells"
b. Hairy cell leukemia belongs to the B-cell type leukemia
c. Immunophenotyping and bone marrow aspiration and biopsy. Asymptomatic patients need "active monitoring." Symptomatic patients are treated with pentostatin and cladribine.

Ans. 3

a. Dark red tongue
b. *Polycythemia rubra vera:* Polycythemia vera (PV) is a stem cell disorder, characterized as a neoplastic marrow disorder. An elevated absolute red blood cell mass is the most prominent feature due to uncontrolled red blood cell production. This is accompanied by increased white blood cell (myeloid) and platelet (megakaryocytic) production also.
c. Increased risk of thrombosis, myocardial infarctions, ischemic strokes, and risk of bleeding.
d. The presence of either all three major criteria or the first two major criteria and the minor criterion.

   The major World Health Organization (WHO) criteria are as follows:
   - Hemoglobin >16.5 g/dL in men and >16 g/dL in women, or hematocrit >49% in men and >48% in women, or red cell mass >25% above mean normal predicted value.
   - Bone marrow biopsy showing hypercellularity for age with trilineage growth (panmyelosis) including prominent erythroid, granulocytic, and megakaryocytic proliferation with pleomorphic, and mature megakaryocytes (differences in size).
   - The presence of *JAK2V617F* or *JAK2* exon 12 mutation.

   The minor WHO criterion is as follows:
   - Serum erythropoietin level below the reference range for normal.

Ans. 4

a. The most likely diagnosis is myelodysplastic syndrome (MDS).
b. Pancytopenia in MDS results from ineffective hematopoiesis in the bone marrow, leading to decreased production of red blood cells, white blood cells, and platelets.
c. One genetic mutation associated with MDS is the deletion of chromosome 5q (del[5q]).

Ans. 5

a. Chronic myeloid leukemia (peripheral blood smear showing left shift with myelocytes, metamyelocytes, and basophilia)
b. t(9;22)
c. Peter C Nowell and David A Hungerford
d. Tyrosine kinase inhibitor (TKI) inhibitor (imatinib, nilotinib, dasatinib, etc.)

Ans. 6

a. Reed–Sternberg (RS) cells
b. Hodgkin's lymphoma

Ans. 7

a. Typical "punched out" lesions characteristic of multiple myeloma.
b. International Staging System (ISS) consisting of serum β-2 microglobulin and serum albumin.

Ans. 8

a. Differentiation syndrome
b. Glucocorticoids, chemotherapy for cytoreduction, and/or supportive measures.

Ans. 9

a. RS cell is seen in Hodgkin's lymphoma.
b. Ann Arbor staging for Hodgkin's lymphoma. The cause of generalized lymphadenopathy—lymphoma, leukemia, human immunodeficiency virus (HIV)/acquired immunodeficiency syndrome (AIDS), systemic lupus erythematosus (SLE), etc.

Ans. 10

a. Superior vena cava obstruction
b.
- Small cell lung cancer
- Nonsmall cell lung cancer
  - Squamous cell carcinoma
  - Adenocarcinomas
  - Large cell carcinomas

Ans. 11

a. The pathological cells in the HPE show a large binucleated cell, with prominent eosinophilic nuclei surrounded by abundant cytoplasm. These are classically known as RS cells.
b. Keeping the clinical picture of Fever, night sweats, and cervical lymphadenopathy in a 20-year-old female with the presence of RS cells in HPE a diagnosis of classical Hodgkin's lymphoma is made.
c. Markers to look for in Hodgkin's lymphoma are cluster of differentiation 15 (CD15), cluster of differentiation 30 (CD30), and paired box 5 (PAX-5). It lacks the classical B-cell markers as it is a mutated B-cell.
d. The staging system to stage the disease is known as the *Ann Arbor staging system*.

Ans. 12

a. This is a case of *lambert-Eaton myasthenic syndrome* as a paraneoplastic manifestation of CA lung (Small cell carcinoma).
b. The classical site affected in the disease process is due to autoantibodies affecting the *presynaptic voltage-gated calcium channel.*
c. HP slide shows malignant epithelial cells composed of small, oval, rounded fusiform cells with scant cytoplasm, irregular borders, fine granular chromatin, and inconspicuous nuclei. Basophilic staining of the vessel wall due to high turnover of tumor cells is known as the "Azzopardi effect."

Ans. 13

a. Auer rods
b. Acute myeloid leukemia
c. Pancytopenia and leukocytosis may also be present.
d. Chemotherapy (daunorubicin, cladribine, and fludarabine), targeted therapy, stem cell transplant, and supportive therapy.

Ans. 14

a. Chronic lymphocytic leukemia (CLL)
b. Smudge cell, basket cell, and Gumprecht shadows.
c. Smudge cells are ruptured CLL B-cells.
d. The lower the percentage of smudge cells worse is the prognosis. About <30% of smudge cells are associated with a poor prognosis in CLL.
e. False

Ans. 15

a.
- Humoral hypercalcemia of malignancy
- Rhabdomyolysis

b. Urine myoglobinuria

c.
- IV 0.9% NaCl bolus
- IV Bisphosphonate

d. Non-Hodgkin's lymphoma

SECTION 8

Nephrology

QUESTIONS

Q1. A 34-year-old female presented with an ultrasonography (USG) showing bilateral large kidneys with multiple cysts and hepatic cysts. Her creatinine is at present 1.4. Her father was a school teacher who also had multiple cysts in both kidneys and died from cerebral hemorrhage at the age of 46 years.
a. What is the diagnosis? *(2 marks)*
b. What are the other complications seen in this disease? *(6 marks)*
c. What are the drugs used in treatment? *(2 marks)*

Q2. A 15-year-old boy presented with reduced urine output with dark urine and swelling of the body for last 3 days. He had history of fever 1 month back with sore throat. His creatinine is at present 1.8 mg/dL, and urine shows 2+ protein, red blood cell (RBC) 20–30/hpf (high-power field), and white blood cell (WBC) 4–6/hpf.
a. What is the possible diagnosis? *(2 marks)*
b. Which organism is involved? *(2 marks)*
c. What are the investigations need to be suggested? *(2 marks)*
d. What treatment needs to be given? *(4 marks)*

Q3. A 7-year-old girl presented with swelling of whole body third time in last 1 year. She has been diagnosed as having nephrotic syndrome, which has responded to steroids in previous episodes.
a. What is the definition of frequent relapse? *(2 marks)*
b. What is partial remission? *(2 marks)*
c. What is complete remission? *(2 marks)*
d. What is steroid-dependent nephrotic syndrome? *(2 marks)*
e. What is steroid-resistant nephrotic syndrome? *(2 marks)*

Q4. A 68-year-old lady presented with history of fever with nausea and anorexia for last 3 days. She is diabetic on insulin and hypertensive but has poor compliance to medications since she lives alone. The CT scan done is given below.

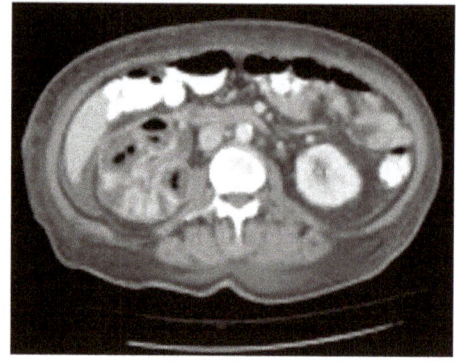

a. What is the diagnosis? (2 marks)
b. What are the clinical presentations? (4 marks)
c. What treatment needs to be given? (4 marks)

Q5. A 39-year-old male from Bengal, known to have kidney stone disease, has been admitted to the accident and emergency department with right renal angle pain. A CT scan with a stone protocol has been performed. Refer to the image below.

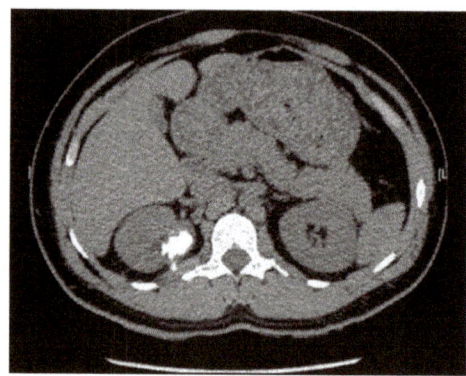

a. What is the most likely diagnosis in this patient? (2 marks)
b. Which organisms are involved? (4 marks)
c. What is the treatment? (4 marks)

Q6. A 64-year-old woman, who has been receiving vancomycin and cefepime for a duration of 10 days, sought nephrology consultation due to an increase in serum creatinine levels, rising from a baseline of 0.6 to 2.4 mg/dL. Her random vancomycin level is measured at 40 ng/mL. Urinalysis reveals traces of blood, 1+ protein, RBC 6–8/hpf, WBC 30–40/hpf, with occasional WBC cast.

a. What is the diagnosis? (2 marks)
b. What classical clinical triad seen? (3 marks)
c. Most common group of drugs involved. (3 marks)
d. Treatment suggested. (2 marks)

Q7. A 78-year-old man was found collapsed on the floor by his caregiver following an inadvertent mechanical fall overnight. He had a medical history of hypertension and dyslipidemia and was undergoing treatment with amlodipine, ramipril, and atorvastatin.

Serum sodium: 157 mmol/L
Serum potassium: 6.0 mEq/L
Blood urea: 9.6 mmol/L
Serum creatinine: 3.71 mg/dL
Adjusted calcium: 8.7 mg/dL
Creatinine phosphokinase (CPK): 14,700 IU/L

a. What is the diagnosis? *(2 marks)*
b. What are the causes? *(4 marks)*
c. How to treat such patient? *(4 marks)*

Q8. A 77-year-old lady underwent coronary angiography followed by percutaneous transluminal coronary angioplasty (PTCA) 2 days back. She had history of chest discomfort and is diabetic and hypertensive. On postoperative day 3 (POD 3), she had rise of serum creatinine to 1.5 mg/dL with no reduction of urine output. The creatinine continued to rise to a level of 1.8 mg/dL till POD 8 after which her creatinine gradually decreased to 1.1 mg/dL on 14th POD.

a. What is the diagnosis? *(2 marks)*
b. Risk factors? *(4 marks)*
c. How this can be prevented? *(4 marks)*

Q9. A 41-year-old man from Assam, a smoker, presents with a 10-day history of low-grade fever, myalgias, cough, shortness of breath, hemoptysis, and decreased oral intake, more recently accompanied by oliguria and a single episode of gross hematuria. Laboratory evaluation reveals a creatinine level of 9 mg/dL, K 5.9 mmol/L, albumin 25 g/dL, hematocrit 30%, white blood cell count 11,500, and platelet count 352,000, hemoglobin (Hb) 7.8 g%, blood pressure (BP) of 140/89 mm Hg, and no edema or skin rash. Urine dipstick reveals 2+protein and 3+ blood. X-ray findings are shown in below image.

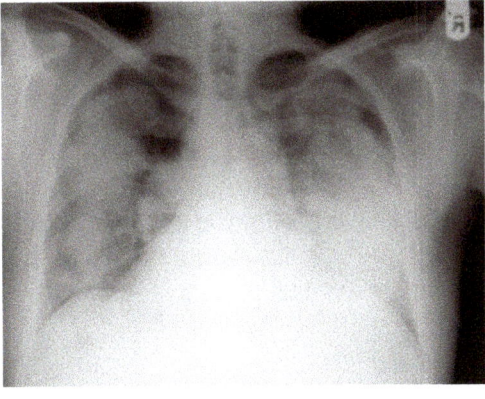

a. What is the diagnosis here? *(2 marks)*
b. What are the most common causes of pulmonary renal syndrome? *(4 marks)*
c. What are the treatment options? *(4 marks)*

Nephrology

Q10. A 55-year-old male with chronic lymphocytic leukemia (CLL) who was initiated on chemotherapy last week presented with seizure in emergency room (ER). On admission, his Hb was 9 g%, total leucocyte count (TLC) 37,000/mL, serum lactate dehydrogenase (LDH) 1,700 U/L, creatinine 3.3 mg/dL, uric acid 11 mg/L, Ca 6.7 mg/dL, Na 130 mmol/L, K 6.4 mEq/L, and PO4 5 mg/dL.
- a. What is the diagnosis? *(2 marks)*
- b. What are the presentations? *(4 marks)*
- c. What are the treatment options? *(4 marks)*

Q11. A 23-year-old male presented with smoky red urine for last 3 days without any pain or dysuria.

He had history of cough and sore throat for last 5 days. He had similar history twice before but did not seek any medical attention.
- a. What is the probable diagnosis? *(2 marks)*
- b. What are the causes of microscopic hematuria? *(4 marks)*
- c. What are the suggested treatments of the cause? *(4 marks)*

Q12. A 21-year-old male from UP presented with severe vomiting and diarrhea for last 2 days with anuria for last 16 hours. He had attended a wedding in his village 2 days back where many more fell ill afterward.
- a. What is the diagnosis? *(2 marks)*
- b. How to identify a prerenal acute kidney injury (AKI)? *(4 marks)*
- c. What is the treatment? *(4 marks)*

Q13. Ramu, a 14-year-old boy, presented with pain and swelling of left leg while playing in the paddy field 1 day back. He was taken to local primary health center (PHC) where he was treated with tetanus and antisnake venom with intravenous fluid (IVF). But since his urine output has decreased from the morning, he has been referred to the apex center.
- a. What types of snakes are most commonly responsible for renal failure? *(2 marks)*
- b. What are the treatment options in this case? *(4 marks)*
- c. What arthropods are responsible for causing AKI? *(4 marks)*

Q14. A 26-year-old female developed anuria on second day postpartum. She had an uncomplicated normal vaginal delivery following an uncomplicated antenatal period. Her reports on admission were: Hb 7.1 g%, TLC 5,600/mL, platelets 70,000/mL, peripheral smear showed schistocytes, LDH 760 U/L, total bilirubin 2.1, aspartate transaminase (AST) 13, and alanine aminotransferase (ALT) 16.
- a. What is the probable diagnosis? *(2 marks)*
- b. What are the treatment options? *(4 marks)*
- c. What are the other causes of AKI in pregnancy? *(4 marks)*

Q15.

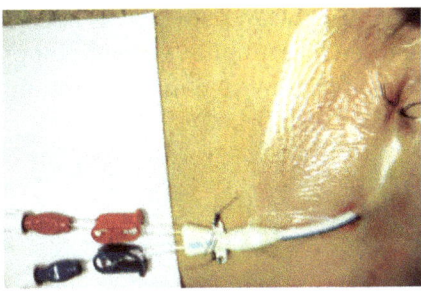

a. What is the name of instrument? (3 marks)
b. What are the indications? (3 marks)
c. What are the complications of the procedure? (4 marks)

Q16.
An 18-year-old girl came to us with chief complaints of flank pain on and off for the last 4 months and frequent passages of tiny stone like substances in urine for the last 10 days. She was also complaining of dryness of the mouth and eyes, fatigue, and joint pain for the last 1 year. X-ray of kidney, ureter, and bladder (KUB) region is shown in the image below. An arterial blood gas analysis showed a pH of 7.21, bicarbonate 15.2 mmol/L, potassium 2.8 mmol/L, sodium 136 mmol/L, and chloride 108 mmol/L, suggesting normal anion gap metabolic acidosis. An early morning urine evaluation showed a urinary pH of 7.2 with a positive urinary anion gap. Serological tests were positive for antinuclear antibody (ANA) and anti-SSA/Ro antibody.

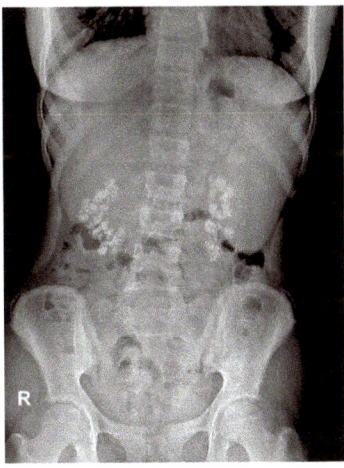

a. What findings are shown in this picture and what is the diagnosis? (2 marks)
b. What are the extraglandular manifestations of this syndrome? (3 marks)
c. What are the investigations to be done to rule out other differential diagnosis of the syndrome? (2 marks)
d. What is the optimal dosage of sodium bicarbonate to be given in patients with Sjögren syndrome with distal renal tubular acidosis (RTA)? (3 marks)

Q17. A 54-year-old man presents to the emergency department with complaints of cough and recurrent hemoptysis for 1 month. On review, he is oliguric and hypertensive and his routine urine examination showed plenty of RBCs, significant proteinuria. His past medical history includes hypertension and recurrent sinusitis. His serum creatinine is 7.2 mg/dL and urinary protein creatinine ratio of 1.22. The image of his chest X-ray is given below.

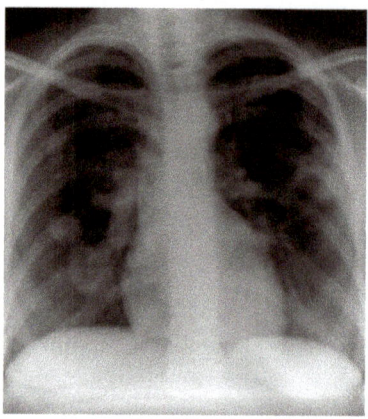

a. What is the most likely underlying diagnosis? *(2 marks)*
b. Write the chest X-ray finding. *(2 marks)*
c. Which type of antineutrophilic cytoplasmic antibody (ANCA) is associated with it? *(3 marks)*
d. Name an investigational drug being tried in it? *(3 marks)*

Q18. A 53-year-old male has been admitted due to worsening peripheral edema over the last 2 months, however feels he had been losing weight before this. He has a 50-pack year smoking history. Laboratory data at admission is given here.

Variable	Value
Hemoglobin, mg/dL	9
Creatinine, mg/dL	1.3
Albumin, g/dL	2.3
24-hour urinary protein quantity, g/24 h	4.2

Lipid profile is suggestive of hyperlipidemia. A chest computed tomography (CT) scan identified a nodule in the medial segment of the right lung lobe. Examination of the renal biopsy under light microscopy indicated slight thickening of the basement membrane and partial absorption of immune complexes. Electron microscopy revealed electron-dense deposits located beneath the epithelium of the glomerular basement membrane.

a. What is the most likely diagnosis? *(2 marks)*
b. Name the antibodies associated with primary membranous glomerulonephritis (MGN). *(3 marks)*
c. Write the condition associated with secondary MGN. *(3 marks)*
d. Write the modified Ponticelli regimen for treatment of primary membranous nephropathy. *(2 marks)*

Q19. Instrument

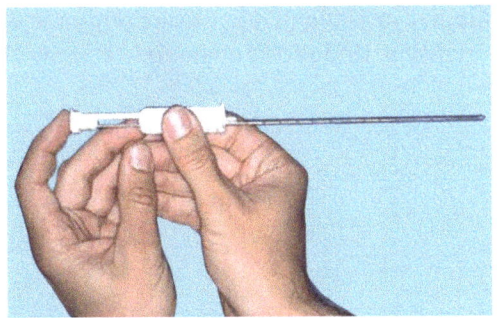

a. Identify the instrument. (2 marks)
b. Name three indications. (3 marks)
c. Name one contraindication. (2 marks)
d. Name three complications. (3 marks)

Q20.
A 65-year-old male, known case of diabetes mellitus (DM) and hypertension for more than 10 years, presented with angina on effort. This has been gradually worsening with the result that he has now angina at rest. Routine investigations revealed a serum creatinine of 1.9 mg% and estimated glomerular filtration rate (eGFR) of 27 mL/min. He has been advised coronary angiography with or without angioplasty.

a. Which renal complication is he likely to get? (2 marks)
b. What are the risk factors associated with the complication? (4 marks)
c. How will you prevent it? Enlist two proven strategies. (4 marks)

Q21.
A 14-year-old boy was evaluated for failure to thrive. His routine investigations suggested hypokalemia. Urine examination suggested a ph. of 6.5. His X-ray of abdomen is shown below.

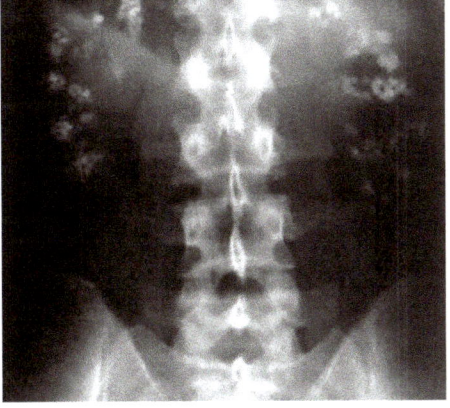

a. Describe the imaging findings. (2 marks)
b. What is the diagnosis? (3 marks)
c. Enumerate three etiologies presenting with the said disorder. (2 marks)
d. List two management steps. (3 marks)

Q22. A 14-year-old girl presented in the emergency with abrupt onset swelling of feet with cola-colored urination. Mother insisting that her urine output is very scanty. Examination revealed presence of hypertension. Urine color of the child is shown below.

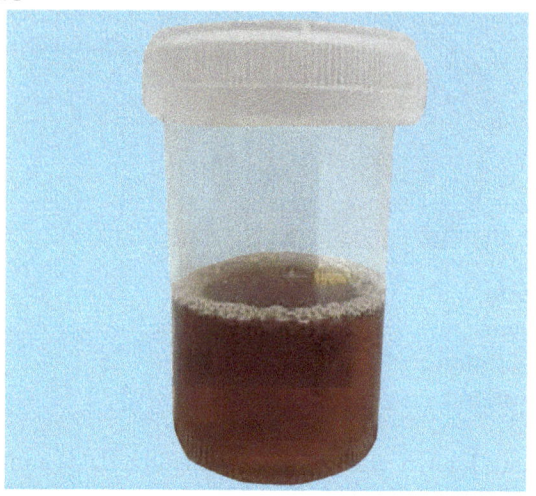

a. What is the diagnosis? (3 marks)
b. Enumerate necessary investigations. (3 marks)
c. What are the treatment options for such a patient? (4 marks)

Q23. A 56-year-old male patient who is known diabetic for last 8 years presented in MOPD with high-grade fever for last 5 days, associated with severe pain over left flank. His complete blood count (CBC) showed TLC 22,000, urine routine examination (RE) showed presence of plenty of pus cells. CT KUB done, and the image is shown below.

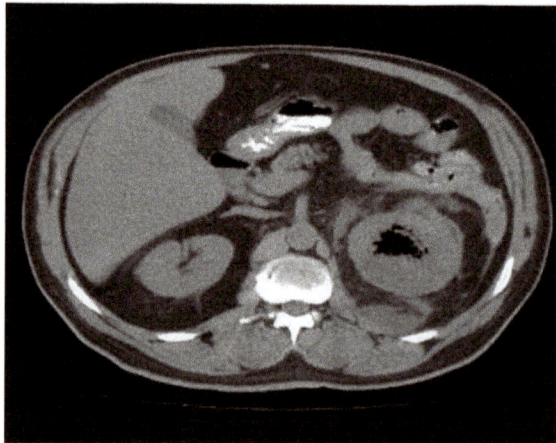

a. What is your diagnosis? (1 mark)
b. What is the most common causative organism? (1 mark)
c. What are the risk factors? (4 marks)
d. How to manage such patient? (4 marks)

Q24. A 13-year-old male patient presented with high-grade fever for last 3 days with dysuria. He had history of repeated urinary tract infection (UTI) in childhood. He underwent micturating cystourethrography (MCU), which is shown below.

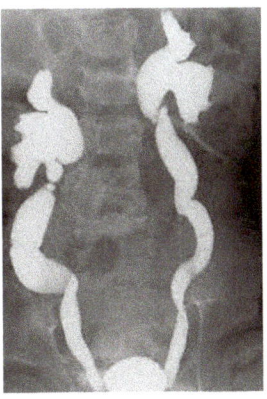

a. Mention your diagnosis. (1 mark)
b. What are the possible presentations? (4 marks)
c. What are the possible complications? (4 marks)

Q25. A 37-year-old male patient without any comorbidity presented with history of gradual onset body swelling with occasional episodes of reddish urination. His urine microscopy is shown below.

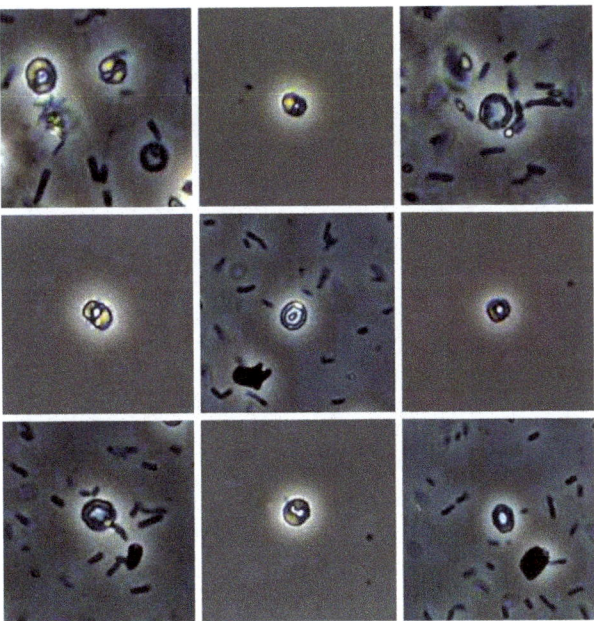

a. What is the likely cause? (1 mark)
b. Mention the common causes of such condition. (4 marks)
c. Enumerate the necessary blood investigations. (5 marks)

Nephrology

Q26. An 82-year-old diabetic male who underwent angioplasty 2 days ago developed sudden onset drop in urine output with bluish coloration of left lower limb. Serum creatinine jumped to 3.7 mg/dL from baseline of 1.3 mg/dL. CBC showed raised TLC with predominance of eosinophils. Image of the lower limb is shown below.

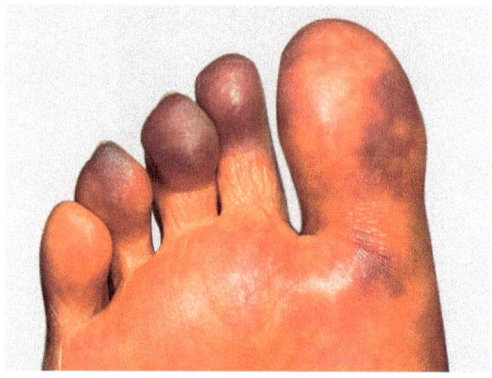

a. What is your diagnosis? (1 mark)
b. What are the risk factors? (3 marks)
c. What are the differential diagnoses? (3 marks)
d. Mention the treatment options. (3 marks)

Q27. A 42-year-old male who is manual labor by profession presented with loose motion with repeated bouts of vomiting for last 10 days. He appeared dehydrated on presentation. His routine investigations showed Hb 12.2 g/dL and serum creatinine 6.7 mg/dL. He underwent renal biopsy due to unexplained renal failure which is shown below.

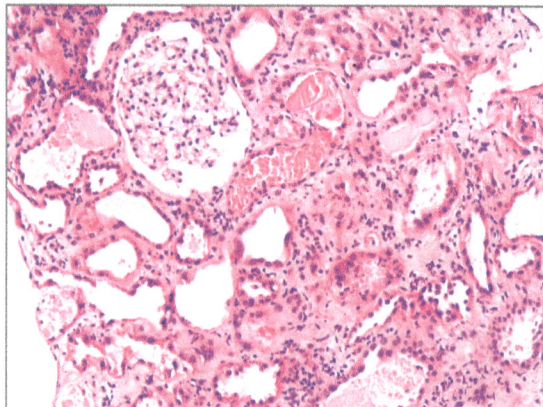

a. What is the diagnosis? (2 marks)
b. What is the likely etiology here? (2 marks)
c. What are the classical clinical features? (4 marks)
d. Name two drugs that can cause similar condition (2 marks)

Q28. A 62-year-old male patient without any comorbidity presented with fatiguability and repeated bouts of vomiting. His blood investigations revealed Hb 6.5 g/dL and serum creatinine of 12.6 mg/dL. He underwent renal biopsy, which is shown below.

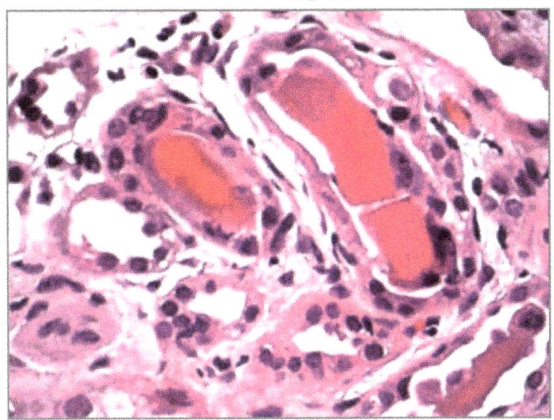

a. What is the histological diagnosis? (2 marks)
b. What is the responsible disease? (2 marks)
c. Describe three classical symptoms. (3 marks)
d. Mention three drugs used in therapy. (3 marks)

Q29. A 23-year-old male patient presented to ER with abrupt onset oliguria for last 2 days. He had history of acute gastroenteritis (AGE) 7 days ago, which was treated conservatively. His blood parameters showed Hb 7.1 g/dL, TLC 7,800, and platelet 35,000 with serum creatinine 4.2 mg/dL. His peripheral blood smear is shown below.

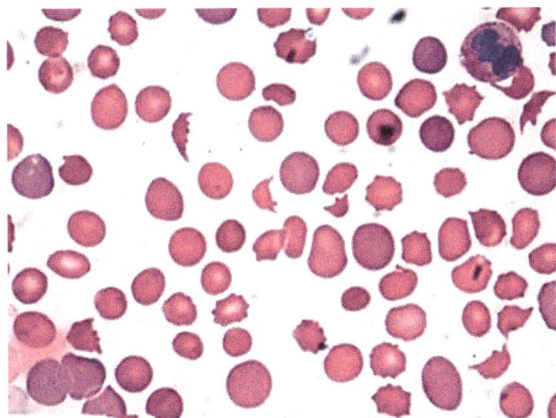

a. What is the syndromic diagnosis? (1 mark)
b. Mention three classical symptoms. (3 marks)
c. Mention three causes. (3 marks)
d. Mention three treatment options (3 marks)

Nephrology

Q30.

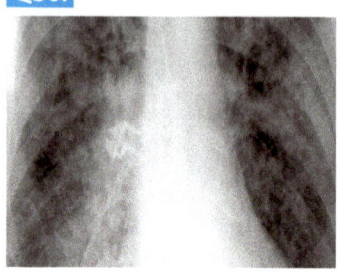
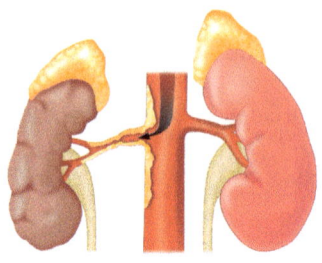
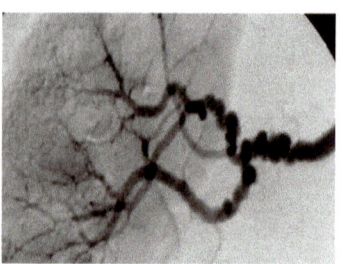

a. Identify the condition. (3 marks)
b. Identify the X-ray finding. (2 marks)
c. Give an important clinical implication of the condition. (2 marks)
d. Treatment of the condition. (3 marks)

Q31. See the image and answer the questions.

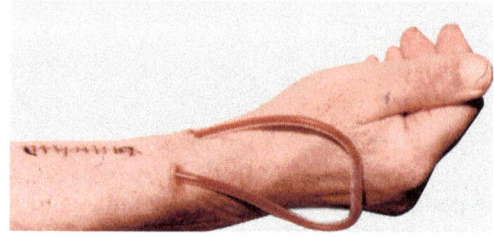

a. Identify the procedure done and its use. (3 marks)
b. Whose name is it described with? (2 marks)
c. Name three methods which have replaced this procedure. (3 marks)
d. Enumerate two complications. (2 marks)

Q32. A 45-year-old man had recurrent nephrolithiasis. Renal function tests and serum calcium measurements were normal.

Investigations:
24-h urinary calcium   8.8 mmol (2.5–7.5)
24-h urinary urate   3.0 mmol (<3.6)
24-h urinary oxalate   0.20 mmol (0.14–0.46)
24-h urinary citrate   0.2 mmol (0.3–3.4)

a. What is the etiology of kidney stone? (3 marks)
b. What is the pathophysiology and how would you treat? (4 marks)
c. What is the most useful therapy to reduce stone formation? (3 marks)

Q33. A 22-year-old man with hypertension presented with a 6-week history of tiredness, ankle swelling, and arthralgia. On examination (O/E), his pulse was 92 beats/min and BP was 150/90 mm Hg. He had bilateral ankle edema. His serum creatinine concentration had been normal 6 months previously. Urinalysis showed blood 2+ and protein 2+.

Investigations:

Hemoglobin	10.3 g/DL (115–165), white cell count 10.5 × 109/L (4.0–11.0)
Platelet count	410 × 109/L (150–400)
Serum creatinine	2.2 mg/dL
eGFR	17 mL/min/1.73 m² (>60)

a. What is the most likely cause of his renal impairment? *(3 marks)*
b. Enumerate three differential diagnoses. *(4 marks)*
c. What further investigations are required? *(3 marks)*

Q34. A 55-year-old female, a case of type 2 DM, end-stage kidney disease (ESKD) on peritoneal dialysis presented with abdominal symptoms like early satiety, anorexia, nausea, vomiting, and altered bowel habit. O/E, she was malnourished. Her CT abdomen is given below.

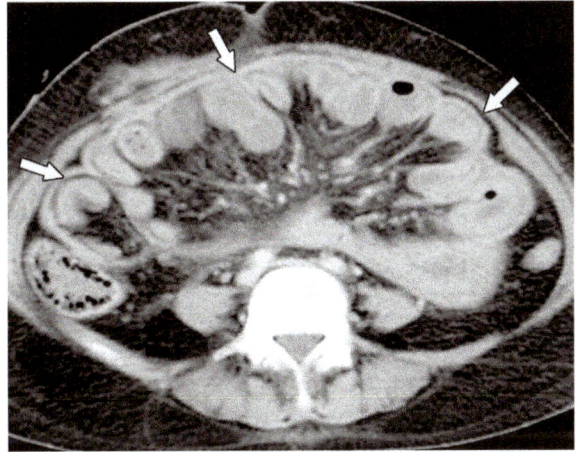

a. What are the findings? *(4 marks)*
b. What is your diagnosis? *(3 marks)*
c. Name three more conditions that can produce this complication. *(3 marks)*

Q35. A 43-year-old truck driver has been referred for the assessment of persistent asymptomatic microhematuria. He last sought medical attention when blood in his urine was initially detected during a Department of Transportation physical examination 9 years ago. Subsequent evaluations included a CT scan of the abdomen and pelvis, cystoscopy with retrograde pyelograms, and urine cytology. Additionally, he was informed about elevated blood glucose levels last year. The patient has never smoked, is not on any medications, and the results of various laboratory tests are provided in the table below. Notably, results for erythrocyte sedimentation rate, antinuclear antibody (ANA) testing, antibodies to myeloperoxidase and proteinase 3, serum protein electrophoresis, and serologies for hepatitis B, hepatitis C, and human immunodeficiency virus are all negative or within normal limits. C3/C4 levels are also normal. Eye and ear examination is normal. No other family history. Renal biopsy is performed.

Component	Finding
Blood pressure, mm Hg	164/94
Pulse, beats/min	76
Weight, kg	92
Height, cm	185
Heart, lungs, and abdomen	Normal
Jugular venous distention	Absent
Pitting edema	Both lower extremities (trace)
Rashes	Absent
Serum creatinine, mg/dL	2.1
Fasting blood glucose, mg/dL	130
Spot urine microalbumin, mg/g	1,586
Urinalysis:	
Blood	3+
Protein	3+
24-h total protein, g	2.1

a. What is most probable diagnosis on renal biopsy? (5 marks)
b. How to differentiate between glomerular and nonglomerular hematuria? (5 marks)

Q36. A 58-year-old woman is being assessed for a rash on her lower extremities persisting for 1 week. She has observed tea-colored urine over the past few weeks and is not on any medications. Her vital signs indicate a temperature of 37.3°C, a pulse rate of 88 beats/min, and a BP of 154/90 mm Hg. Palpable purpura is evident on both legs and feet. Other examination findings are unremarkable. Laboratory results reveal a creatinine level of 2.8 mg/dL. The erythrocyte sedimentation rate is 80 mm/h. Tests for ANA, antibodies to double-stranded DNA, myeloperoxidase, and proteinase 3 are negative. The C4 complement level is low, and cryoglobulin testing is positive. Urinalysis indicates proteinuria (2+) and hematuria (3+). Microscopic examination of urine shows 31–40 erythrocytes per HPF and 3–10 leukocytes per HPF.
a. Which of the following viruses is most likely to be associated with this disorder? (3 marks)
 (i) Epstein-Barr virus; (ii) Cytomegalovirus; (iii) Human immunodeficiency virus; (iv) Parvovirus B_{19}; (v) Hepatitis C virus (HCV)
b. What is most probable glomerular finding on renal biopsy? (3 marks)
c. Classify cryoglobulinemia. (4 marks)

Q37. A 60-year-old woman presents with a maculopapular rash, fever, and fatigue and reports decreased urine output. Laboratory tests reveal a serum creatinine level of 3.8 mg/dL (baseline, 1.0 mg/dL). She has peripheral eosinophilia, and urine eosinophils are detected. Her history is notable for recent antibiotic exposure starting 10 days ago for an upper respiratory tract infection.
a. What is the probable diagnosis? (5 marks)
b. What are the renal biopsy findings? (5 marks)

Q38.

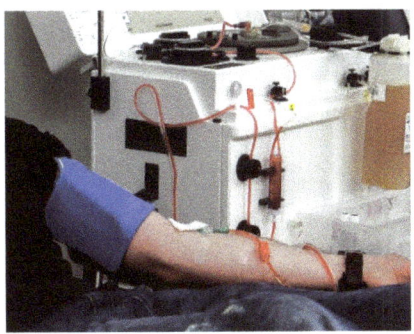

a. Name the procedure. (5 marks)
b. Enumerate its uses. (5 marks)

Q39. A 70-year-old male known case of HTN and DM and CKD, and is not on hemodialysis. Creatinine 5.3 mg/dL, serum Na^+ 131 mEq/L, and serum K^+ 7.3 mEq/L

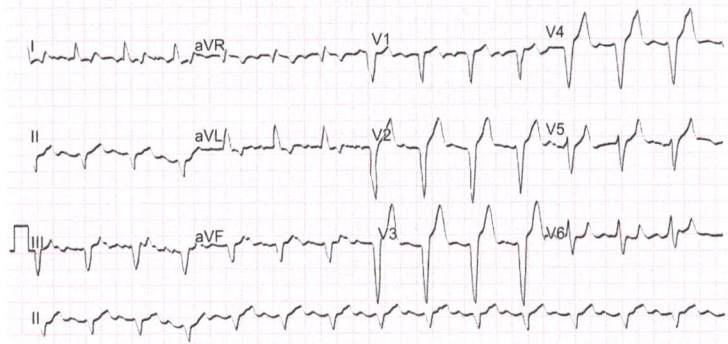

a. Identify the ECG finding. (5 marks)
b. Drug and its dosage used for membrane stabilizing action in this condition. (5 marks)

Q40. Hypertensive patient presenting with flank pain and hematuria.

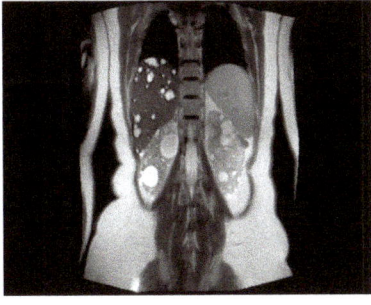

a. Name the condition and the genes involved. (5 marks)
b. Extrarenal sites/clinical features of the above condition. (5 marks)

Q41. A 40-year-old male weighing 60 kg was admitted in the hospital with complicated UTI was found to have *Escherichia coli* in his blood culture/sensitivity (C/S), which was sensitive to meropenem. Initially, the physicians started him on injection meropenem 1 g intravenous (IV) every 8 hourly. Subsequently, the patient developed sepsis and his serum creatinine levels increased to 2.5 mg/dL.

a. Does this patient require any dose adjustments in drug therapy? Why? *(2 marks)*
b. Mention the commonly used formula for the calculating the necessary pharmacokinetic (PK) parameter *(2 marks)*
c. What is the dose adjustment necessary for this patient? Justify. *(3 marks)*
d. Mention three examples of other drugs requiring dose adjustment based on the same PK parameter. *(3 marks)*

Q42. A researcher is planning to conduct an observational study on 180 patients to understand the relationship between urinary KIM-1 (kidney injury molecule-1) levels and lupus nephritis. The researcher plans to include patients between 12 and 60 years of age with biopsy-proven lupus nephritis irrespective of the severity of the disease. As per the study protocol, urine samples and blood samples will be collected at baseline, 2 weeks, 4 weeks, 6 weeks, and 12 weeks in patients undergoing treatment as per standard treatment guidelines. No active intervention is planned as part of the study. Based on the above details, answer the following questions:

a. What type of risk does this study involve? *(2 marks)*
   i. Less than minimal risk
   ii. Minimal risk
   iii. Minor increase over minimal risk or low risk
   iv. More than minimal risk or high risk
b. What are the potential benefits of the study to the participant? *(2 marks)*
   i. No direct benefit to the participant
   ii. Direct benefit in the form of monitoring lupus nephritis activity
c. As this study involves vulnerable population (adolescents aged 12–17) what type of consent is applicable? *(2 marks)*
   i. Written informed consent from parents and written informed assent from adolescents to be taken
   ii. Oral consent from parents and written informed assent from adolescents
   iii. As this study comes under the purview of biomedical research, waiver of consent can be obtained from ethics committee.
   iv. Waiver of consent can be obtained as study is observational.
d. Ethics committee approval was obtained for 180 patients, after interim analysis it was found that the existing sample size is inadequately powered and the recalculated sample size found to be 240. Can the researcher recruit more than 180 patients on the basis of existing approval?
e. What is your opinion on inclusion of vulnerable population (adolescents aged 12–17)? *(2 marks)*
   i. Yes, inclusion is justified as onset of lupus nephritis is in adolescents, and this is an observational study with minor increase over minimal risk.
   ii. No, adolescents should not be included.

Q43. You get a call to attend a 26-year-old diabetic lady admitted in orthopedics ward for severe backache and fever. O/E, she had tenderness over lumbar area, more to the right. Look at the image of her CT KUB.

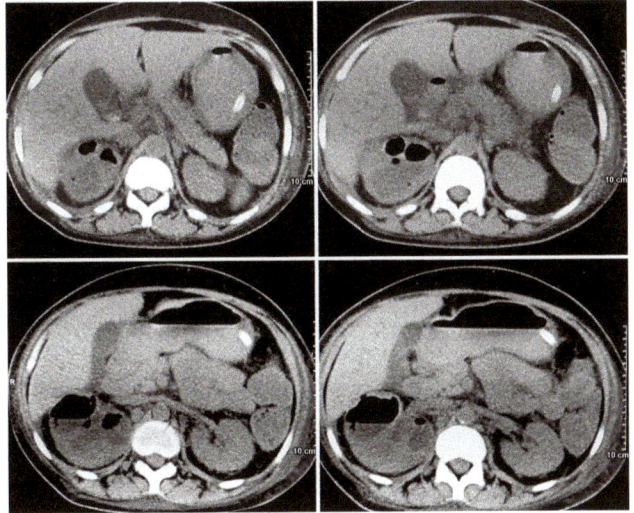

a. What is the diagnosis? (3 marks)
b. What is the most common causative agent? (3 marks)
c. Name 2 modalities for the treatment of this condition. (4 marks)

Q44. A 60-year-old lady presented with bilateral loin pain for 3 days. O/E, she had hypertension and bilateral palpable flank masses. Her investigations were as follows: Hb 17.7 g%; creatinine 3.2 mg%; urine routine microscopic examination: pus cells 10/hpf; and RBC 10–12/hpf.
a. Name two investigations you would like to do next. (3 marks)
b. Write three possible causes of loin pain. (4 marks)
c. What do you expect to find in liver? (3 marks)

Q45. A 78-year-old male, a former smoker with a history of 40 pack-years, presents with weakness and a cough that includes blood. He currently uses an ipratropium bromide inhaler. Upon physical examination, his vital signs are within normal range, his jugular venous pressure is normal, and there is no observed edema. Laboratory results indicate sodium levels of 123 mEq/L, potassium levels of 3.8 mEq/L, bicarbonate levels of 24 mEq/L, serum urea nitrogen at 12 mg/dL, and serum creatinine at 0.9 mg/dL.
a. What should you obtain next? (4 marks)
   i. Serum osmolality value
   ii. Urine osmolality value
   iii. Thyrotropin and morning cortisol values
   iv. CT scan of the chest
   v. Magnetic resonance imaging of the brain
b. What is pseudohyponatremia and its causes? (3 marks)
c. Enumerate three causes of euvolemic hyponatremia. (3 marks)

ANSWERS

Ans. 1
a. Autosomal dominant polycystic kidney disease
b. Liver cyst, intracranial aneurysms, epididymal cyst, and mitral valve prolapse
c. Vaptans, somatostatin analogues, angiotensin-converting enzyme inhibitor/angiotensin receptor blocker (ACEI/ARB)

Ans. 2
a. Infection-related glomerulonephritis (GN)/post streptococcal GN
b. Nephritogenic strains of Group A beta hemolytic streptococci
c. Urine analysis, serum complement C3, C4, culture of throat or wound, antistreptolysin O (ASO) titer
d. Antibiotic therapy, diuretics, salt, and water restriction, antihypertensives

Ans. 3
a. Two or more relapse in last 6 months and three or more relapse in consecutive 12 calendar months
b. Urine protein–creatinine ratio (uPCR) >0.2 but <2 mg/mg or >20 and <200 mg/mmol, and, if available, serum albumin ≥3 (children)

   Reduction of proteinuria to between 0.21 g/day and 3.4 g/day ± decrease in proteinuria of ≥50% from baseline (adults)
c. uPCR <0.2 mg/mg or <20 mg/mmol or negative or trace dipstick on three or more consecutive occasions (children). Reduction of proteinuria to ≤0.20 g/day and serum albumin >3.5 g/dL (adults)
d. Relapses during therapy with prednisone or prednisolone (either at full dose or during tapering) or within 15 days of prednisone or prednisolone discontinuation
e. Lack of complete remission at 4 weeks of therapy with daily prednisone or prednisolone at standard dose (children). Persistence of proteinuria despite prednisone therapy, 1 mg/kg/day for 16 weeks (adults).

Ans. 4
a. Emphysematous pyelonephritis
b. Fever, pyuria, flank pain, tachycardia, and dysuria
c. Supportive treatment, antibiotics, relief of obstruction, drainage of gas/purulent material

Ans. 5
a. Staghorn calculi
b. *Proteus, Pseudomonas, Providencia, Klebsiella,* and *Morganella*
c. Prolonged antibiotic treatment. Relieve of obstruction with percutaneous nephrostomy (PCN). Stone removal with PCNL, lithotripsy, or both. Prevention of recolonization of urea splitting organisms with antibiotic prophylaxis.

Ans. 6

a. Acute interstitial nephritis
b. Fever, rashes, and eosinophilia
c. Antimicrobial agents, nonsteroidal anti-inflammatory drugs (NSAIDs), and proton pump inhibitors
d. Withdrawal of drug, corticosteroids

Ans. 7

a. Rhabdomyolysis
b. Muscle injury/ischemia trauma; pressure necrosis, electric shock, burns, acute vascular disease, seizures, excessive exercise, and heat exhaustion

   Toxins: Alcohol, cocaine, heroin, amphetamines, ecstasy, phencyclidine, and snakebite

   Drugs: Statins, fibrates, zidovudine, neuroleptic malignant syndrome, azathioprine, theophylline, lithium, and diuretics

   Electrolyte disorders: Hypophosphatemia, hypokalemia, and hyperosmolar states

   Infections viral: Influenza, HIV, coxsackievirus, Epstein-Barr virus, and COVID-19

   Bacterial: Legionella, Francisella, Streptococcus pneumoniae, Salmonella, Staphylococcus aureus

   Familial: McArdle disease

c.
   - Aggressive IV fluid administration (target urine output 200–300 mL/h)
   - Prevention of compartment syndrome
   - Administration of mannitol
   - Treatment of hypocalcemia and other electrolyte abnormality
   - Hemodialysis

Ans. 8

a. Contrast-induced nephropathy
b. Older age group (>75 years), preexisting kidney disease, diabetic nephropathy, concurrent nephrotoxic drugs, dehydration, high-osmolar contrast medium (approximately 2,000 mOsm/kg)
c. Drugs to stop 48 hours before and reassess 48 hours after procedure based on creatinine:
   - NSAIDs
   - Metformin
   - Diuretics if feasible
   - ACEI/ARB
   - Avoid repeated use of iodinated contrast for next 72 hours if feasible

   And hydration with:
   - Isotonic saline 3 mL/kg/h × 1 h before examination then 1 mL/kg/h × 6 h or
   - Isotonic saline 1 mL/kg/h × 12 h before examination then 1 mL/kg/h × 12 h

   Use of low-osmolar contrast medium (600–800 mOsm/kg), or iso-osmolar contrast medium (290 mOsm/kg) (preferred).

Ans. 9

a. Small vessel vasculitis
b. Vasculitis, Goodpasture syndrome, systemic lupus erythematosus (SLE), other nonimmune causes like lung infection, paraquat poisoning, and hypervolemia with cardiac failure
c. Glucocorticoids, rituximab, cyclophosphamide, plasma exchange, and azathioprine

Ans. 10

a. Tumor lysis syndrome
b. Seizure, arrhythmia, tetany, and AKI
c. Rehydration, measures to reduce K^+, xanthine oxidase inhibitors, hemodialysis, and correction of electrolyte abnormality

Ans. 11

a. Synpharyngitic nephritis/immunoglobulin A (IgA) nephropathy
b. *Hematuria:* UTIs, renal stone disease, urothelial malignancy, renal cell carcinoma, sickle cell anemia, Alport syndrome, thin basement membrane disease, exercise, and glomerulonephritis.
c. Supportive management, BP control with ACEI/ARB, sparsentan, target-release budesonide, and steroids

Ans. 12

a. Prerenal AKI
b. Prerenal AKI clinically presents with dehydration, hypotension, or hemorrhage, having volume loss leading to concentrated urine, with no past history of renal injury. *Laboratory studies:* Fractional excretion of sodium (FENa) <1%, fractional excretion (FE) of urea <35%, Una—<20 mmol/L, proteinuria—nil/trace, no cast or few hyaline cast.
c. Volume resuscitation with IVF, control of vomiting, diarrhea, antibiotics, and oral rehydration solution where possible, dialysis.

Ans. 13

a. Viperidae group, sea snakes, and the Colubridae group
b. Rehydration with IVF, supportive management, local wound treatment and avoidance of compartment syndrome, treatment with adequate dosage of AVS, antibiotics, supportive management, and hemodialysis
c. Bees, caterpillar, spider, and scorpions

Ans. 14

a. Thrombotic microangiopathy
b. Adequate fluid resuscitation, blood transfusion, plasma exchange, hemodialysis, and eculizumab in case of hemolytic uremic syndrome (HUS).
c. Vomiting (hyperemesis), incomplete or infected complicated abortion, abruptio placentae, postpartum hemorrhage, preeclampsia, HELLP (hemolysis, elevated liver enzymes and low platelets) syndrome, puerperal sepsis, fatty liver of pregnancy, and pyelonephritis.

Ans. 15

a. Nontunneled hemodialysis catheter
b. Acute need to establish vascular access for hemodialysis
c. Bleeding, infection, and injury to adjacent artery or nerve

Ans. 16

a. X-ray of KUB region showed multiple clusters of tiny radiopaque stones in bilateral renal region suggesting medullary nephrocalcinosis. On the basis of normal anion gap metabolic acidosis, hypokalemia, positive urinary anion gap, and an alkaline urinary pH, the diagnosis is distal RTA. Therefore, Sjögren syndrome-related type I RTA with medullary nephrocalcinosis and hypokalemia is the diagnosis.
b. The extraglandular manifestations of Sjögren syndrome are as follows:
   - Nonspecific:
     - Arthralgia or arthritis
     - Raynaud's phenomenon
   - Accumulation of periepithelial lymphocytes:
     - Interstitial lung disease—most common type is nonspecific interstitial pneumonia (NSIP)
     - RTA—distal (type 1) RTA
     - Primary biliary cirrhosis
   - Immune complex mediated:
     - Small vessel vasculitis—presents as cutaneous palpable purpura
     - Glomerulonephritis with cryoglobulinemia
     - Peripheral neuropathy
   - Lymphoma:
     - Extranodal marginal zone B-cell lymphoma of mucosal-associated lymphoid tissue (MALToma)
c. Primary Sjögren syndrome is diagnosed if:
   - Ocular examinations reveal keratoconjunctivitis sicca.
   - Oral assessments show dryness of the oral mucosa, and/or
   - The patient's serum demonstrates reactivity with immunoglobulins, Ro/SS-A, and/or La/SS-B autoantigens.
   - Labial biopsy is essential for diagnostic and prognostic purposes.
d. Individuals with RTA should be administered oral sodium bicarbonate (0.5–2 mmol/kg in four divided doses).

Ans. 17

a. The presence of upper respiratory tract signs points toward granulomatosis with polyangiitis (GPA) in a patient with rapidly progressive glomerulonephritis
b. Chest X-ray showed some reticulonodular shadows
c. GPA is primarily associated with PR3-ANCA (proteinase 3-antineutrophil cytoplasmic antibody)

d. Avacopan (a C5a receptor inhibitor) was recently investigated in a randomized trial as an alternative to glucocorticoids in patients of GPA receiving induction with either cyclophosphamide or rituximab.

Ans. 18

a. This is a case of secondary membranous nephropathy due to probable underlying lung cancer. The weight loss, heavy smoking history, and computed tomography (CT) findings plus the new development of membranous nephropathy all point to lung cancer.
b. Membranous nephropathy is split into two main causes—primary and secondary. Primary membranous nephropathy is commonly associated with anti-PLA2R antibodies and antithrombospondin type 1 domain containing 7A (THSD7A) antibodies.
c. The condition associated with secondary MGN are:
   - Malignancy such as solid tumors (lung, colon, breast, and kidney)
   - *Infections:* Hepatitis B or C, Haemophilus influenzae type b, malaria, syphilis, and schistosomiasis
   - *Autoimmune diseases:* SLE, sarcoidosis, and inflammatory bowel disease (IBD)
   - *Drugs:* NSAIDs, captopril, gold, penicillamine, lithium, and clopidogrel
d. Modified Ponticelli regimen (mPR), consisting of cyclical steroids and cyclophosphamide
   - Months 1, 3, and 5:
     - IV methylprednisolone 500 mg/day for 3 days
     - Oral prednisolone 0.5 mg/kg/day for 27 days
   - Months 2, 4, and 6: Oral cyclophosphamide 2 mg/kg/day

Ans. 19

a. Tru-cut kidney biopsy needle
b. Unexplained acute or rapidly progressive renal failure:
   - Nephrotic syndrome and significant non-nephrotic proteinuria
   - Persistent glomerular hematuria
   - Systemic diseases with renal involvement
c. Small kidneys, abnormal coagulopathy, and uncontrolled hypertension
d. Hematuria, hematoma, and pain

Ans. 20

a. Contrast-associated AKI
b. Risk factors for contrast-induced AKI include chronic kidney disease (CKD), diabetes, heart failure, advanced age, volume depletion, hypotension, use of concurrent nephrotoxic medications, and use of a large-volume or high-osmolality contrast agent.
c. The recommended approach for reducing the risk for contrast-induced kidney injury is to administer IVFs and then use low-osmolar or iso-osmolar contrast media, rather than high-osmolar contrast media.

Ans. 21

a. Nephrocalcinosis
b. RTA type 1 (distal RTA)

c. Mutations of genes that encode the chloride-bicarbonate exchanger (AE1), SLE, and Sjögren syndrome
d. Potassium citrate/alkali therapy

Ans. 22

a. Acute postinfective glomerulonephritis
b. Urine routine examination (RE) and microscopic examination (ME), 24 hours urine protein, creatinine, C3, C4, and ASO titer
c. Fluid restriction, diuretics, anti hypertensive, and steroid in special cases

Ans. 23

a. Emphysematous pyelonephritis left kidney
b. *Escherichia coli*
c. Diabetes, immunosuppressed state, urinary obstruction, and old age
d. Antibiotic, drainage of collection, managing obstruction, and nephrectomy

Ans. 24

a. Bilateral hydronephrosis (HDN) due to probably vesicoureteral reflux (VUR)
b. Recurrent UTI, failure to thrive, nephrotic syndrome, CKD, and asymptomatic patient detected on screening
c. Anemia, failure to thrive, reflux nephropathy, pyelonephritis, growth retardation, and CKD

Ans. 25

a. Dysmorphic RBC due to glomerular hematuria
b. Pauci-immune glomerulonephritis (PIGN), membranoproliferative glomerulonephritis (MPGN), SLE, focal and segmental glomerulosclerosis (FSGS), ANCA vasculitis, IgA nephropathy
c. Serum urea, creatinine, liver function test (LFT), electrolytes, ANA by Hep-2, anti-MPO and PR3, and C3, C4

Ans. 26

a. Atheroembolic renal disease
b. Older age, diabetes, atherosclerotic disease, and CKD
c. ANCA vasculitis, cryoglobulinemia, and contrast-induced nephropathy
d. Heparin, thrombectomy, and dialysis

Ans. 27

a. Acute tubular necrosis
b. Dehydration due to diarrhea and vomiting
c. Sudden rise in serum creatinine, maintained urine output with absence of edema/hypertension
d. Aminoglycosides and cisplatin

Ans. 28

a. Myeloma cast nephropathy
b. Multiple myeloma
c. Bone pain, anemia, and renal failure
d. Steroid, cyclophosphamide, and bortezomib

Ans. 29

a. Microangiopathic hemolytic anemia
b. Anemia, thrombocytopenia, and AKI
c. Infection, SLE, and pregnancy
d. Plasma exchange, eculizumab, and dialysis

Ans. 30

a. Renal artery stenosis
b. Flash pulmonary edema (in bilateral cases)
c. To be investigated for in cases of resistant hypertension
d. Renal artery stenting

Ans. 31

a. AV shunt created for hemodialysis
b. Belding scribner
c. AV fistula, AV graft, and internal jugular vein catheter
d. Bleeding and infection

Ans. 32

a. *Possible etiology:* Hypercalciuria: Although the serum calcium measurements are normal, the elevated 24-hour urinary calcium excretion (8.8 mmol) suggests that the patient may have hypercalciuria and hypocitraturia. The low 24-hour urinary citrate excretion (0.2 mmol) indicates hypocitraturia, which can promote stone formation as citrate inhibits the crystallization of calcium salts in the urine.
b. *Pathophysiology:* The combination of hypercalciuria and hypocitraturia can contribute to stone formation. Hypercalciuria increases the concentration of calcium in the urine, making it more likely to form calcium-containing stones. Hypocitraturia reduces the inhibitory effect of citrate on stone formation, further promoting crystallization.
c. *Treatment:*
   - *Dietary modification:* The first step in managing this patient's kidney stones is dietary modification. Encourage the patient to reduce dietary sources of calcium and oxalate and increase fluid intake to maintain high urine volume, which can help prevent stone formation.
   - *Citrate supplementation:* Since the patient has hypocitraturia, citrate supplementation may be beneficial. Potassium citrate can help increase urinary citrate levels, which inhibits stone formation.

- *Thiazide diuretics:* In cases of persistent hypercalciuria despite dietary changes and citrate supplementation, thiazide diuretics (e.g., hydrochlorothiazide) can be considered.
- *Lifestyle and hydration:* Lifestyle changes, including maintaining a healthy weight and reducing salt intake, can also be helpful in preventing stone recurrence. Adequate hydration is crucial to maintain a high urine volume.

Ans. 33

a. Given these clinical and laboratory findings, the most likely cause of his renal impairment is IgA nephropathy. IgA nephropathy, also known as Berger's disease, is characterized by the deposition of IgA immune complexes in the glomeruli of the kidneys. It often presents with episodic hematuria and proteinuria.
b. Differential diagnosis (D/d) could be crescentic glomerulonephritis, membranoproliferative glomerulonephritis, and membranous nephropathy which can also cause renal impairment and may present with some similar features, the combination of hematuria, proteinuria, and the patient's age make IgA nephropathy the most likely diagnosis in this case.
c. Further diagnostic tests, including a kidney biopsy with light microscopy and immunofluorescence, may be necessary to confirm the diagnosis and assess the extent of kidney damage.

Ans. 34

a. Peritoneal enhancement, peritoneal thickening, calcification, bowel tethering, bowel wall thickening, signs of bowel obstruction, and loculated collection
b. Encapsulating peritoneal sclerosis (EPS)
c. (1) Autoimmune diseases, (2) sarcoidosis, and (3) peritoneal and intra-abdominal malignancies, intraperitoneal chemotherapy, and abdominal surgery

Ans. 35

a. IgA nephropathy
b. *Glomerular hematuria:*
   - Hematuria in glomerular conditions often presents as "smoky" or cola-colored urine.
   - Microscopic examination of urine may reveal RBC casts, indicating bleeding from the glomeruli.
   - Glomerular diseases are commonly associated with proteinuria due to the compromised glomerular filtration barrier.

   Nonglomerular hematuria:
   - Hematuria in nonglomerular conditions may present as bright red or pink urine.
   - Passage of clots suggests bleeding from the upper urinary tract (e.g., kidneys and ureters).
   - Nonglomerular hematuria may be associated with pain, especially if originating from the bladder or urethra.
   - Infections causing nonglomerular hematuria may be accompanied by positive urine cultures.

Ans. 36

a. (v) Cryoglobulinemia can develop in patients with asymptomatic hepatitis C infection, and this can cause a vasculitis involving small vessels (skin).
b. Membranoproliferative glomerulonephritis
c. *Brouet classification criteria:*
   - Type I cryoglobulinemia involves monoclonal immunoglobulins (IgG, IgM, IgA, or free Ig light chains) arising from protein-secreting monoclonal gammopathies like monoclonal gammopathy of undetermined significance (MGUS) or B-cell malignancies.
   - Type II features a mix of monoclonal IgM (or IgG/IgA) with rheumatoid factor, often linked to HCV infection or autoimmune diseases.
   - Type III comprises a blend of polyclonal IgG and IgM, commonly associated with autoimmune disorders or infections, especially HCV. Atypical cases, like type II–III or biclonal cryoglobulins, may represent transitional stages without a clear pathogenic link.

Ans. 37

a. Acute interstitial nephritis
b. The primary histological alterations involve interstitial edema and a substantial interstitial infiltrate, predominantly composed of T lymphocytes and monocytes. Additionally, the presence of eosinophils, plasma cells, and neutrophils may be observed. The characteristic "tubulitis" lesion is identified when inflammatory cells invade the tubular basement membrane (TBM).

Ans. 38

a. Plasmapheresis
b. Conditions associated with renal failure include Guillain-Barré syndrome, myasthenia gravis, chronic inflammatory demyelinating polyneuropathy, hyperviscosity in monoclonal gammopathies, thrombotic thrombocytopenic purpura, Goodpasture syndrome (except in cases dependent on dialysis where there is no diffuse alveolar hemorrhage), HUS (atypical, resulting from an autoantibody targeting factor H), and fulminant Wilson disease.

Ans. 39

a. Tall T waves seen in hyperkalemia
b. 10 mL of 10% calcium gluconate infused intravenously over 10 minutes

Ans. 40

a. Autosomal dominant polycystic kidney disease (ADPKD) due to mutation in *PKD1* and *PKD2* genes.
b. Liver cysts, intracranial aneurysm/subarachnoid hemorrhage, diffuse arterial dolichoectasia, mitral/tricuspid valve prolapse, colonic diverticae, and abdominal wall hernia

Ans. 41

a. Yes. The major route of elimination of meropenem is renal and as his renal clearance is altered which might expose the patient to high concentration of meropenem leading to toxicity.

b. Cockroft-Gault equation for estimating GFR:

$$\frac{[140 - \text{age (years)}] \times \text{ideal weight (kg)}}{([\text{creatinine (mg/dL)}] \times 72)}$$

*For women, multiply by 0.85
c. His eGFR = 33.33 mL/min, as per the above formula. For injection meropenem, the dosing recommendations (as per drug label) are:

Creatinine clearance (mL/min)	Dose for UTI	Dosing interval
>50	1 g	Every 8 hours
26–50	Recommended dose	Every 12 hours
10–25	One-half recommended dose	Every 12 hours
<10	One-half recommended dose	Every 24 hours

His dose has to be adjusted to injection meropenem 1 g IV every 12 hours.
d. Other drugs needing dose adjustments as per clearance: Aminoglycosides (amikacin), vancomycin, colistin, and anticoagulants like enoxaparin, etc.

Ans. 42

a. (iii) Minor increase over minimal risk or low risk
b. (ii) Direct benefit in the form of monitoring lupus nephritis activity
c. (i) Written informed consent from parents and written informed assent from adolescents to be taken.
d. No. As the ethics committee approval was taken on a calculated sample size of 180 patients, it is unethical to recruit more patients than the approved sample size by the ethics committee.
If the researcher wants to recruit more patients based on recalculated sample size, then ethics committee approval is required for the amended protocol, which includes the recalculated sample size.
e. (i) Yes, inclusion is justified as onset of lupus nephritis is in adolescents, and this is an observational study with minor increase over minimal risk.
Source: ICMR. National ethical Guidelines for Bio-medical and health research involving Human Participants 2017. [online] Available from https://main.icmr.nic.in/sites/default/files/guidelines/ICMR_Ethical_Guidelines_2017.pdf [Last accessed January, 2024].

Ans. 43

a. Emphysematous pyelonephritis of the right kidney (RK)
The image shows enlarged RK, gas formation suggestive of emphysematous pyelonephritis of the RK.
b. E. coli
Escherichia coli is the most common organism that causes the emphysematous pyelonephritis.
c. IV antibiotics, drainage of pus, and nephrectomy
Three recommended modalities of the treatment for emphysematous pyelonephritis are IV antibiotics, drainage of pus, and nephrectomy if not better.

Ans. 44

a. *USG of abdomen and urine culture and/or blood culture:* This is a case of ADPKD. Cystic kidney disease can cause polycythemia. With available tests, next line of investigation would be to confirm polycystic kidney disease and rule out possible pyelonephritis with demonstration of fat stranding on USG or CT KUB and isolation of bacteria on cultures.
b. *Bleeding into cyst, cyst infection, and mechanical backache:* In a case of ADPKD, possible causes of loin pain are bleeding into cyst, cyst infection, and mechanical backache
c. *Cysts:* In a case of ADPKD, liver cysts are common association.

Ans. 45

a. (i) Serum osmolality value
The patient's presentation raised suspicion for lung cancer-associated syndrome of inappropriate antidiuretic hormone secretion (SIADH). To confirm hypo-osmolar hyponatremia, it is essential to assess serum osmolality. Additionally, checking urine osmolality is crucial to confirm the presence of arginine vasopressin (AVP), where concentrated urine (lack of maximally diluted urine) indicates the presence of AVP. To rule out other potential causes of hyponatremia, investigations for hypothyroidism and adrenal insufficiency are warranted. The presence of AVP in a patient with normal intravascular volume, low serum osmolality, and the absence of other known AVP-stimulating factors suggest ectopic AVP production. Considering the patient's history, a high-resolution CT scan of the chest is recommended to assess for lung cancer, a possible source of AVP.
b. Regarding hyponatremia without hypotonicity, it is termed as pseudohyponatremia. This can occur in patients with hyperglycemia or those who have accumulated exogenous effective osmoles like mannitol, sucrose, maltose, sorbitol, glycine, or radiocontrast. In cases of extreme hyperlipidemia or hyperproteinemia, autoanalyzers may measure the serum sodium concentration as low, leading to a laboratory artifact known as "pseudohyponatremia." However, direct sodium-selective electrodes used by blood gas analyzers and certain point-of-care devices will measure the sodium concentration as normal in such instances.
c. SIADH, drug-induced hyponatremia, and hypothyroidism

SECTION 9

Cardiology

QUESTIONS

Q1. A 17-year-old girl was seen in the outpatient with progressive dyspnea and palpitations of 2 years duration. She gave a past history of (H/O) joint pains. On examination (O/E), a mid-diastolic rumble with presystolic accentuation was auscultated in the mitral area.
a. Enumerate two more findings to illustrate the severity of the lesion. (3 marks)
b. What are the typical findings on the X-ray of a chest posterior-anterior (PA) and lateral view? (4 marks)
c. Enumerate three complications of the lesion. (3 marks)

Q2. A 30-year-old woman presents to the cardiology clinic with frequent palpitations and episodes of dizziness on exertion. She has no prior medical history. Her father passed away at the age of 34 years by sudden cardiac death. Her 12-lead electrocardiogram (ECG) at rest shows:

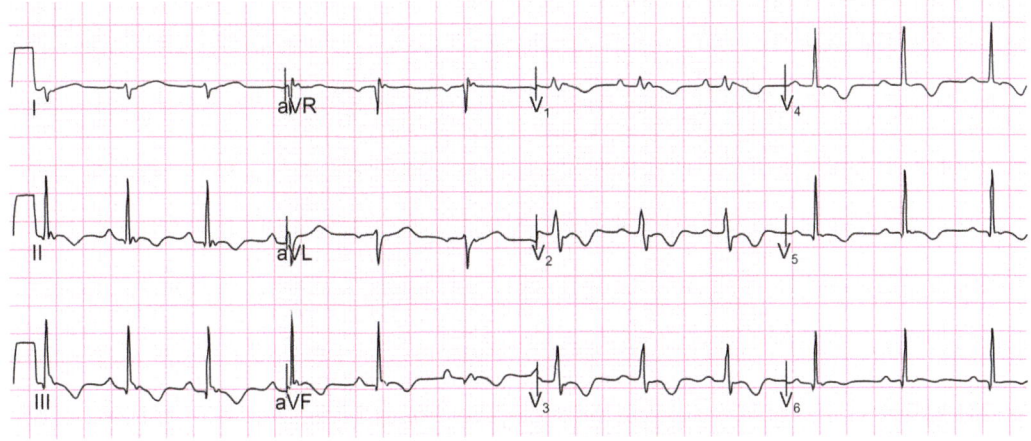

A 24-hour Holter monitor shows evidence of frequent premature ventricular complexes and runs of nonsustained ventricular tachycardia.
a. Write the ECG finding. (3 marks)
b. Name the condition. (2 marks)

c. What is the most likely underlying pathological process? *(2 marks)*
d. Outline the treatment and management options available. *(3 marks)*

Q3. See the image and answer the questions.

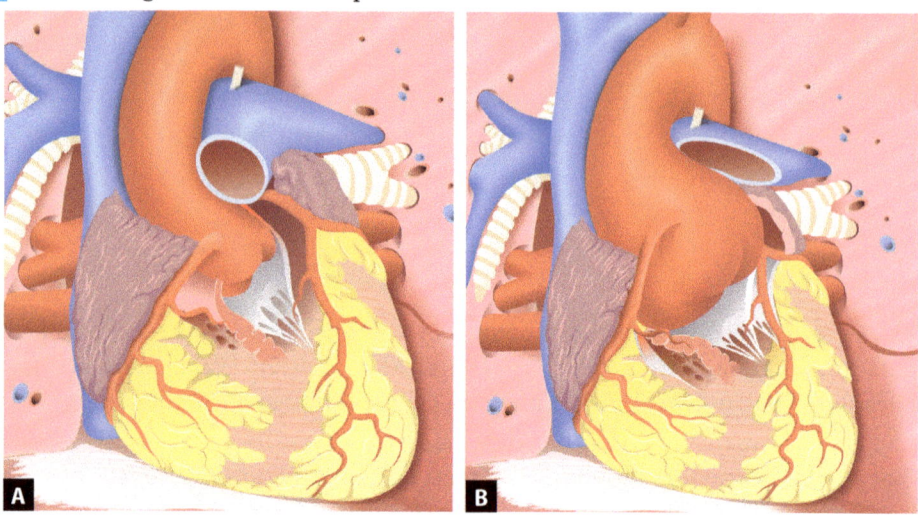

a. What is the abnormality and its diagnosis (Dx)? *(2 marks)*
b. Enumerate three cardiac/aortic findings. *(3 marks)*
c. Enumerate three skeletal and eye signs. *(2 marks)*
d. Enlist two differential diagnoses (D/D). *(3 marks)*

Q4. A young female patient in her early 20s, presented to the hospital with new-onset chest pain and uncontrolled hypertension (HTN). She was found to have blood pressure (BP) in the 200s/100s. Her investigations revealed a high ESR and CRP. Her imaging study is given below.

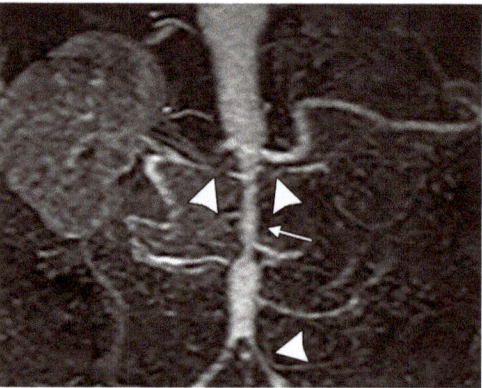

a. Name the imaging study done. *(2 marks)*
b. What are the findings? *(2 marks)*
c. What is the diagnosis? *(2 marks)*
d. How will you manage? *(4 marks)*

Cardiology

Q5. A 46-year-old white male diabetic (type 2 diabetes mellitus) patient presented to the hospital with fatigue and dyspnea. He had an H/O chronic back pain for which he takes ibuprofen. The patient was febrile with a BP of 140/98 mm Hg and heart rate (HR) around 150 beats/min. Heart sounds were distant and no murmur or rub was noted. Pulses were irregularly irregular. The patient had mild jugular venous distension, but the inspiratory decrease in systolic BP was not exaggerated. Breath sounds were decreased at the bases with faint crackles. The rest of his physical examination was normal.

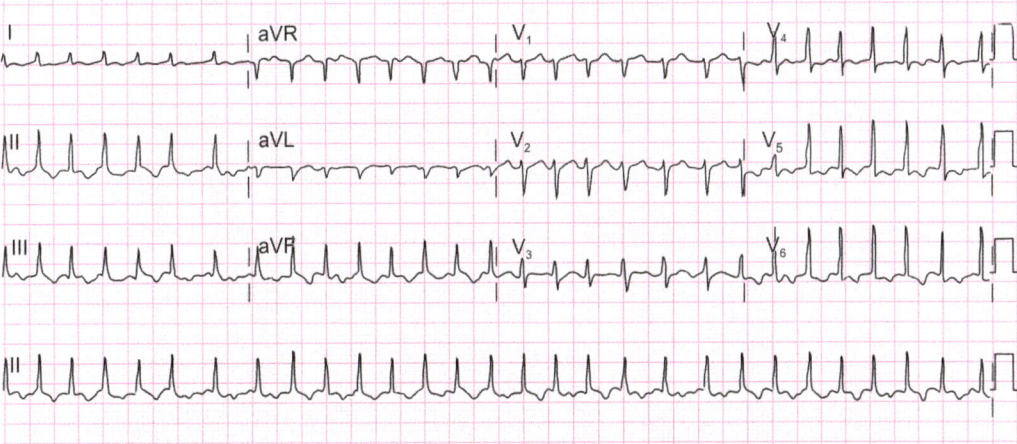

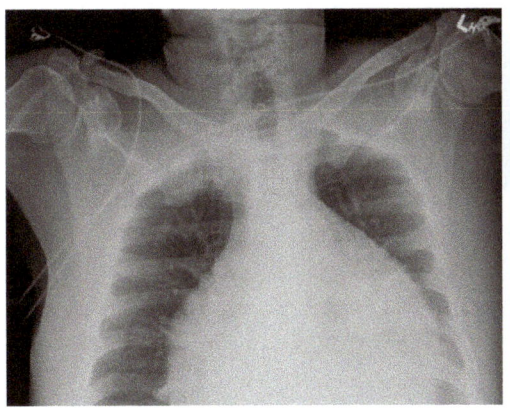
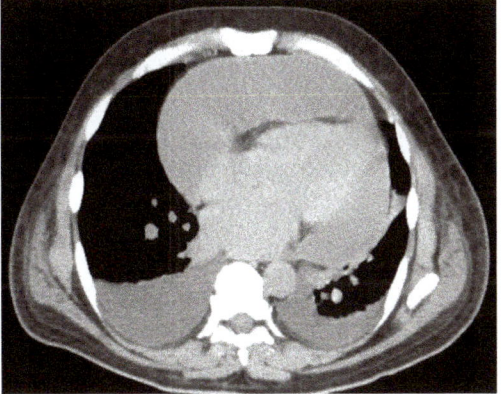

a. What is the diagnosis? (3 marks)
b. How will you confirm? (2 marks)
c. Which organism is commonly grown? (1 mark)
d. How will you manage? (4 marks)

Q6. A 24-year-old male presented with H/O palpitations and breathlessness of 4 years duration. On examination, his BP was 180/50 mm of Hg. His height was 180 cm.
a. What is the cardiac diagnosis? (2 marks)
b. Enumerate four specific general physical findings associated with this condition. (4 marks)

c. Enumerate three other associations of this syndrome. (3 marks)
d. Mention one complication. (1 mark)

Q7. A 21-year-old lady presented to emergency room (ER) with a headache. She had long-standing resistant HTN with lower limb fatigue on walking. Her upper limb BP was 230/110 mm Hg but her lower limb BP was 100/60.

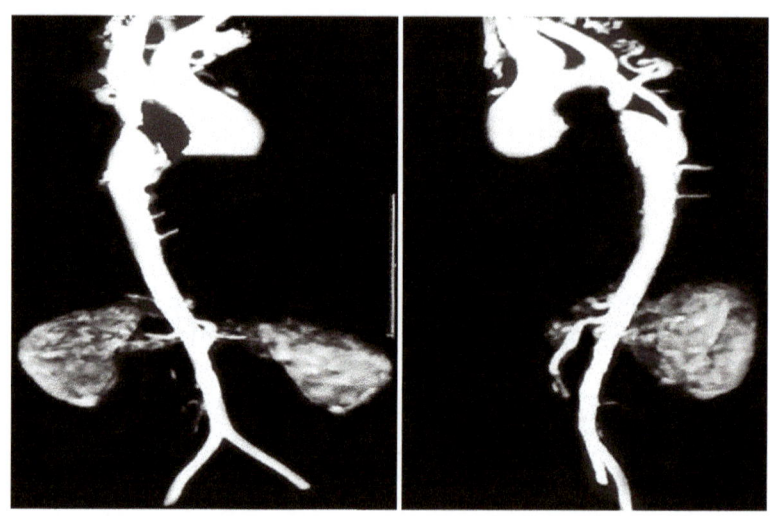

a. What is the pathological finding in this magnetic resonance (MR) aortography? (4 marks)
b. Diagnose the disease. (2 marks)
c. Name the chest X-ray sign of this disease. (2 marks)
d. Enumerate the corrective management. (2 marks)

Q8. A 70-year-old gentleman presented to the ER with repeated blackouts. An urgent ECG was done.

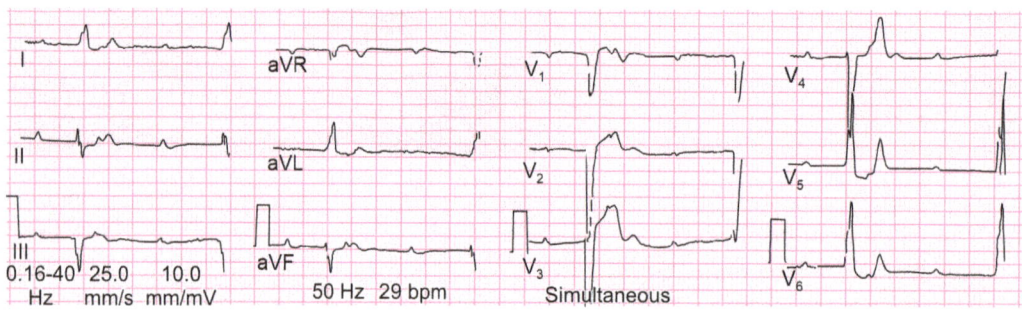

a. Identify the primary ECG abnormality. (2 marks)
b. What is the diagnosis? (2 marks)
c. Justify your diagnosis. (3 marks)
d. Highlight the management strategy. (3 marks)

Q9. A 35-year-old male presented to the ER with palpitation and respiratory distress. He had a H/O embolic cerebrovascular accident (CVA) 2 years back. Chest X-ray and ECG were done.

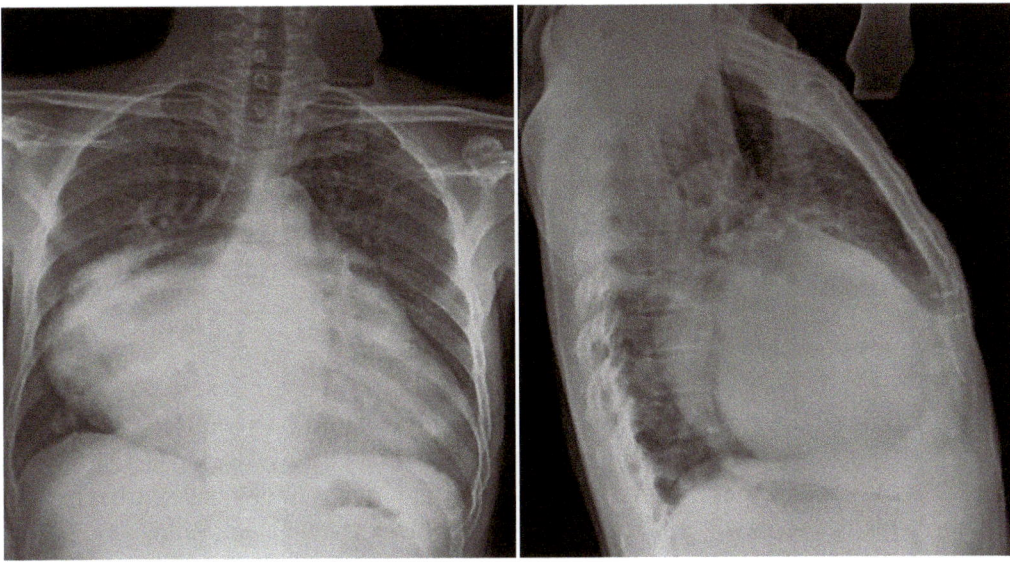

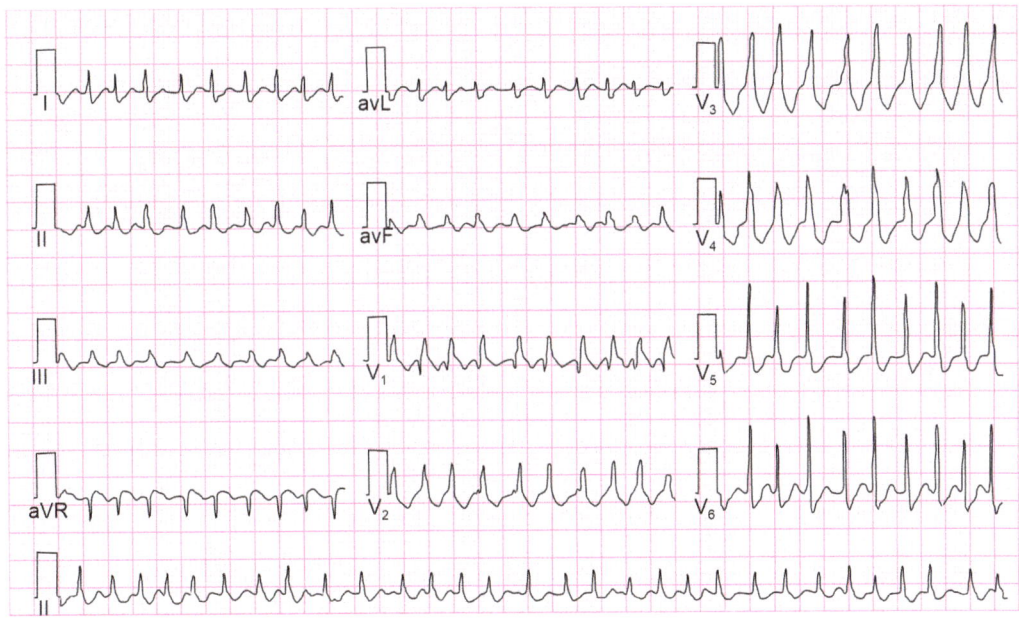

a. What are the abnormal findings of the chest X-ray? (3 marks)
b. Diagnose the ECG. (3 marks)
c. Enumerate the possible complications of this disease. (4 marks)

Q10.

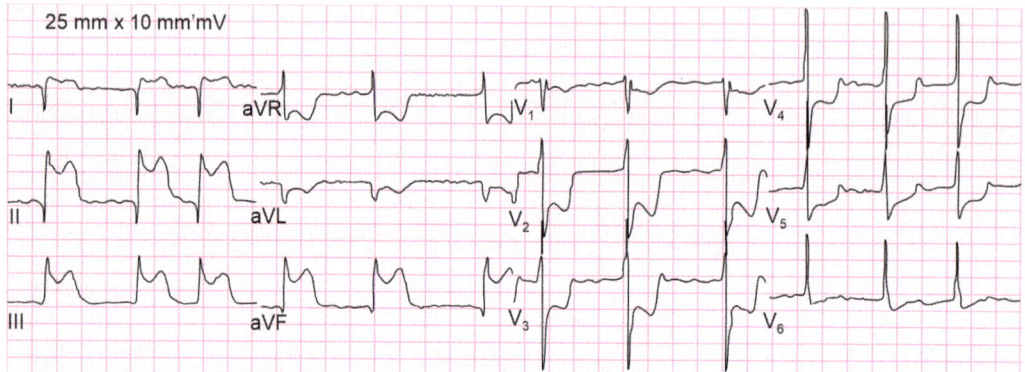

a. Identify the ECG. (10 marks)

Q11. Mr Gautam presents to the emergency department with a 1-month H/O increasing shortness of breath (SOB) on exertion and orthopnea. He reports waking up at night feeling breathless and needing to use extra pillows to sleep comfortably. Additionally, he has noticed swelling in his legs, especially in the ankles, which has been gradually worsening.

a. What is the provisional diagnosis? (3 marks)
b. What will be the possible ECHO and laboratory findings? (3 marks)
c. What drugs can be used for management? (4 marks)

Q12.

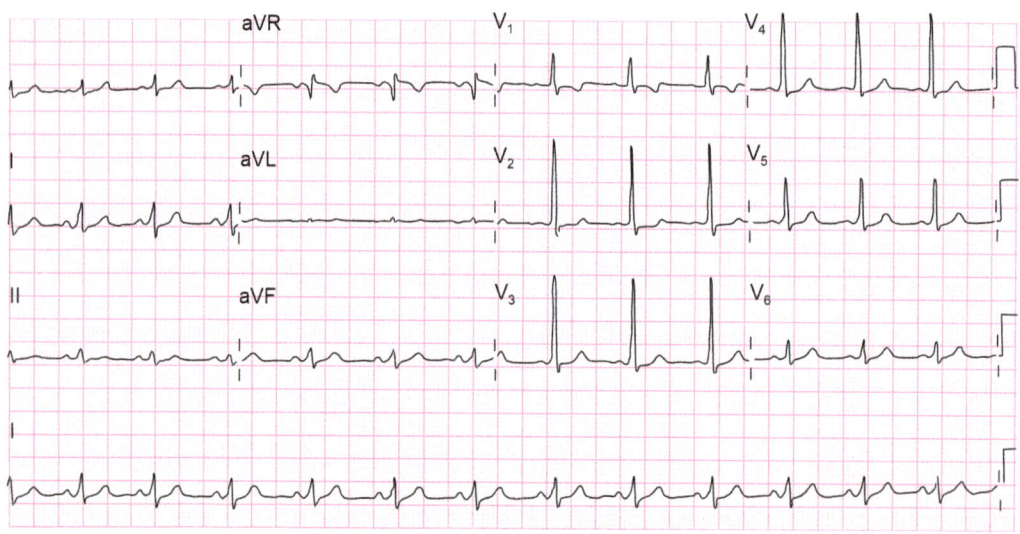

a. Which syndrome is depicted in the given ECG? (5 marks)
b. Treatment of choice for the given syndrome. (5 marks)

Q13. A 60-year-old female with an old known case of (K/C/O) HTN and diabetes mellitus (DM) female with past-H/O left middle cerebral artery (MCA) CVA and bedridden since 7 months. Complaints of (C/O) acute onset chest pain and breathlessness. On examination, tachycardia, regular rhythm, auscultation of the cardiovascular system (CVS), and respiratory system (RS) were normal.

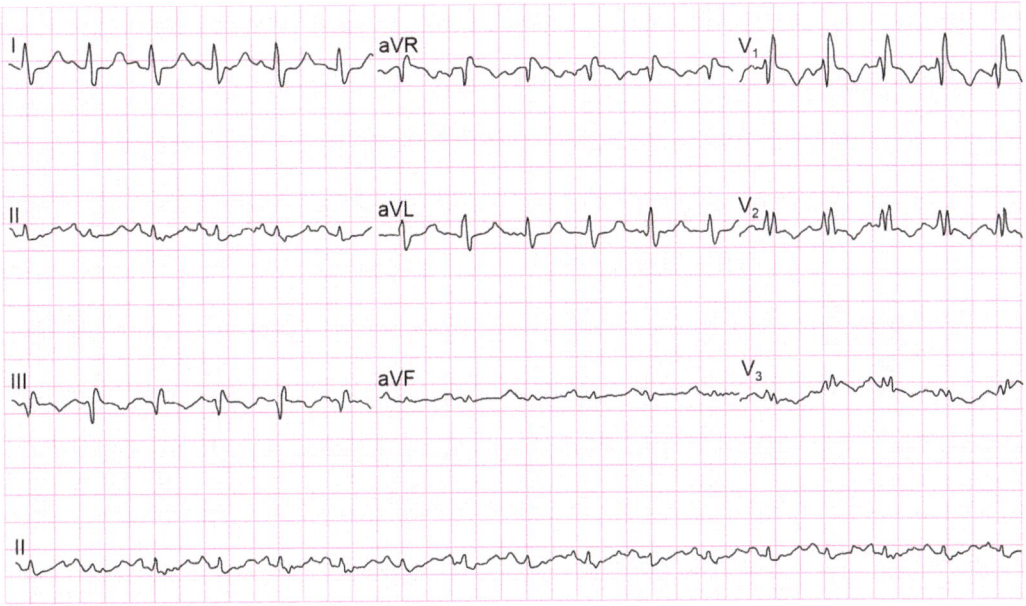

a. Identify the findings seen on ECG and diagnosis of the condition. (5 marks)
b. Discuss the ECHO sign seen in this condition. (5 marks)

Q14.

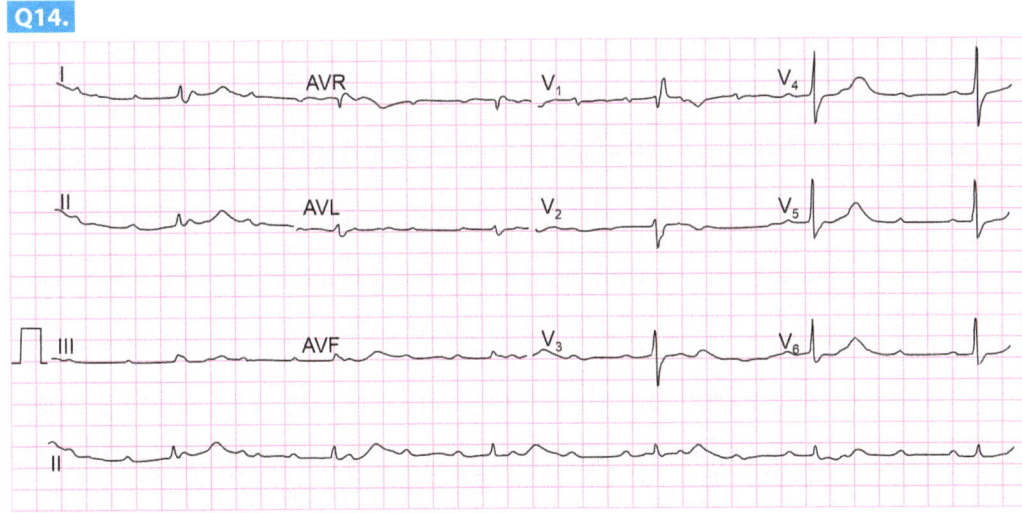

a. Identify the condition seen on the ECG. (5 marks)
b. Discuss the treatment for the condition. (5 marks)

Q15.

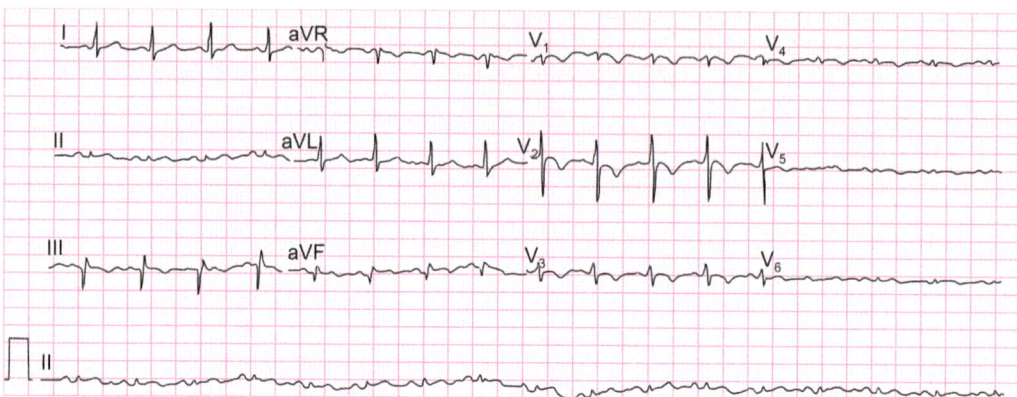

a. Identify the ECG. (5 marks)
b. Discuss the treatment in a tertiary care center. (5 marks)

Q16.
A young woman presented with C/O arm claudication, Raynaud's phenomenon. On examination, her left side brachial pulse was found to be feeble with discrepancies in the upper limb BP readings. Laboratory findings showed elevated erythrocyte sedimentation rate (ESR) with mild anemia.

a. What is the most probable diagnosis? (5 marks)
b. Treatment of the above condition. (5 marks)

Q17.
A 35-year-old female presented with C/O chest pain of insidious onset, gradually progressive, exaggerated on lying down, and relieved with sitting and leaning forward. She is a nonsmoker and has no risk factors for coronary artery disease (CAD). She is a known C/O rheumatoid arthritis on irregular medications. Electrocardiogram recordings are shown below.

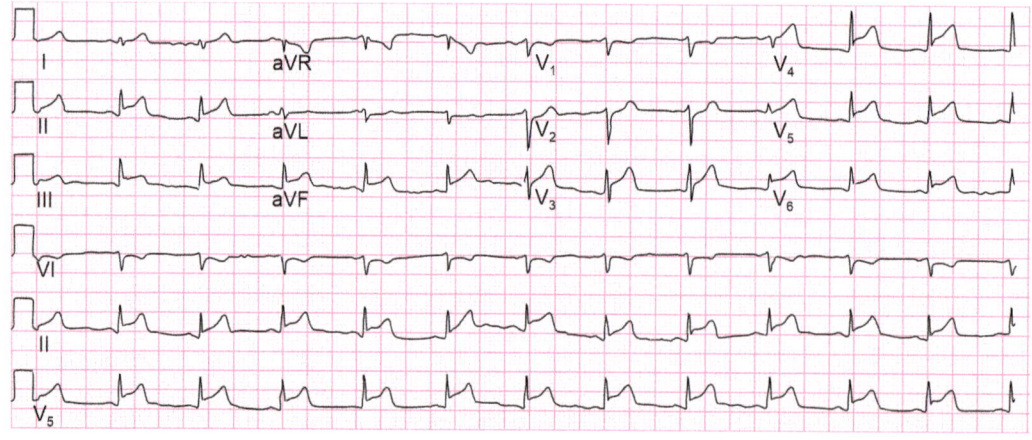

a. Read the ECG. (5 marks)
b. Discuss the provisional diagnosis and management. (2 marks + 3 marks)

Q18.

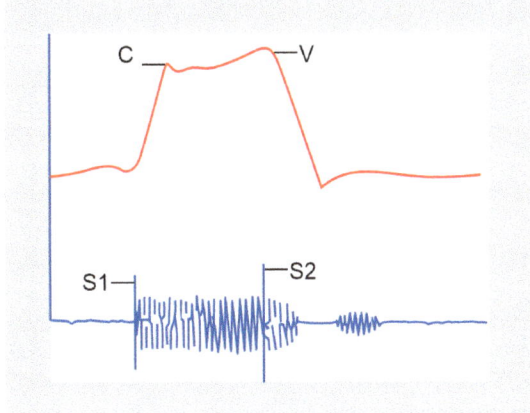

a. Identify the abnormalities in the jugular venous pressure (JVP) wave pattern. *(5 marks)*
b. Give your diagnosis. *(2 marks)*
c. What are the clinical findings do you expect in this condition? *(3 marks)*

Q19.
A 19-year-old male came to Srirama Chandra Bhanj Medical College & Hospital (SCBMCH) casualty with severe chest pain for 3 hours, sudden in onset and gradually progressive and tearing in nature with radiation to the back.

On examination:
- *General appearance:* Pale, weight—70 kg, height—180 cm, PR—130/min, thready
- *BP:* 80/40 mm Hg
- *CVS:* Heart sounds muffled
- *Chest:* Bilateral (B/L) vesicular breath sound (VBS)+
- *Urine output (U/O):* Nil since last 90 minutes
- Urgent ECG and contrast-enhanced computerized tomography (CECT) thorax done which shows the following:

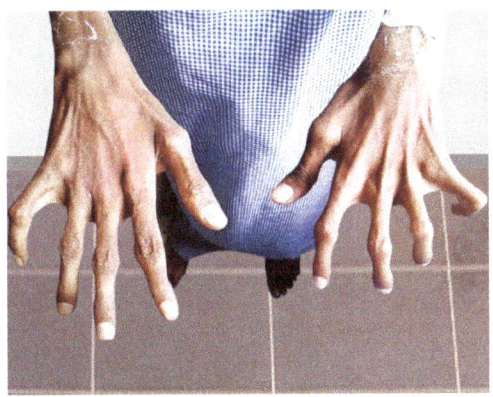
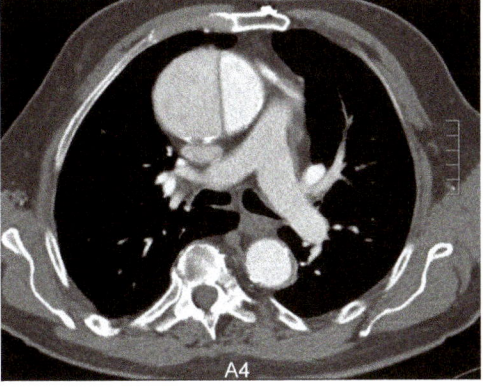

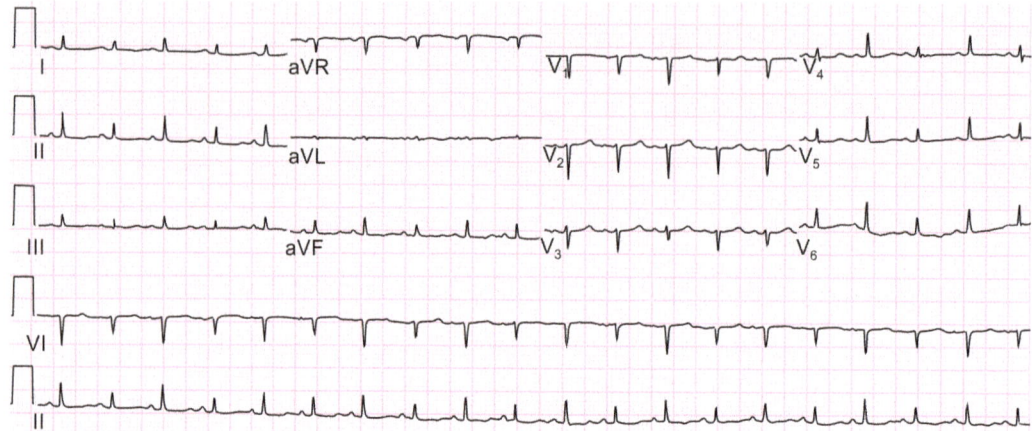

a. Read the ECG and CECT thorax. (3 marks)
b. What is your diagnosis and what is the gene involved? (4 marks)

Q20. A 20-year-old medical graduate was playing basketball with his colleagues. On attempting a shot he suddenly collapsed and was rushed to the casualty. No H/O any cardiac respiratory illness in the past. His maternal uncle has H/O sudden cardiac death.

On examination:
- Patient unresponsive
- Pulse rate (PR) is not palpable
- BP is not recordable

On auscultation: Breathe sound (BS) +nt heart sounds +nt

i. The patient was intubated in view of airway compromise, lines were established, and intravenous (IV) fluids and drugs were started and managed at the cardiology intensive care unit (ICU). Two-dimensional (2D) ECHO showed.

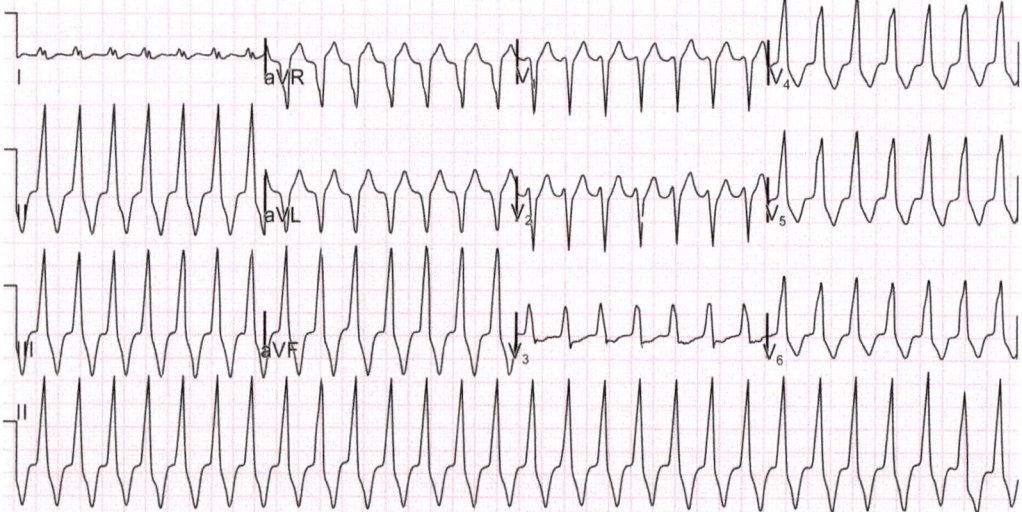

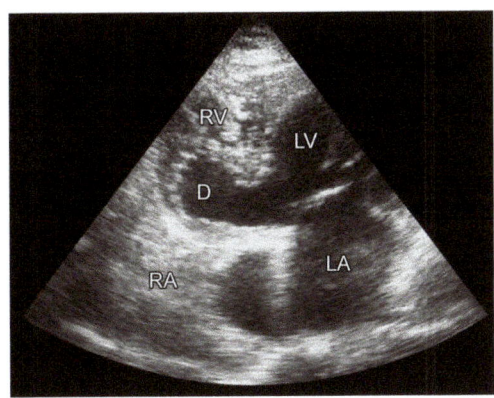

a. Read the ECG and abnormality in a 2D ECHO. (2 marks)
b. What is the diagnosis and gene involved? (3 marks)
c. What is the treatment? (3 marks)

Q21. A 25-year-old female C/O sudden onset weakness of the left upper limb and lower limb for the last 3 hours with facial deviation to right on attempted smiling. The weakness was severe at onset but has improved to a bit extent over the last 2 hours. She has had H/O shortness of breath on doing regular household activities for the last 1 year.

She gave H/O fever with multiple migratory joint pain when she was 10 years old for which she was treated with injectable medications.

On examination:
- HR: 132/min
- PR: 110/min
- BP: 118/60 mm Hg
- CVS: S1, S2 mid-diastolic murmur (MDM) at apex plantar—left side (Babinski positive)

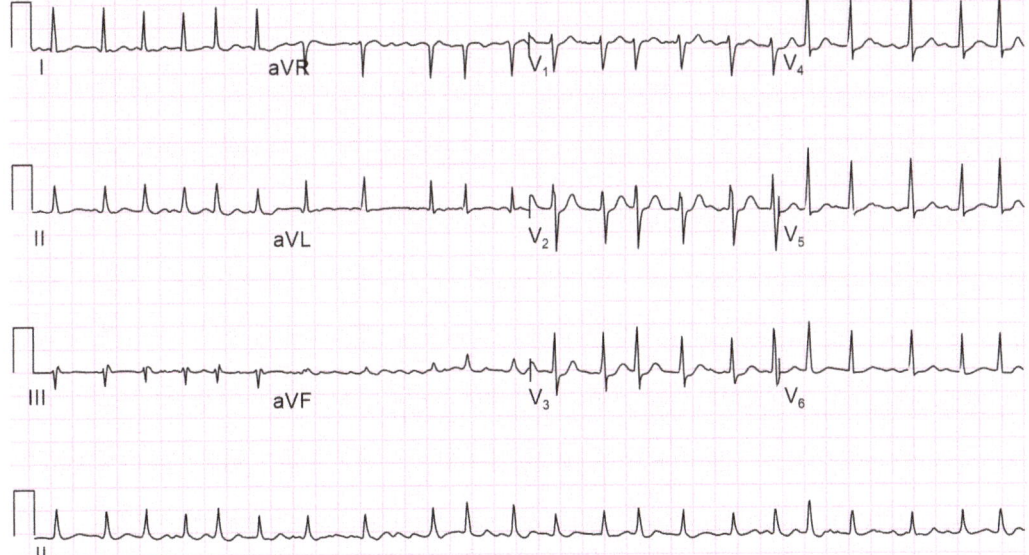

150 Cardiology

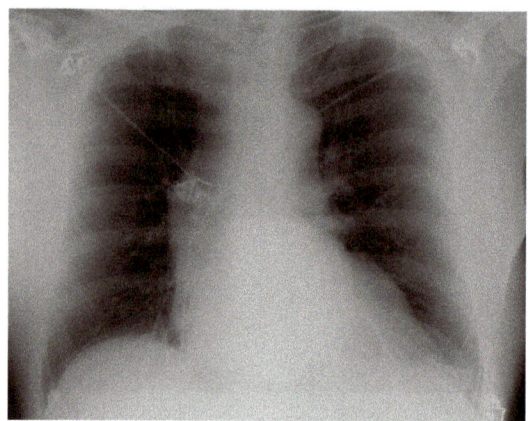

a. Read the ECG. (3 marks)
b. Read the X-ray. (3 marks)
c. What is your diagnosis? (4 marks)

Q22. Mrs Rai, a 62-year-old female with an H/O HTN and hyperlipidemia, presents to the emergency department with severe chest pain that began approximately 2 hours ago. The patient describes the pain as a crushing sensation in the center of her chest that radiates down her left arm. She also reports feeling nauseous and light-headed. The pain started while she was at rest and has not improved.

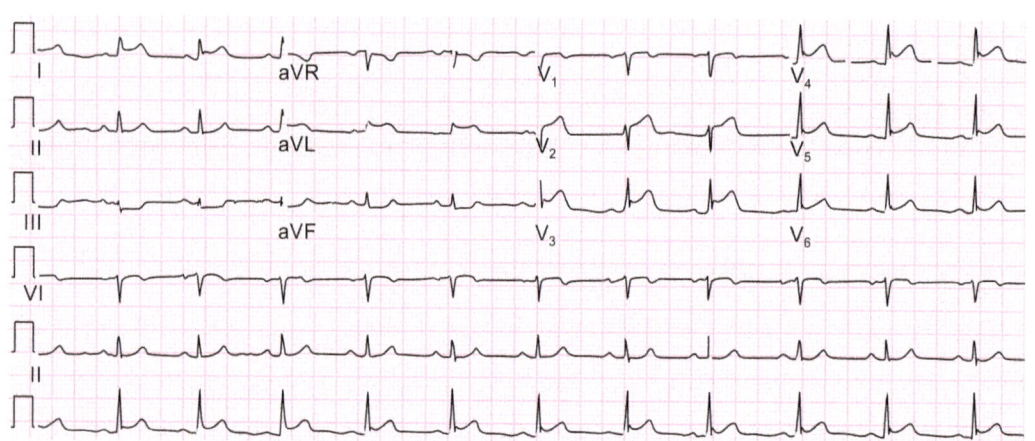

a. What is the diagnosis? (3 marks)
b. What are the drugs used to manage this condition? (3 marks)
c. Name two D/D of this condition. (3 marks)

Q23. A previously healthy 21-year-old man is brought to the emergency for the evaluation of an episode of unconsciousness that suddenly happened while playing football 30 minutes ago. He was not shaking and regained consciousness after about 30 seconds. Over the past 3 months, the patient has had several episodes of shortness of breath while exercising as well as sensations of a racing heart. He does not smoke or drink alcohol. He takes no medications. His vital signs are within normal limits. On mental status examination, he is oriented to person, place, and time. Cardiac examination shows a systolic ejection murmur that increases with the Valsalva maneuver and standing and an S4 gallop. The remainder of the examination shows no abnormalities. An ECG shows a deep S wave in lead V1 and tall R waves in leads V5 and V6.

a. What is your diagnosis? *(2 marks)*
b. What will be his echocardiography findings? *(4 marks)*
c. Explain the findings on auscultation. *(2 marks)*
d. What is the management in brief? *(2 marks)*

Q24.

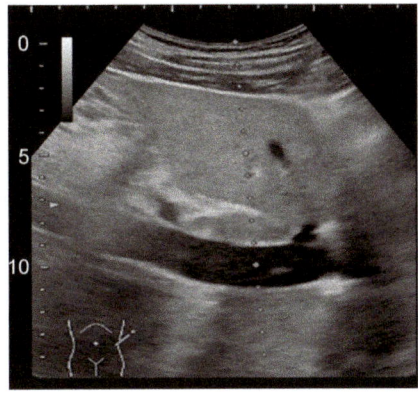

a. What is the structure labeled here? *(2 marks)*
b. Why do we need to evaluate it? *(3 marks)*
c. How does it help in diagnosis? *(5 marks)*

Q25.

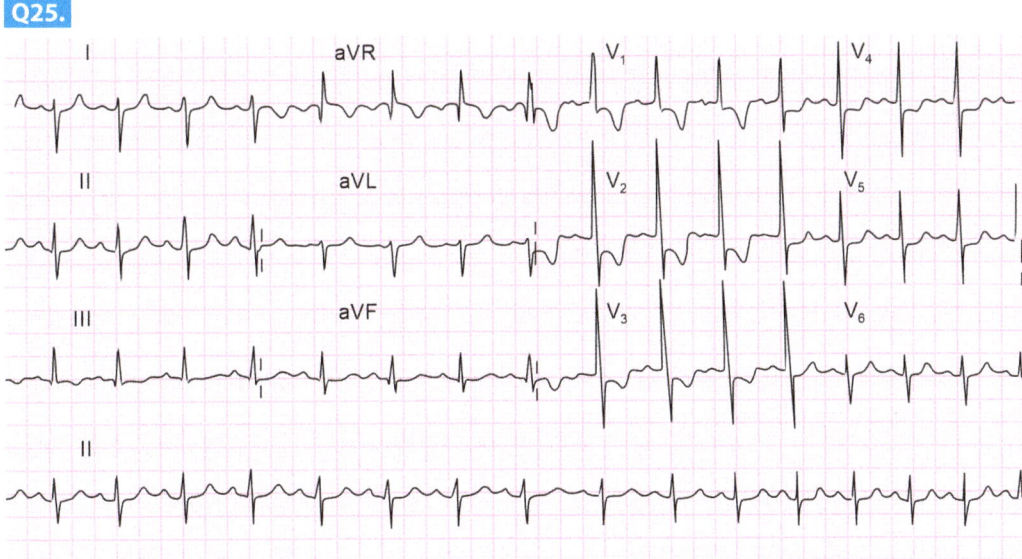

a. Mention the important ECG findings. *(2 marks)*
b. What is the ECG diagnosis? *(1 mark)*
c. List three important D/D for these ECG changes. *(3 marks)*
d. List four important findings on general examination. *(4 marks)*

Q26. A 35-year-old female with aortic incompetence (AI) has a BP of 140/60 in the right upper limb and 170/68 in the right lower limb.
a. What is this sign known as? *(1 mark)*
b. In healthy individuals, what is the maximum difference between systolic BP of the upper and lower extremities? *(1 mark)*
c. What is the difference between systolic BP of the upper and lower extremities in severe AI? *(1 mark)*
d. What is de Musset's sign in AI? *(1 mark)*
e. What is the most common cause of chronic AI? *(1 mark)*

Q27. A 34-year-old female, residing in India, presents with an irregularly irregular pulse with a pulse deficit of 26/min and a grade 4 pansystolic murmur maximally heard at the apex and transmitted to the left axilla. She C/O fatigue, exertional dyspnea, orthopnea, and palpitations. There is no H/O chest pain.
a. What is the likely diagnosis? *(1 + 1 = 2 marks)*
b. Enlist two common causes leading to this condition. *(1 + 1 = 2 marks)*
c. Name two common complications of this condition. *(0.5 + 0.5 = 1 mark)*

Q28. A 73-year-old farmer has come to the hospital with a past H/O stable angina. He uses nitroglycerin (0.4 mg sublingually) approximately three times per month. His HR is 90 beats/min, and his BP is 132/72 mm Hg. He had undergone a stent placement in his coronary arteries 5 years back. His low-density lipoprotein (LDL) cholesterol level is 134 mg/dL. His medications include a tablet aspirin (75 mg), tablet lisinopril (20 mg daily) for HTN, and tablet atorvastatin (40 mg daily).
a. Is there a need for any other antianginal drugs now? Justify. *(4 marks)*
b. Explain the role of tablet aspirin and tablet atorvastatin in this case. *(3 marks)*
c. Rewrite his prescription with appropriate drugs. *(3 marks)*

Q29. A 65-year-old man presented with reduced exercise tolerance for 3 weeks, worsening of shortness of breath at rest, body swelling, and chest discomfort for 72 hours duration. His clinical examination showed elevated JVP, bibasal fine end-inspiratory crepitations, and sacral and moderate bilateral pedal edema.

His respiratory rate was 30, SpO$_2$ 94 on 2 L/min O$_2$, PR was 140 and BP was 80/50. The ECG findings are shown below.

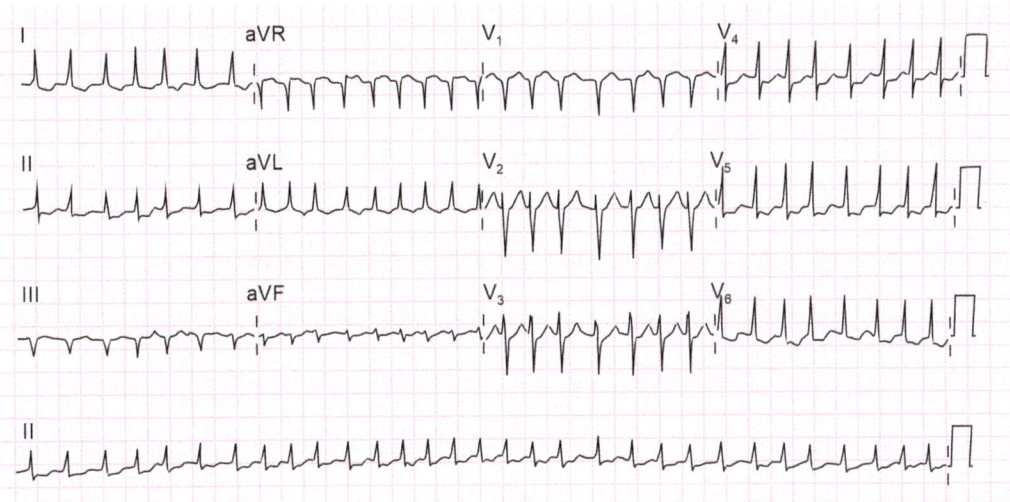

a. What is an ECG diagnosis? (2 marks)
b. What is the underlying diagnosis? (2 marks)
c. State the three immediate treatment options that can be used in emergency settings. (3 marks)
d. State three medications that can be used in the long-term management of this patient if his echocardiogram showed an ejection fraction (EF) of 25%. (3 marks)

Q30. A 35-year-old underwent a medical check-up for the job. He gave a family H/O CAD. His eye examination is shown below.

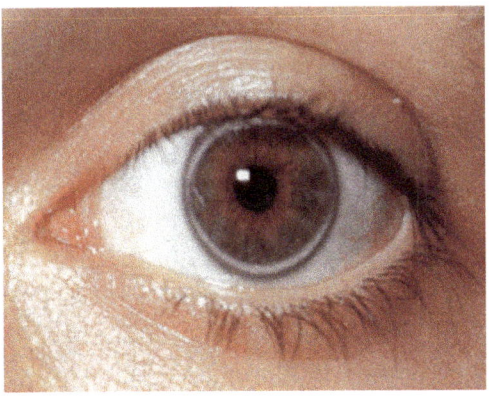

a. Identify the abnormality. (2 marks)
b. Name at least one more associated abnormal finding in general physical examination (GPE). (3 marks)
c. What does it predispose to? (2 marks)
d. Name two drugs to manage. (3 marks)

Q31.

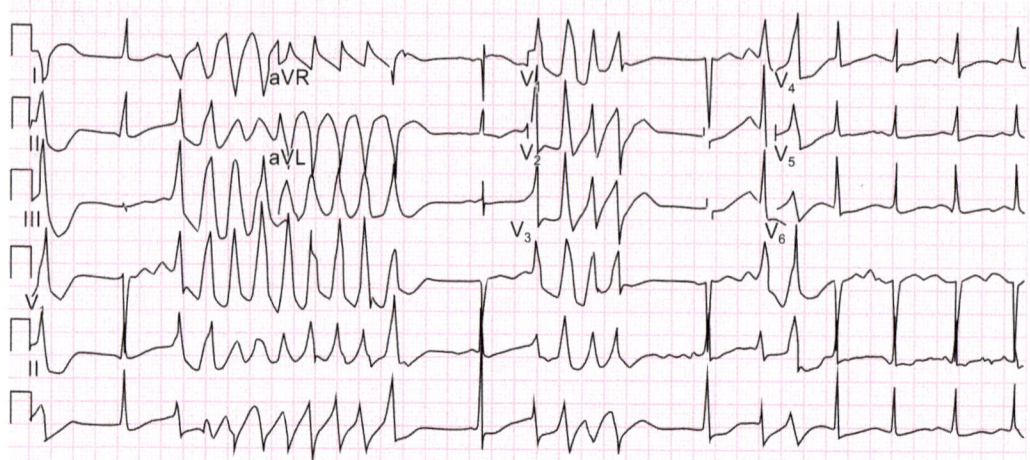

a. Identify the ECG. (5 marks)
b. Which electrolyte abnormality can lead to the above ECG? (5 marks)

Q32.

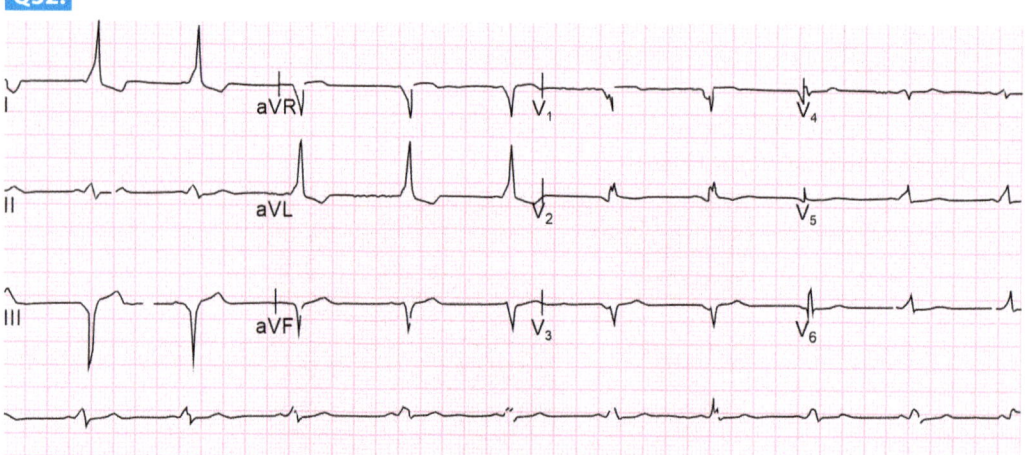

a. Identify the ECG and the characteristic finding. (5 marks)
b. Identify the condition. (5 marks)

Q33.

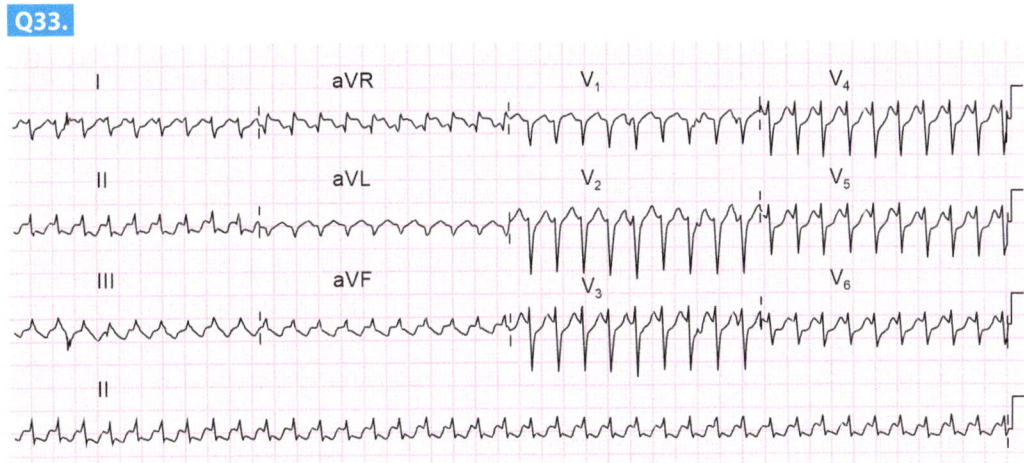

a. Identify the ECG. (5 marks)
b. Treatment of the given condition. (5 marks)

Q34.
A 26-year-old male was brought to the ER in a gasping condition following a road traffic accident. Initial evaluation excluded tension pneumothorax, major vessel rupture, and cardiac tamponade. There was a soft decrescendo systolic murmur over the apical area and lung bases were full of rales. A screening echocardiography was done.

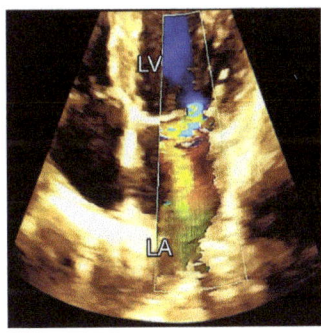 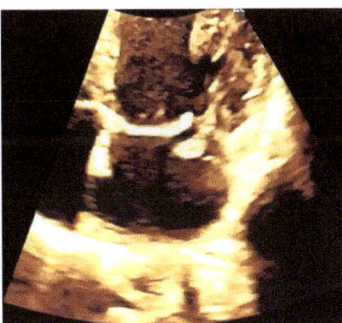 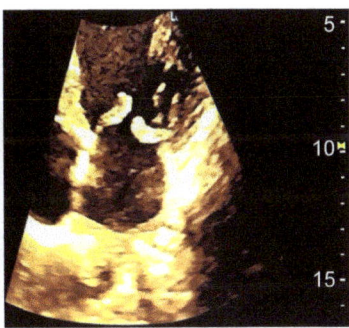

a. What are the pathological findings? (4 marks)
b. Enumerate the common causes. (4 marks)
c. What is the management? (2 marks)

Q35.

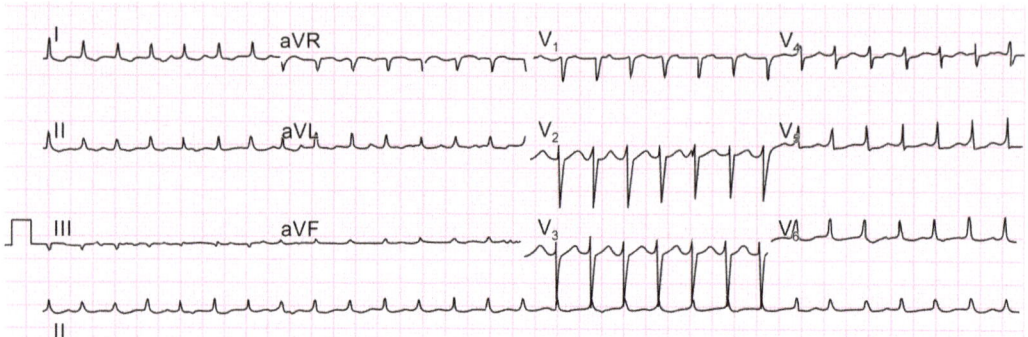

a. Identify the ECG findings. (3 marks)
b. Enumerate the drug of choice in hemodynamically stable patients. (3 marks)
c. Enumerate the drug of choice in hemodynamic instability. (3 marks)

Q36.
A 54-year-old human immunodeficiency virus (HIV) patient on dolutegravir, tenofovir, and emtricitabine; and PCP prophylaxis was found to have the ECG changes during routine testing.

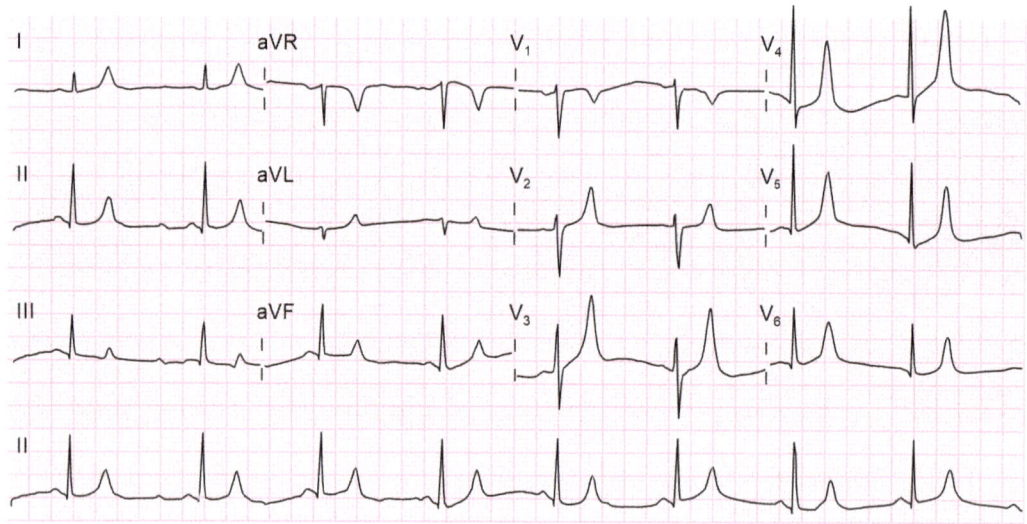

a. Name the causative drug that produces the ECG abnormality. (3 marks)
b. How will you manage this condition? (4 marks)
c. Mention two other important side effects of that drug. (3 marks)

ANSWERS

Ans. 1

a. Opening snap (OS) S2 difference. An opening snap that almost immediately follows S2 indicates severe mitral stenosis and the length of the murmur.
b. Straightening of left heart border, double contour due to enlarged LA, Kerley B lines, colonel's mustache, elevation of the left main bronchus, and splaying of the carina.
c. Congestive heart failure, pulmonary HTN, Ortner's syndrome, atrial fibrillation, and pulmonary embolization.

Ans. 2

a. ECG of a patient with demonstrating:
   - T-wave inversion in precordial and inferior leads, without right bundle branch block (RBBB) pattern.
   - Epsilon wave in V1
   - Localized widening of QRS in V1–2
b. Arrhythmogenic right ventricular dysplasia (ARVD)
c. Replacement of right ventricular free wall myocardium with fibrous and fatty tissue.
d. *Management:*
   - *Drugs:* Sotalol is the most widely used antiarrhythmic.
   - Catheter ablation to prevent ventricular tachycardia.
   - Implantable cardioverter-defibrillator

Ans. 3

a. Panel A depicts a normal-sized aortic root. In contrast, panel B shows a markedly dilated aortic root-Marfan syndrome
b. Aortic regurgitation, aortic dissection, and mitral valve prolapse (MVP)
c. Arachnodactyly (wrist and thumb sign), pectus deformity, and ectopia lentis
d. Homocystinuria and Ehlers–Danlos types

Ans. 4

a. Coronal maximum intensity projection (MIP) three-dimensional (3D) MR angiogram.
b. Narrowing of the abdominal aorta (arrow). The narrowing starts below the celiac trunk and is associated with stenosis of the renal arteries (top arrowheads) and the left common iliac artery (bottom arrowheads).
c. Type IV Takayasu arteritis
d. The two most important aspects of treatment are (1) controlling the inflammatory process and (2) controlling HTN. Critical stenotic lesions should be treated by angioplasty or surgical revascularization during periods of remission.

Ans. 5

a. Purulent pericarditis.
b. CT of chest and culture/sensitivity (C/S) of the pericardial aspirate.
c. *Streptococcus pneumoniae*

Ans. 6

a. Aortic regurgitation
b. Corrigan pulse, Hill's sign, pistal-shot sign, and de Musset's sign
c. High-arched palate, ectopia lentis, and pectus excavatum
d. Dissection of aorta and bacterial endocarditis

Ans. 7

a. Abrupt focal narrowing at the juxta ductal portion of the arch of the aorta near the origin of the left subclavian artery.
b. Juxta ductal coarctation of the aorta.
c. "Figure of 3" sign
d. Coarctoplasty (endovascular coarctation stenting or surgical correction)

Ans. 8

a. Atrioventricular (AV) dissociation
b. Complete heart block
c. P and QRS are not related to each other, the atrial rate is more than the ventricular rate. Low ventricular escape rate.
d. Temporary pacemaker insertion, reversal of any possible reversible cause of complete heart block (CHB), and permanent pacemaker implantation if the cause is irreversible.

Ans. 9

a. Abnormal findings of the chest X-ray are as follows:
   - Increased CT ratio.
   - Double contouring of the right border of the heart (double bubble sign).
   - Right ventricular (RV)-type apex with RV enlargement as per lateral view
   - The fullness of pulmonary bay and left atrial (LA) appendage prominence.
   - Splaying of carina with horizontal left main bronchus
   - "Walking man sign." (It results from posterior displacement of the left main bronchus such that it no longer overlaps the right bronchus in lateral projection. The left and right bronchus thus appears as an inverted "V", mimicking the legs of a walking man)
   - Upper lobe venous prominence.
b. Irregular narrow complex tachycardia with RBBB and without any distinct P wave; suggestive of (S/O) atrial fibrillation with right bundle branch block and fast ventricular rate.
c. The patient is suffering from severe mitral stenosis and the possible complications are as follows:
   - Pulmonary edema
   - Pulmonary HTN
   - Right heart failure
   - Atrial fibrillation
   - LA thrombus

- Embolism
- Dysphagia
- Hemoptysis
- Ortner's syndrome

Ans. 10

a. IWMI

Ans. 11

a. Congestive heart failure
b. *Laboratory findings:* Elevated N-terminal pro-brain natriuretic peptide (NT-proBNP), ECHO-elevated right ventricular systolic pressure (RVSP) with decreased EF/normal EF.
c. Diuretics and angiotensin-converting enzyme (ACE) inhibitors/β-blockers.

Ans. 12

a. Wolff–Parkinson–White (WPW) syndrome
b. Radiofrequency ablation

Ans. 13

a. S1Q3T3 pattern seen in pulmonary embolism
b. *McConnell's sign:* Hypokinesis of the RV free wall with normal or hyperkinetic motion of the RV apex.

Ans. 14

a. Complete heart block
b. Permanent pacing

Ans. 15

a. Posterior wall myocardial infarction (MI)
b. Pregnancy-associated acute myocardial infarction (PAMI)

Ans. 16

a. Takayasu arteritis
b. *Glucocorticoid therapy:* 40–60 mg/day
   Surgical correction and or arterioplastic approach to stenosed vessels

Ans. 17

a. This is a 12-lead ECG showing:
   - *PR:* 75/min
   - *Rhythm:* Regular
   - *Axis:* Normal
   - P-wave, QRS complex, and T-wave of normal morphology
   - ST-segment elevated with concavity upward, down-sloping of TP segments (Spodick sign), and PR segment depression in leads II, III, aVF, and V3–V6.
   - ST-segment depression and PR segment elevation in V1 and R side of the heart (aVR)

b. Keeping the clinical history in the background with the nature of chest pain and the H/O improperly controlled RA with the above ECG findings our provisional diagnosis is *acute pericarditis*.
Management: Nonsteroidal anti-inflammatory drugs (NSAIDs) to control chest pain. Treat the underlying cause leading to acute pericarditis disease-modifying antirheumatic drugs (DMARDs).

Ans. 18

a. JVP has five waves [three positive waves (a, c, and v) and two negative waves (x and y descent)]. In the above tracing the x descent is absent and there is a large premature v wave k/a *Lancisi sign* which suggests that the pressure are rising prematurely in the right atria during the right ventricular contraction(possible only when a regurgitant jet of blood travels from the right ventricle to atria during systole).
b. Considering a Lancisi sign on JVP tracing with the concomitant tracing of a pansystolic murmur on heart sound tracing a clinical diagnosis of *tricuspid regurgitation (TR)* can be made.
c. Although less common Isolated TR is associated with a clinical finding of *pan-systolic murmur at the tricuspid area*, but more commonly occurs due to RVH due to underlying pulmonary HTN secondary to left ventricular failure (LVF)/lung pathology which may be associated with a complaint of palpable/loud P_2, parasternal heave, and laterally displaced apex.

Ans. 19

a. The 12-lead ECG reads an HR is 130/min; sinus and regular rhythm with alternate high and low voltage QRS complex S/O "electrical alternans." All other waves, segments, and intervals are normal. The CECT thorax reveals the ascending aorta to have a false lumen (not taking the dye) and a true lumen (taking the dye) and the false lumen being larger than the true lumen all S/O "aortic dissection."
b. With the given clinical history and examination findings of Arachnodactyly and height of 180 cm, muffled heart sounds with ECG evidence of electrical alternans, and CECT evidence of Aortic dissection a provisional diagnosis of *Marfan syndrome with aortic dissection and pericardial effusion is made*. The gene most commonly involved is fibrillin.

Ans. 20

a. The 12-lead ECG shows wide complex tachycardia (ventricular rate 250/min) with QRS complex being a positive complex and T-wave being a negative wave S/O ventricular tachycardia. The 2D ECHO shows *banana-shaped left ventricular cavity* S/O hypertrophy of interventricular septum.
b. From the H/O sudden collapse during outdoor activities with ECG showing VT and 2D echo showing IVS hypertrophy with past H/O sudden cardiac death in family members a Dx of *hypertrophic cardiomyopathy (HCM)* is made. The gene involved is the β-myosin heavy chain gene.
c. *Management:* Placement of implantable cardioverter defibrillator (ICD) device for prevention of further recurrence.

Ans. 21

a. The 12-lead ECG shows irregularly irregular rhythm without any P-wave and ventricular rate of 140/min so our diagnosis is *atrial fibrillation with fast ventricular rate*.
b. The chest X-ray (PA view) shows a *double atria shadow* which is S/O LA enlargement.
c. Our clinical diagnosis is *rheumatic heart disease (mitral stenosis) with atrial fibrillation with fast ventricular rate, cardioembolic CVA with left-sided hemiparesis* evidenced by H/O migratory joint pain with fever in the past treated with injectables with MDM at the apex and LA enlargement on X-ray with sudden onset left sided weakness with extensor plantar on the left side to be confirmed with noncontrast computed tomography (NCCT) brain/magnetic resonance imaging (MRI) brain and 2D ECHO.

Ans. 22

a. Acute anterolateral wall MI
b. Antiplatelets, anticoagulants, antihypertensives, antihyperlipidemic, opioids, and fibrinolytic drugs
c. Acute pericarditis and hyperkalemia

Ans. 23

a. Hypertrophic cardiomyopathy
b. Systolic anterior motion of mitral valve with interventricular septal hypertrophy
c. During the Valsalva strain phase, and standing, because of decreased preload, the blood volume in the left ventricular cavity decreases and it causes an increase in the intensity of the murmur. During rapid filling phase reverberation of the left ventricular wall causes an S4 heart sound.
d. β-blockers, septal myectomy, or ablation.

Ans. 24

a. Inferior vena cava (IVC)
b. To estimate fluid status, determine fluid requirement, evaluate right heart dysfunction, and monitor prognosis
c. To evaluate the collapsibility of IVC to suggest a clue for diagnosing right heart dysfunction

Ans. 25

a. Right axis deviation, tall R wave in V_1-V_3, deep S-wave in V_4-V_6, right ventricular strain pattern, tall R in aVR
b. Right ventricular hypertrophy
c. True posterior infarct, RBBB, WPW syndrome, and dextrocardia
d. Cyanosis, clubbing, raised JVP, lower extremity edema, and polycythemia

Ans. 26

a. Hill's sign
b. 20 mm Hg
c. >60 mm Hg

d. To and fro nodding of the head synchronous with carotid pulsation or heartbeat
e. Rheumatic

Ans. 27

a. Mitral regurgitation with atrial fibrillation.
b. Rheumatic fever/dilated cardiomyopathy/infective endocarditis
c. Heart failure and thromboembolic stroke

Ans. 28

a. Given his resting HR, β-blocker can be prescribed, also a long-acting nitrate as a second-line drug as he uses sublingual nitroglycerin sublingual (NTG) around three times a month.
   - Tablet metoprolol 50 mg BD; isosorbide dinitrate (ISDN) 10 mg OD to be added
b. Aspirin 75 mg to be added to prevent MI and stroke, and atorvastatin 40 mg to achieve non-high-density lipoprotein (non-HDL) cholesterol reduction >40% [National Institute for Health and Care Excellence (NICE) guidelines].
c. Tablet metoprolol 50 mg BD:
   - Tablet isosorbide dinitrate (ISDN) 10 mg OD
   - Tablet aspirin 75 mg OD
   - Tablet atorvastatin 40 mg OD

   Continue all the drugs for 2 weeks, sublingual nitroglycerin 0.5 mg for immediate pain relief as and when needed, review after 2 weeks.
   Advice: Cessation of smoking, alcohol abstinence. Patient to be advised for stress testing after review.

Ans. 29

a. Atrial fibrillation with rapid ventricular rhythm
b. Cardiogenic shock with acute pulmonary edema
c.
   - IV amiodarone
   - IV inotropes adrenalin, noradrenalin, and metaraminol
   - IV Frusemide (low dose)
d.
   - *Sacubitril:* Valsartan angiotensin receptor/neprilysin inhibitor (ARNI)
   - Spironolactone mineralocorticoid receptor antagonists (MRAs)
   - Bisoprolol β-blockers

Ans. 30

a. Arcus juvenilis
b. Xanthelasma
c. CAD
d. Statins and ezetimibe

Ans. 31

a. TDP
b. Hypokalemia and hypomagnesemia

Ans. 32
a. Delta wave
b. WPW syndrome

Ans. 33
a. Paroxysmal supraventricular tachycardia (PSVT)
b.

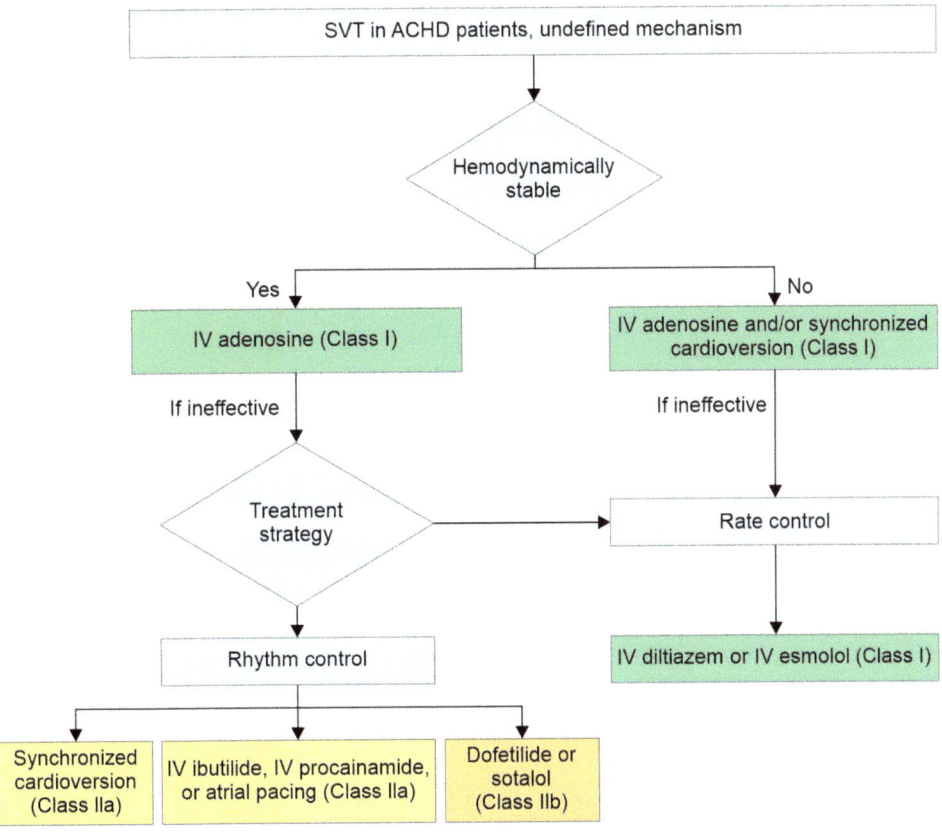

Ans. 34
a. Improper closure of the posterior mitral leaflet causes flail mitral leaflet leading to severe acute mitral regurgitation due to rupture chordae following the road traffic accident.
b. *Causes of chordal rupture are:*
   - Trauma
   - Myxomatous
   - Endocarditis
   - Spontaneous rupture
c. Immediate thoracotomy and repair of the mitral valve apparatus.

Ans. 35

a. PSVT
b. Lidocaine
c. Cardioversion

Ans. 36

a. *ECG abnormality:* Tall T wave
b. *Treatment:* Insulin-dextrose, nebulized α-2 agonist, potassium binding resin, bicarbonate supplementation if there is associated acidosis, and hemodialysis in refractory cases.
c. *Side effect:* AKI and bone marrow suppression.

SECTION 10: Gastroenterology

QUESTIONS

Q1. A 26-year-old female presented with severe and recurrent abdominal pain worsening after meals, typically located in the epigastric area (upper central abdomen) and the right upper quadrant. Nausea and vomiting abdominal bloating and fullness. She admitted to be trying to lose weight. Examination revealed a body mass index (BMI) of 14 and epigastric tenderness. A plain X-ray of the abdomen was suggestive of an enlarged stomach.
a. What is the diagnosis? *(2 marks)*
b. How would you confirm? *(4 marks)*
c. How would you manage? *(4 marks)*

Q2. A 70-year-old male experiencing bladder outlet obstruction from benign prostatic hyperplasia and chronic constipation, and currently using a urethral (Foley) catheter, presented with a concern about a purplish discoloration observed in his urine collection bag.

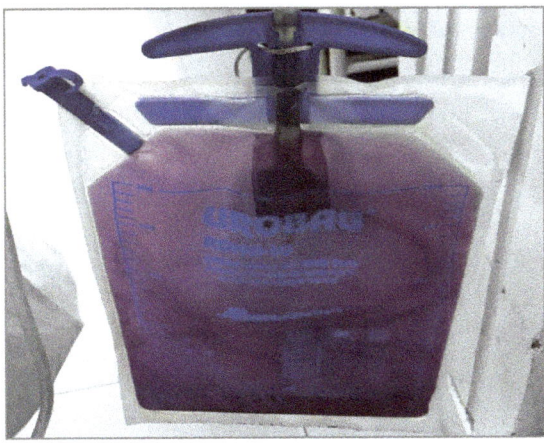

a. What is the diagnosis? *(2 marks)*
b. What causes it? *(3 marks)*
c. What is the management for it? *(5 marks)*

Q3.

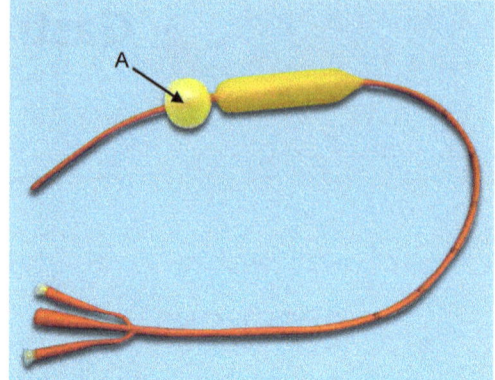

a. Identify the image. (2 marks)
b. What are the indications of using this? (3 marks)
c. What is the use of part A? (5 marks)

Q4.
A 26-year-old male presented with frequent diarrhea and flatulence. He denied any weight loss but complained of (C/O) gastrocolic reflex.

a. Describe the Rome criteria for this diagnosis. (2 marks)
b. Where is the tenderness most likely in irritable bowel syndrome (IBS)? (3 marks)
c. What does "FODMAP" stand for? (5 marks)

Q5.
A 32-year-old male presented with bloody diarrhea, pain abdomen, fever, and weight loss of 6 weeks duration.

a. Define this condition and name its two types. (2 marks)
b. Describe three differences between the two. (3 marks)
c. Describe three complications. (5 marks)

Q6.

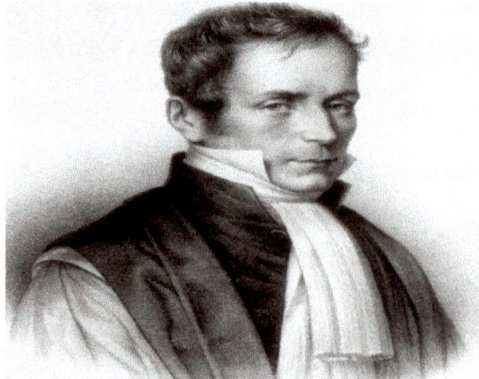

a. Who is he? (5 marks)
b. What is his contribution? (5 marks)

Q7.

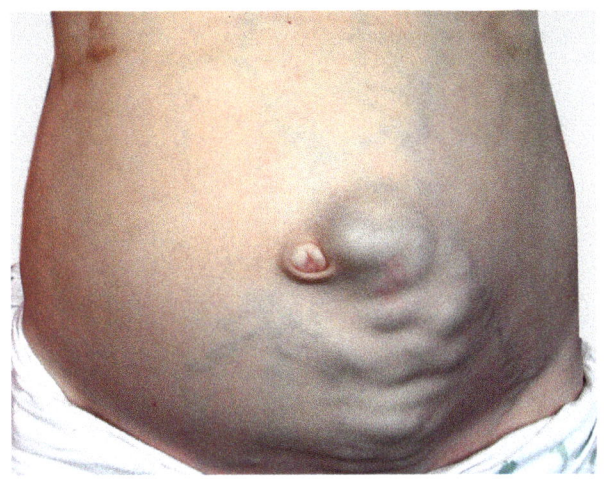

a. What are the auscultation findings? (3 marks)
b. What is the syndrome? (7 marks)

Q8.
A 55-year-old smoker and alcoholic has presented with severe abdominal pain, hematemesis, and fatigue. On examination, pulse rate (PR)—120/min, blood pressure (BP)—80 systolic, respiratory rate (RR)—2/min, and temperature—99 °F. On gastroscopy, the above finding is seen as shown in the image below.

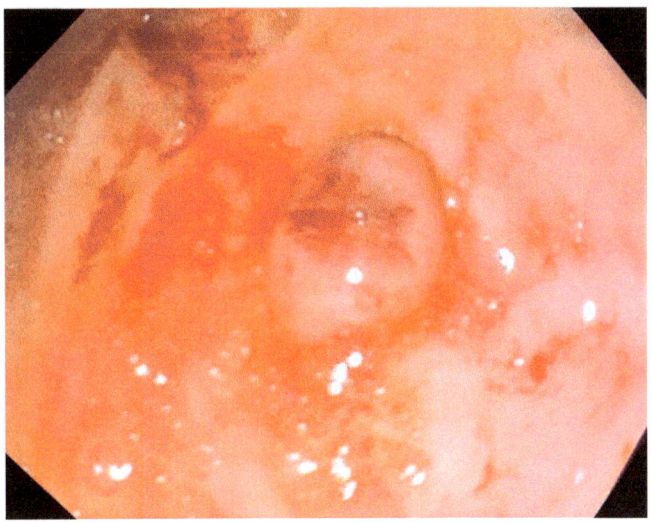

a. Name the lesion depicted in the picture. (2 marks)
b. Name the causes of this lesion. (2 marks)
c. List the physical findings that reveal the volume status of this patient. (3 marks)
d. Enumerate the treatment modalities in this patient. (3 marks)

Q9. A 45-year-old male patient has presented with a burning sensation in his abdomen. The image reveals a finding observed during gastroscopy.

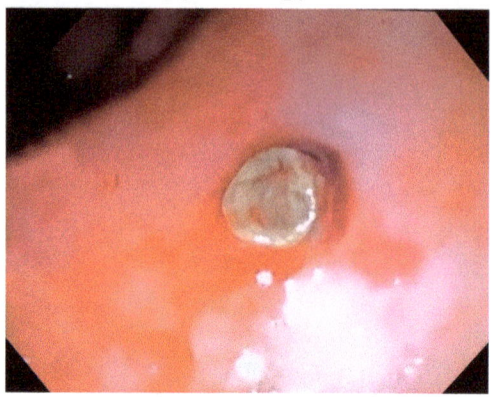

a. Name the lesion in the picture. *(2 marks)*
b. List risk factors causing this lesion. *(2 marks)*
c. List the danger signs associated with this lesion. *(3 marks)*
d. Enumerate the drugs used to treat the infection leading to this lesion. *(3 marks)*

Q10. Mrs Roy presents to the clinic with a complaint of persistent epigastric pain. She describes the pain as a burning sensation that typically occurs 1-2 hours after meals and is relieved by antacids. She has also noticed a decrease in appetite and unintentional weight loss over the last month. She denies any vomiting or black, tarry stools.

a. What is the provisional diagnosis? *(3 marks)*
b. What will be the upper gastrointestinal (GI) endoscopy findings? *(4 marks)*
c. What will be the management? *(3 marks)*

Q11. A 50-year-old male presented with complaints of dysphagia, regurgitation, and chest pain. X-ray of barium swallow revealed the following:

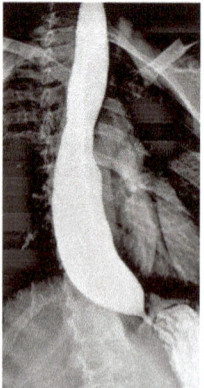

a. Identify the condition. *(5 marks)*
b. Discuss the treatment of the given condition. *(5 marks)*

Gastroenterology

Q12. A 40-year-old female presented with complaints of generalized weakness, shortness of breath following exertion, and difficulty in swallowing. General examination and routine investigations were done; additionally, a videofluoroscopic swallow study was done for her. Shown below are the findings of the same.

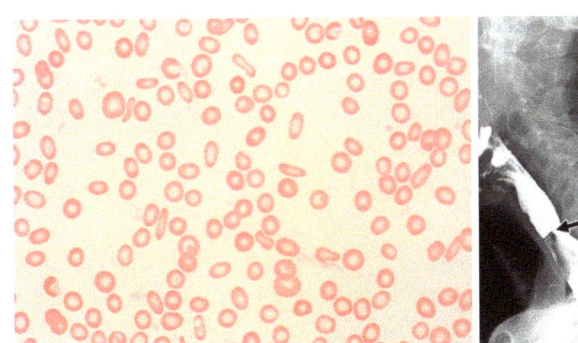
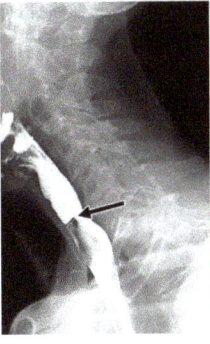
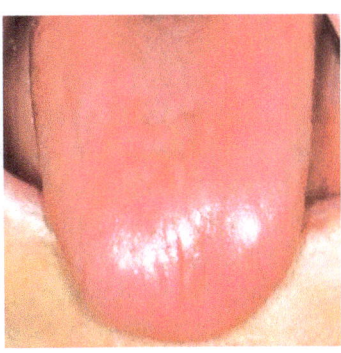

a. Name the syndrome. *(3 marks)*
b. Discuss the cardinal symptoms associated with the syndrome. *(2 marks)*
c. Which endoscopic procedure might be required in the treatment? *(3 marks)*
d. Discuss the malignancies associated with this condition. *(2 marks)*

Q13. A 35-year-old male presented in the outpatient department (OPD) with low-grade fever and pain abdomen for 1 month. He had high-risk sexual behavior on history. The examination revealed hepatosplenomegaly. The image below displays the computed tomography (CT) scan of the abdomen.

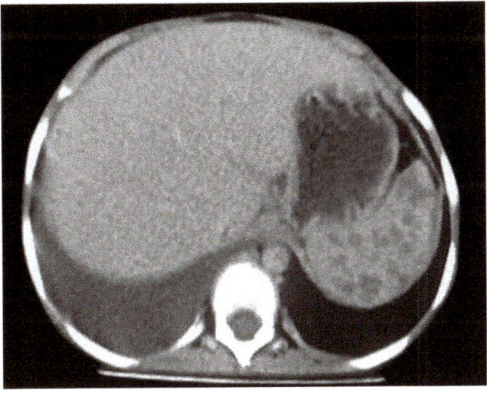

a. Point out the findings. *(1 mark)*
b. Enumerate the differentials. *(3 marks)*
c. How will you confirm the diagnosis? *(3 marks)*
d. How will you manage the case? *(3 marks)*

ANSWERS

Ans. 1

a. Superior mesenteric artery (SMA) syndrome is a rare condition that involves compression of the third portion of the duodenum between two arteries—(1) the abdominal aorta (AA) and (2) the SMA.
b. An abdominal CT scan with contrast reveals constriction of the third portion of the duodenum due to compression by the SMA, resulting in dilation of the proximal duodenal segment. Ultrasound with a Doppler is employed to measure the aortomesenteric (AO) angle and AO distance. The normal AO angle typically falls between 45 and 60°, whereas in this patient, the AO angle measured 18°.
c. The management approach for this syndrome involves (1) rectifying electrolyte imbalances, (2) alleviating obstruction through nasogastric tube decompression, and (3) providing nutritional support. If there is no improvement, corrective surgery is considered.

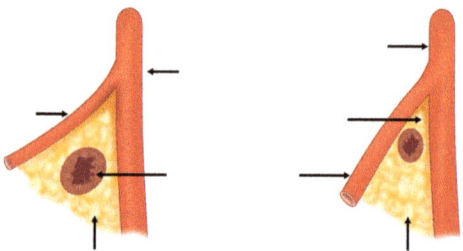

Superior mesenteric artery syndrome

Ans. 2

a. Purple urine bag syndrome (PUBS) is a rare condition primarily found in individuals with chronic catheterization and constipation, often associated with bacterial urinary infections, particularly *Escherichia coli*, which produce sulfatase/phosphatase.
b. The purple coloration in the urine results from a combination of indigo and indirubin, derived from tryptophan metabolites. Tryptophan undergoes metabolism in the GI tract by gut bacteria, producing indole, which is absorbed into the portal circulation. In the liver, indole is converted into indoxyl sulfate. The majority of indoxyl sulfate is excreted in the urine, where it is further transformed into indoxyl-by-indoxyl sulfatase produced by specific bacteria.
c. PUBS is generally a benign process.

Ans. 3

a. Sengstaken-Blakemore tube
b. Indications—upper GI bleeding, e.g., esophageal varices bleeding.
c. It is a gastric balloon, which is used in gastric bleed.

Ans. 4

a. The Rome IV criteria, used for diagnosing irritable bowel syndrome, stipulate that individuals must have experienced recurring abdominal pain for a minimum of 1 day/

week over the past three months. This pain should be linked to two or more of the following conditions:
- Connected to defecation, with the possibility of its intensity being heightened or unaffected by the act of defecation.
- Correlated with alterations in stool frequency.
- Linked to changes in stool form or appearance.

b. Right lower quadrant
c. FODMAP is an acronym representing fermentable oligosaccharides, disaccharides, monosaccharides, and polyols. These are types of short-chain carbohydrates or sugars that the small intestine has limited absorption capacity for.

Ans. 5

a. Inflammatory bowel disease (IBD) is an idiopathic disease caused by a dysregulated immune response to host intestinal microflora. Crohn's disease and ulcerative colitis (UC).
b. Crohn's can affect mouth to anus while UC rectum, skip lesions in Crohn's, continuous in UC, and pancolitis in UC.
c. Stricture, toxic megacolon, and malignancy.

Ans. 6

a. René Laennec, a French physician, and musician.
b. Invention of the stethoscope described the understanding of peritonitis and cirrhosis.

Ans. 7

a. and b. The term *Cruveilhier–Baumgarten syndrome* is used for cases of portal hypertension due to any cause in which a loud venous murmur can be heard over the upper abdomen.

Ans. 8

a. Bleeding peptic ulcer
b. Helicobacter pylori (*H. pylori*) infection, nonsteroidal anti-inflammatory drugs (NSAIDs), smoking, and alcohol.
c. Tachycardia, low pulse volume, hypotension, cold and clammy extremities, and low jugular venous pressure (JVP)
d. Proton pump inhibitors, *H. pylori* eradication therapy, and endoscopic measures, such as hemoclip, epinephrine injections, and cautery.

Ans. 9

a. Peptic ulcer
b. *Helicobacter pylori* infection, smoking, alcohol, and NSAIDs.
c. Weight loss, iron deficiency anemia, hematemesis, anorexia, and Virchow's node.
d. Amoxicillin, clarithromycin, and pantoprazole

Ans. 10

a. Peptic ulcer disease
b. Duodenal ulcer ± bleeding and rapid urease test (RUT) are positive.
c. Proton pump inhibitors and anti-*pylori* treatment.

Ans. 11

a. Achalasia cardia
b. Reducing lower esophageal sphincter (LES) pressure by means of pharmacological therapy, pneumatic balloon dilation, or LES myotomy by means of submucosal endoscopy, or laparoscopic surgery.

Ans. 12

a. Plummer–Vinson syndrome
b. Postcricoid dysphagia, esophageal web, and iron deficiency anemia.
c. Endoscopic bougie dilation
d. Squamous cell cancer antigen (CA) of the esophagus

Ans. 13

a. Multiple hypodense lesions in the spleen.
b. Multiple abscesses or granuloma in the spleen. Causes may be tuberculosis (TB), pyogenic abscess, melioidosis, etc.
c. USG or CT-guided FNA from the spleen and aspirate material for cytology, gram stain and culture/sensitivity (C/S), cartridge-based nucleic acid amplification test (CBNAAT), fungal stain and C/S, and special culture for *Burkholderia pseudomallei*.
d. If TB—antitubercular drugs [four fixed-dose combination (4-FDC)]
    - If pyogenic or melioidosis—long-term IV antibiotics according to culture sensitivity.
    - If histoplasma or other fungus- antifungal preferably amphotericin B.

SECTION 11

Hepatology

QUESTIONS

Q1. A 45-year-old male patient has presented with complaints of gradual distension of the abdomen and a previous history of (H/O) recurrent jaundice. His eyes on examination (O/E) can be seen in the image.

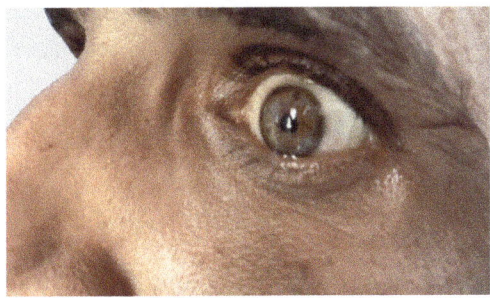
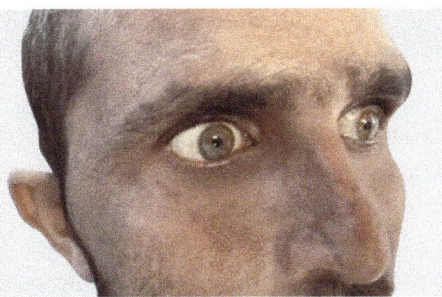

a. Name the finding on the eye examination of this patient. (2 marks)
b. List the findings on the general examination of this patient. (3 marks)
c. Enumerate the per abdominal findings of this patient. (3 marks)
d. Name three investigations used to diagnose this chronic disease. (2 marks)

Q2.

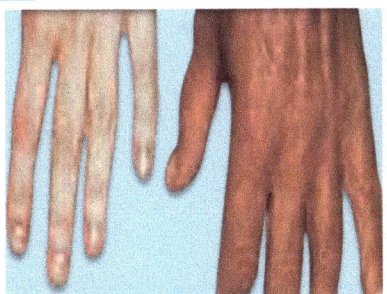
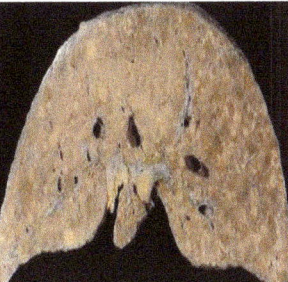
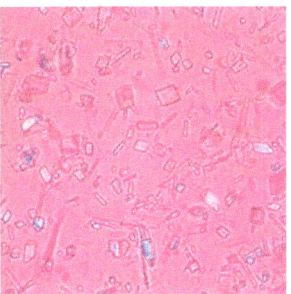

Image A   Image B   Image C

a. Identify the disease and chromosomal abnormality involved. (2 marks)
b. Identify the type of crystals deposited and the site. (4 marks)
c. Identify the skin condition shown in Image A. (4 Marks)

Q3. A 28-year-old housewife presented to her physician with painless progressive swelling of the upper abdomen without fever or weight loss. On examination, she was having hepatomegaly without any enlargement of the spleen or lymph nodes. A routine blood workup revealed eosinophilia. Ultrasound (USG) and computed tomography (CT) of the abdomen were done.

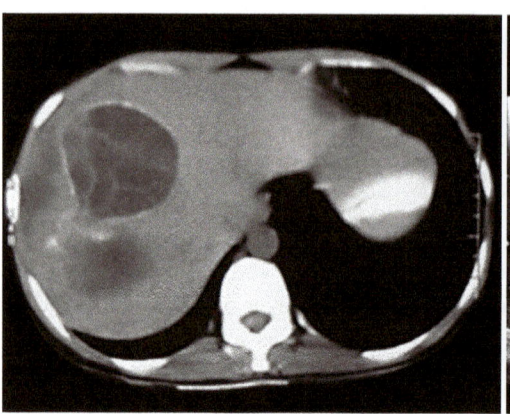
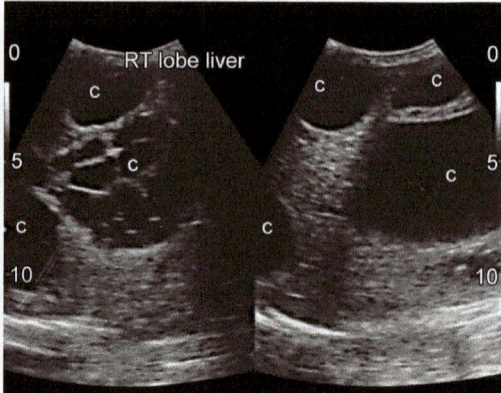

a. What are the pathological findings? (4 marks)
b. Name the causative agents. (2 marks)
c. What is the management? (2 marks)
d. Enumerate the organ involvement in this disease. (2 marks)

Q4. A 69-year-old male while being evaluated for unexplained fever and weight loss was found to have five times normal elevated serum alkaline phosphatase (447 IU/L) n = 44–147.
a. Name three hepatobiliary possibilities that need to be evaluated further. (5 marks)
b. Name three nonhepatic causes of elevated alkaline phosphatase. (3 marks)
c. Name two causes of low alkaline phosphatase. (2 marks)

Q5. During the rounds for evaluating liver cases, the resident was asked about the workup for a patient with positive hepatitis B surface antigen (HBsAg).
a. Name two markers/tests for evaluating disease activity in such a case. (4 marks)
b. Name two tests to evaluate chronicity. (3 marks)
c. Name two drugs to treat chronic hepatitis due to hepatitis B infection. (4 marks)

Q6. A 30-year-old patient on an oral contraceptive pill presented with sudden onset abdominal distension and pain right upper abdomen. A first-year-old resident O/E demonstrated tender hepatomegaly with ascites.
a. What is a likely diagnosis in this lady? (4 marks)
b. Discuss three other etiological causes for this diagnosis. (3 marks)
c. Suggest three investigations to confirm the diagnosis. (3 marks)

Q7. A 30-year-old male was undergoing routine USG abdomen as a part of a health checkup. His USG of the liver (image representative) showed some abnormality. (See arrow in image)

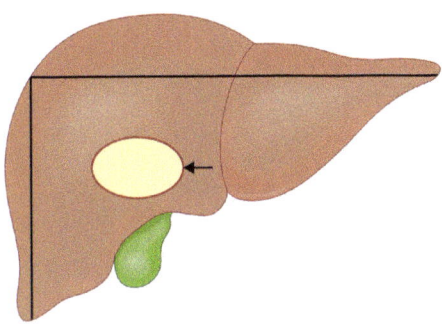

a. Enumerate three differential diagnoses (D/D) of such a lesion in the liver. (3 marks)
b. What is Caroli's disease? How does it present? (4 marks)
c. How do you manage Caroli's disease? (3 marks)

Q8. A 50-year-old male presented with H/O fatigue, and loss of sexual drive. He was recently diagnosed with type 2 diabetes mellitus (T2DM). O/E he was dark-skinned and had hepatomegaly.
a. What further investigations would you do to corroborate and confirm the diagnosis? (2 marks)
b. What is the diagnosis? (3 marks)
c. How will you manage? (5 marks)

Q9.

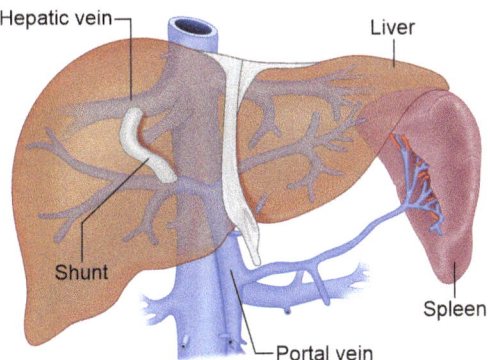

a. What is this? (2 marks)
b. In which condition it is performed? (3 marks)
c. List the complications associated with the condition. (5 marks)

Q10. A 30-year-old ethanol abuser for 10 years was seen in the outpatient department (OPD) with H/O jaundice. During the examination, the following findings were observed in the image given below. In addition, he had evidence of fluid in the abdomen.

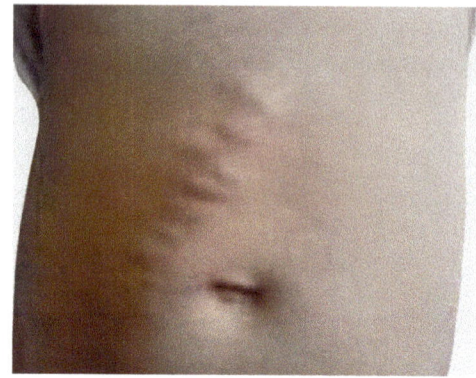

a. What will be the auscultatory signs? (2 marks)
b. Name the syndrome. (2 marks)
c. Suggest three more investigations to confirm the diagnosis. (3 marks)
d. List three complications of this disease complex. (3 marks)

Q11. Sarah reports feeling increasingly unwell over the past week. She initially experienced generalized fatigue and loss of appetite, followed by the development of nausea and dark urine. In the last few days, she noticed yellow discoloration of her skin and sclera, prompting her to seek medical attention. She denies abdominal pain, fever, or recent travel. Sarah works as a restaurant server. She occasionally consumes alcohol on social occasions but denies any illicit drug use. There is no known H/O liver disease in her family. Liver function test (LFT) shows hyperbilirubinemia with severe transaminitis.

a. What is the provisional diagnosis? (4 marks)
b. What laboratory and radiological investigations will you send for workup? (2 marks)
c. What will be the management? (4 marks)

Q12.

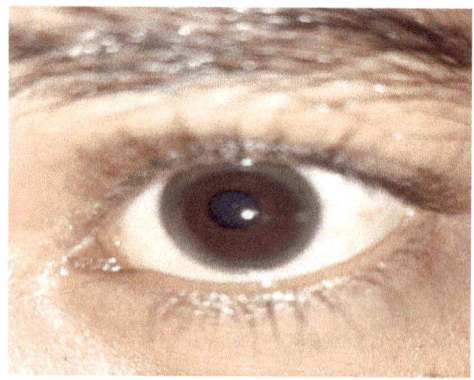

a. What is the most likely diagnosis? (3 marks)
b. Which genes are involved? (3 marks)
c. Discuss the gold standard test for the diagnosis. (2 marks)
d. What are the treatment options available? (2 marks)

Q13. A patient with chronic hepatitis B has the following serology:
- *HBsAg:* Positive
- *Anti-HBc (IgG):* Positive
- *Hepatitis B envelope Antigen (HBeAg):* Positive
- *Anti-HBe:* Negative
- *Hepatitis B virus (HBV) deoxyribonucleic acid (DNA):* >2 × 10^4 copies/mL
- *Alanine aminotransferase (ALT):* 500 IU

a. Name the phase of the disease. *(4 marks)*
b. Will you treat it or not? If yes name the antivirals used. *(3 marks)*
c. Name the directly acting antiviral used for treatment of hepatitis C. *(3 marks)*

Q14.

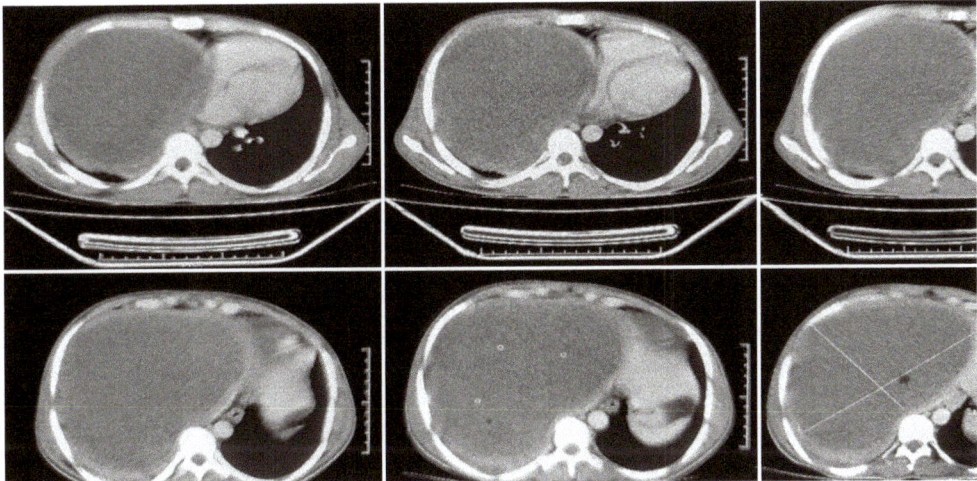

a. What is the diagnosis? *(2 marks)*
b. What is the probable etiology from imaging? *(2 marks)*
c. How will the patient present? *(2 marks)*
d. What is the next line of treatment? *(4 marks)*

Q15. A 53-year-old male diagnosed with cirrhosis of the liver (COL) presents with complaints of malaise, fatigue, one episode of hematemesis and melena, swelling of legs, and progressive distension of the abdomen for the last 5 days. On examination, he has gynecomastia, spider angioma, caput medusae, moderate nontender splenomegaly, and ascites.

a. What is the probable cause of gastrointestinal (GI) bleeding in this case? *(1 mark)*
b. The serum-ascites albumin gradient (SAAG) is >11g/L. What is the cause of the ascites? *(1 mark)*
c. What are the components of the Child–Pugh classification of prognosis of COL? *(2.5 marks)*
d. What is the other score used for assessing the prognosis in COL? *(0.5 mark)*

Hepatology

ANSWERS

Ans. 1
a. Kaiser-Fleischer ring
b. Parotid enlargement, gynecomastia, absence of axillary and pubic hair, testicular atrophy, clubbing, spider nevi, and Dupuytren's contracture.
c. Shrunken liver, splenomegaly, fluid thrill, and shifting dullness
d. USG abdomen, serum ceruloplasmin, and 24-hour urinary copper levels.

Ans. 2
a. Hemochromatosis, *HFE* gene on CHR 6
b. Calcium pyrophosphate crystal deposition in joints
c. Bronze diabetes

Ans. 3
a. Multiple well-defined nonenhancing hypodense cystic lesions of varying sizes involving predominantly the right lobe of the liver, one of which has a cart-wheel appearance. Overall suggestive of a hepatic hydatid cyst.
b. Hydatid disease is a zoonotic parasitic infection primarily caused by either *Echinococcus granulosus* or *Echinococcus multilocularis*, the latter leading to the formation of multilocular cysts.
c. A combination of preoperative albendazole therapy, surgical intervention, and postoperative albendazole therapy proves to be an effective regimen. Albendazole plays a role in inhibiting the development of hydatid cysts after intraperitoneal inoculation of protoscolices.
d. The liver is the most commonly affected site, accounting for 59–75% of cases, followed by the lungs (27%), kidneys (3%), bones (1–4%), and the brain (1–2%). Other infrequently affected sites include the heart, spleen, pancreas, omentum, ovaries, parametrium, pelvis, thyroid, orbit, retroperitoneum, and muscles.

Ans. 4
a. Sclerosing cholangitis, cholangiocarcinoma, hepatic tuberculosis, and sarcoidosis.
b. Osteomalacia, Paget's disease, and chronic kidney disease (CKD–MBD).
c. Malnutrition, Wilson's disease, and hypothyroidism.

Ans. 5
a. HBeAg, high-HBV DNA, and elevated ALT.
b. FibroScan and liver biopsy
c. Adefovir and entacavir

Ans. 6
a. Oral contraceptive steroids (OCS) as the cause of hepatic vein thrombosis (Budd–Chiari syndrome)
b. Protein C/S deficiency, renal cell carcinoma, and myeloproliferative disorder.
c. Doppler USG, magnetic resonance imaging (MRI), and hepatic venography.

Ans. 7

a. Simple hepatic cyst, hydatid cyst, and biliary cystadenoma.
b. Caroli disease, recognized as congenital communicating cavernous ectasia of the biliary tree, is an uncommon hereditary condition characterized by the segmental enlargement of significant intrahepatic bile ducts.
    Patients commonly exhibit episodes of recurrent bacterial cholangitis, manifesting as abdominal pain, fevers, chills, and jaundice, akin to the symptoms seen in ascending cholangitis. Additionally, pruritis is frequently reported, arising from hyperbilirubinemia due to intrahepatic cholestasis.
c. Antibiotics for cholangitis, endoscopic retrograde cholangiopancreatography (ERCP)/ percutaneous transhepatic cholangiography (PTC) with stent placement.

Ans. 8

a. LFT, transferrin saturation, and ferritin levels (>60% in men and 50% in women with high serum ferritin levels). Magnetic resonance imaging is a useful noninvasive technique for quantifying hepatic iron overload.
b. Examination of HFE mutations is pivotal for diagnosis- Hemochromatosis
c. Chelation therapy or phlebotomy depending on the underlying causes and liver transplantation.

Ans. 9

a. Transjugular intrahepatic portosystemic shunt (TIPS) is a widely accepted percutaneous approach for reducing portal hypertension.
b. The primary clinical indications for employing transjugular intrahepatic portosystemic shunts encompass instances of intractable variceal hemorrhage and unresponsive ascites.
c. Spontaneous bacterial peritonitis, hepatorenal syndrome, and hepatic encephalopathy.

Ans. 10

a. Venous hum
b. Cruveilhier Baumgarten syndrome
c. UGI endoscopy, USG of abdomen, LFT, and ascitic tap.
d. Spontaneous bacterial peritonitis, hepatic encephalopathy, and hepatorenal syndrome.

Ans. 11

a. Viral hepatitis
b. Hepatitis A virus (HAV), HBsAG, hepatitis C virus (HCV), hepatitis E virus (HEV), dengue NS1/IgM, and USG WA.
c. No specific drug treatment, supportive medications

Ans. 12

a. Wilson's disease
b. ATP 7B on chromosome 13.

c. Liver Biopsy—Gold standard for diagnosis
d. *Treatment:* Copper chelation therapy (penicillamine), and liver transplantation.

Ans. 13

a. Immune active phase.
b. Treatment should be given, antivirals used-pegylated interferon, lamivudine, entecavir, and tenofovir.
c. Sofosbuvir, velpatasvir, ledipasvir, and glecaprevir.

Ans. 14

a. Liver abscess
b. Amebic liver abscess
c. Pain in the right upper quadrant and fever.
d. Pigtail catheter drainage, metronidazole, and empiric antibiotics.

Ans. 15

a. Esophageal varix
b. Portal hypertension
c. Encephalopathy, bilirubin, albumin, prothrombin time, and ascites
d. Model for end-stage liver disease (MELD)

Section 12: Neurology

QUESTIONS

Q1. During the rounds the resident was asked to evaluate the reflexes of lower limbs (LLs) presenting with paresthesias. He observed brisk (++) knee jerk, absent ankle jerk, and extensor planter response.
a. What is this neurological condition? *(4 marks)*
b. Enumerate four causes. *(3 marks)*
c. Enlist four investigations to elucidate the etiology. *(3 marks)*

Q2. A 38-year-old man, who is human immunodeficiency virus (HIV) positive, is presented to the emergency department with confusion and drowsiness. He has been complaining of headaches for a number of days. On examination, heart rate is 92 beats/min, blood pressure (BP) is 108/76 mm Hg, and temperature is 37.2°C. He is confused giving a Glasgow Coma Scale (GCS) score of 14. There is no photophobia or neck stiffness.

His infectious diseases consultant reports that he is prescribed highly active antiretroviral treatment (HAART) but he has poor compliance and frequently misses clinic sessions.

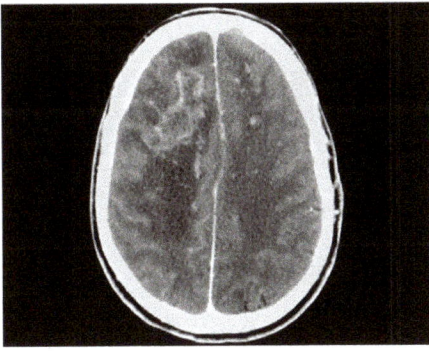

A contrast-enhanced computed tomography (CECT) brain is requested:
a. State abnormalities in the image. *(2 marks)*
b. What is the most likely diagnosis? *(3 marks)*
c. What is the differential diagnosis for this condition? *(2 marks)*
d. Write treatment. *(3 marks)*

Q3. See the image and answer the questions.

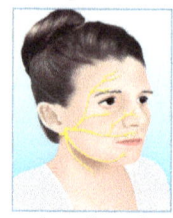
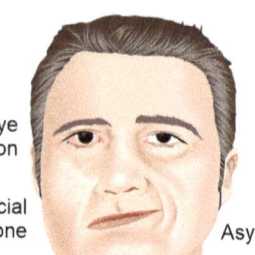

a. Where is the lesion? Which part is affected the most? (3 marks)
b. Enumerate three differential diagnoses. (3 marks)
c. Enumerate the management in three steps. (4 marks)

Q4.

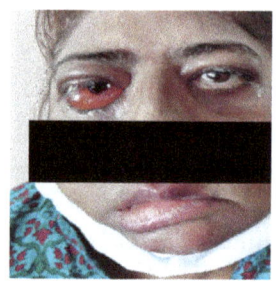

Describe findings in the picture? (10 marks)

Q5. A 40-year-old known case of (c/o) hypertension (HTN) presented with acute-onset headache and vomiting.

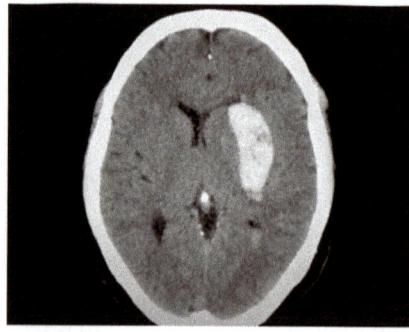

a. What is your diagnosis? (2 marks)
b. Mention site of given condition. (2 marks)
c. What is intracerebral hemorrhage (ICH) score? (3 marks)
d. What are the management strategies? (3 marks)

Q6. A 40-year-old female presented with acute-onset headache.

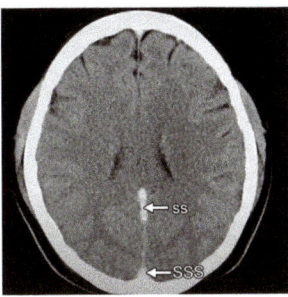

a. What is the diagnosis? (3 marks)
b. What are the four risk factors? (3 marks)
c. What are the treatment options? (4 marks)

Q7.

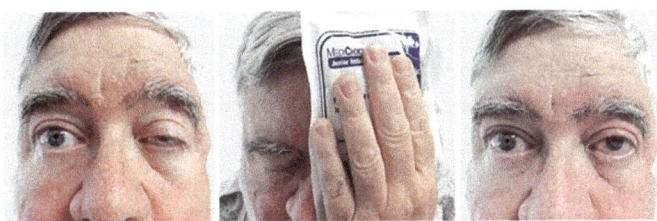

a. Name the test and inference. (2 marks)
b. What is the diagnosis? (2 marks)
c. Name three antibodies. (3 marks)
d. Name the classification system of the condition. (3 marks)

Q8. An immunocompromised 32-year-old man with poor compliance to art presented to emergency department with complaints of intense headache, seizures, and altered sensorium. A noncontrast computed tomography (NCCT) brain was immediately done and the image is shown below.

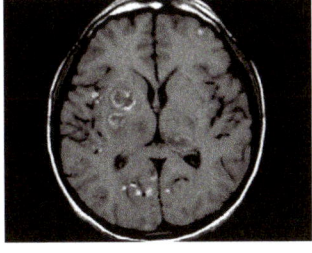

a. Identify the diagnosis and the causative organism. (2 marks)
b. What are the differential diagnoses? (2 marks)
c. Name the drugs used for treatment. (2 marks)
d. Mention any two criteria to suspect treatment failure in a person on art. (4 marks)

Q9.

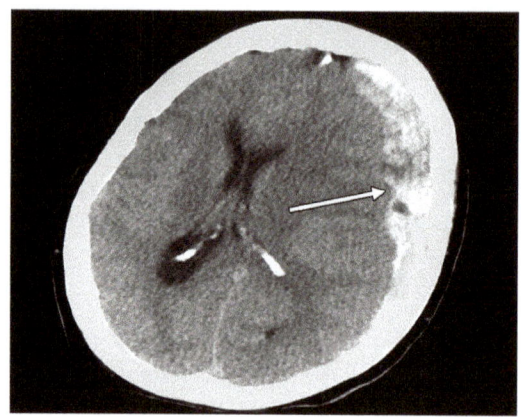

a. Name the type of brain hemorrhage. (5 marks)
b. What is main pathology of the type of brain? (5 marks)

Q10. A 60-year-old patient comes with history of (H/O) hemiparesis which developed suddenly while he was doing his household chores. He reached a regional geriatric center which provides tertiary level care within 3 hours of his onset of symptoms. His BP on presentation was 170/100 mm Hg and he was also a known diabetic which was well controlled with oral hypoglycemic agent (OHA). CT scan done in the emergency department which showed an infarct involving the right basal ganglia.
a. Mention three causes of ischemic stroke. (3 marks)
b. Mention two differential diagnoses of stroke. (2 marks)
c. Mention the treatment modality specific to his presentation and the drug used for the same. (3 marks)
d. Name two to three indications and contraindications for the procedure. (2 marks)

Q11. Mrs R, a 76-year-old lady, who is living alone presented to the clinic with her son in law, with short-term memory loss. She was able to give a detailed history, but struggled with details throughout her life and at times inaccurate. Her main hobby was cooking and reading newspapers. Nowadays she is facing difficulty in completing the tasks. She is also not able to remember any major events from the newspaper. She is also forgetting scheduled family meetings like going to temple or shopping and going for a wedding. She once went to the nearby shop, forget her ways to return back to the home.
a. What is the most probable diagnosis? (1 mark)
b. Which is the most important investigation that you will do to confirm your diagnosis? (1 mark)
c. Name two drugs which are used in treatment. (2 marks)
d. Mention three causes of dementia in elderly. (3 marks)
e. Name three nutritional deficiencies causing dementia. (3 marks)

Q12. A 26-year-old woman exhibited asymmetrical pupils. The right pupil was larger than the left and showed no response to light, either directly or consensually. During accommodation, the right pupil exhibited slow reactivity, eventually becoming smaller than the left pupil.
a. What is the best description of this type of pupillary abnormality? (3 marks)
b. What is the association of this feature with deep tendon reflexes?
   What is that condition known as? (3 marks)
c. What is the underlying cause of this condition? (4 marks)

Q13. A 35-year-old obese woman presented with symptoms of recurrent sudden-onset most intense headache peaking immediately to maximal intensity over seconds to minutes (thunderclap headache.) This was associated with vomiting, photophobia, phonophobia, confusion, and blurred vision. She had recently delivered a healthy baby 3 months back. There was no family H/O such attacks. She was being treated as migraine.
a. What is the name of this condition? (3 marks)
b. What is the diagnostic feature on imaging? (2 marks)
c. What is a close differential diagnosis? How does it differ? (3 marks)
d. Name one drug to manage this condition. (2 marks)

Q14. A 65-year-old female patient presented with occasional headache of recent onset.

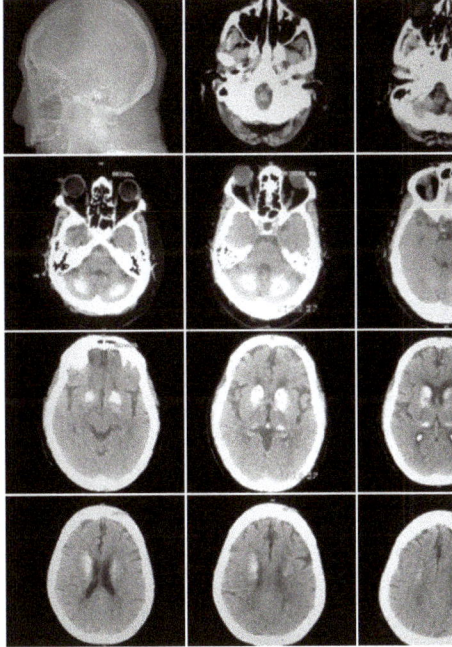

a. What is the diagnosis? (1 mark)
b. Mention other sites of CT scan changes. (2 marks)
c. What is the treatment? (3 marks)
d. What are the four differential diagnoses? (4 marks)

Q15. A 15-year-old boy has presented with complaints of progressive weakness of all four limbs along with fasciculations for the past 2 years. His hands can be seen in the image below. There are no complaints involving the sensory system or bowel/bladder system.

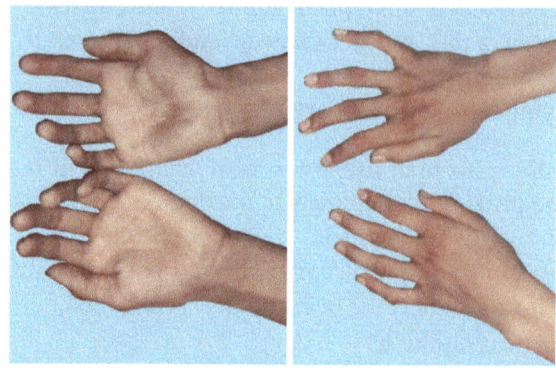

a. What is the finding in the image? (2 marks)
b. List the other physical findings in the nervous system. (6 marks)
c. Enumerate two differential diagnoses. (2 marks)

Q16.

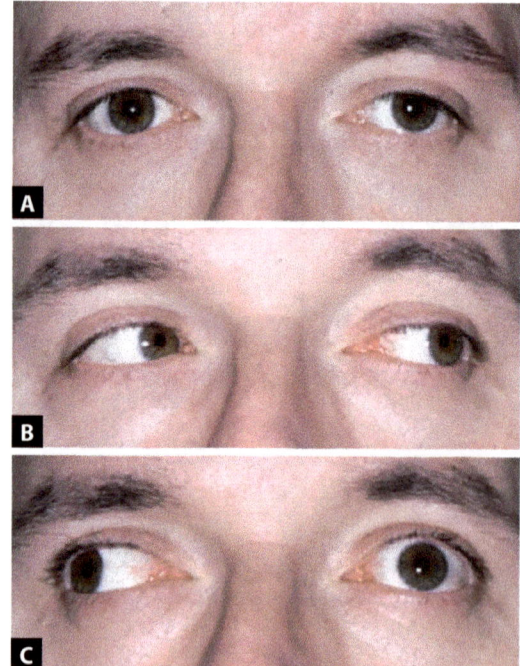

a. Describe ocular abnormality. (3 marks)
b. What is the diagnosis? (3 marks)
c. Mention site of lesion. (4 marks)

Neurology

Q17. Emily is brought to the neurology clinic by her husband with a H/O recurrent episodes over the last 6 months. According to her husband, Emily experiences sudden episodes where she becomes unresponsive, stares blankly, and exhibits rhythmic, repetitive movements of her arms and legs. Each episode lasts for about 2 minutes, and afterward, Emily is confused and fatigued. The episodes occur without warning and seem to happen both during wakefulness and sleep. Her husband also notes occasional loss of bladder control during these episodes.

a. What is the provisional diagnosis? *(3 marks)*
b. How will you confirm the diagnosis? *(3 marks)*
c. What other investigations should be suggested? *(4 marks)*

Q18. Mr Anand presents with a 6-month H/O progressive difficulty in initiating movements, resting tremors, and stiffness in his limbs. His family reports that he has become slower in his daily activities. They also observe a reduced arm swing on one side and a tendency to favor one leg while standing.

Mini-mental state examination (MMSE) reveals no cognitive impairment. Cranial nerve examination is unremarkable. Reflexes are normal, and there is no sensory loss.

a. What is the provisional diagnosis? *(3 marks)*
b. What is the typical gait in this disorder? *(3 marks)*
c. What is the drug of choice? *(4 marks)*

Q19. A 56-year-old man complains of gradual bending of his right middle finger for 6 months duration. It has begun with a firm lump in the palm of his hand.

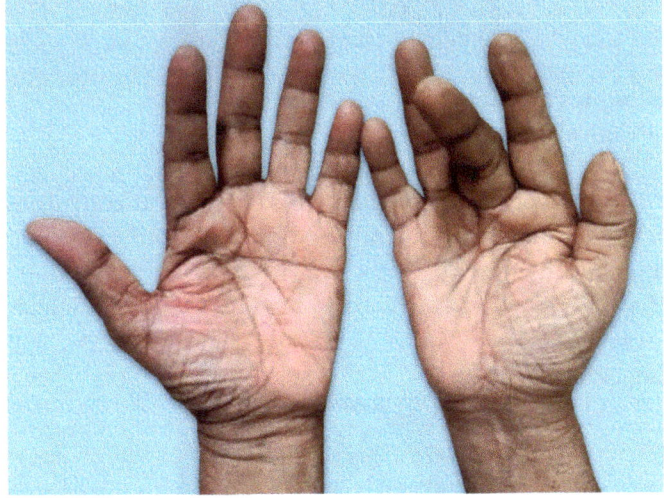

a. What is the abnormality seen in the image? *(2 marks)*
b. What is the diagnosis? *(2 marks)*
c. What are the associations of this condition? *(4 marks)*
d. What is the treatment? *(2 marks)*

Q20.

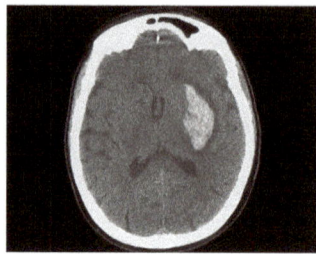

a. Describe the CT findings. *(3 marks)*
b. List any two absolute contraindications for thrombolytic therapy. *(3 marks)*
c. List the indications for thrombolytic therapy. *(4 marks)*

Q21.

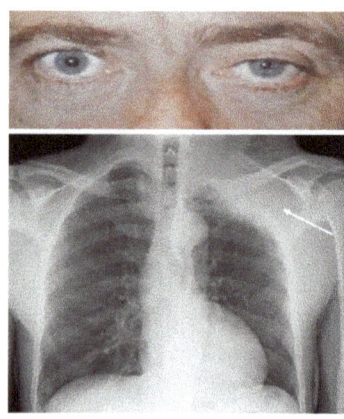

a. Identify the following condition. *(5 marks)*
b. Enumerate the clinical features of the same. *(5 marks)*

Q22.
A 40-year-old male patient presented with episodes of convulsions and impaired cognition for 3 months. He has positive family H/O similar disorder.
a. Read the findings in NCCT brain. *(3 marks)*
b. What is your diagnosis? *(2 marks)*
c. How you will evaluate such a case? *(3 marks)*
d. What are the genes involved? *(2 marks)*

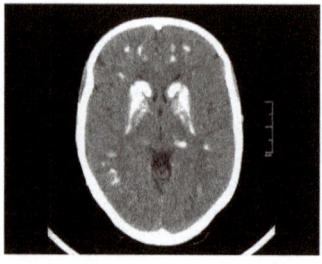

Q23. A 37-year-old man was admitted with chief complain of insidious onset weakness of bilateral LL, gradually progressive and leading to complete weakness and sensory loss over 3 days. Past H/O pulmonary tuberculosis (PTB) completed antituberculosis drug (ATD).

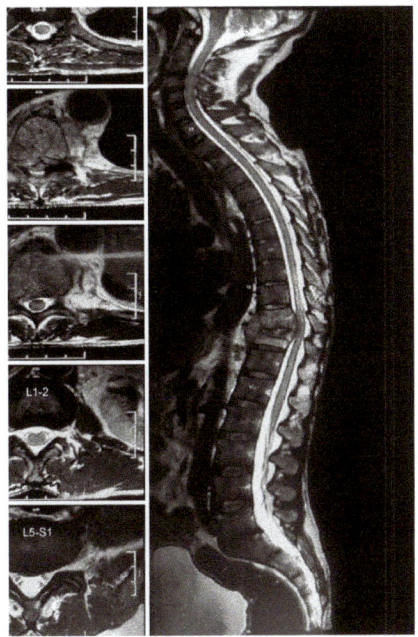

a. Read the given picture. (4 marks)
b. What is your diagnosis? (3 marks)
c. How will you manage? (3 marks)

Q24. A 60-year-old male presented with H/O repeated fall and forgetfulness.

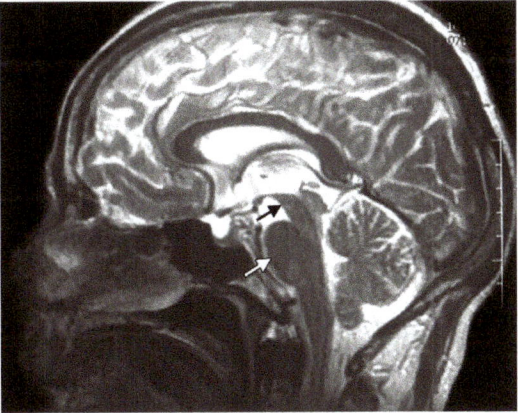

a. Name the disease. (5 marks)
b. Discuss magnetic resonance imaging (MRI) sign. (5 marks)

Q25. A 26-year-old female presented to the casualty with H/O headache, vomiting, and seizures (two episodes) since 6 hours. At admission BP was 170/98 mm Hg. She was having bilateral pitting pedal edema, oral ulcer, butterfly shaped malar rash. Urine routine examination (R/E) revealed 3+ proteinuria.

On further evaluation, she was having anemia [autoimmune hemolytic anemia (AIHA)], raised urea, and creatinine. Antinuclear antibody (ANA) Hep-2 revealed 3+ homogenous with anti-Sm and double-stranded deoxyribonucleic acid (dsDNA) positivity leading to the diagnosis of systemic lupus erythematosus (SLE).

Her NCCT brain at onset was as follows:
a. Read the CT scan. *(5 marks)*
b. What is your diagnosis? *(5 marks)*

Q26. A 23-year-old female is complaining of severe headache since 2 days which is associated with projectile vomiting and at present she is c/o blurring of vision.

She has been married for 3 years and has been taking oral contraceptive pills (OCPs) for contraception. CECT brain was done which showed the following image.

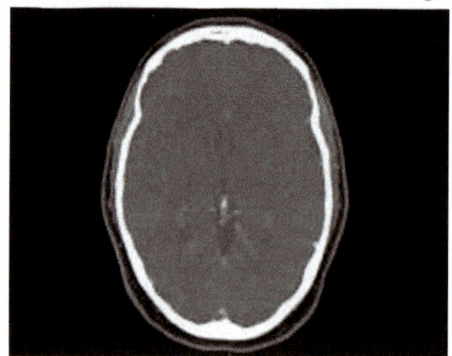

a. Read the CT scan of brain. *(3 marks)*
b. What is your diagnosis? *(4 marks)*
c. How will you manage the case? *(3 marks)*

Q27. A 72-year-old female who presented with a progressive gait disturbance characterized by shuffling and difficulty initiating movement, urinary incontinence with urgency and frequency, cognitive decline manifesting as forgetfulness, and executive dysfunction. MRI imaging findings revealed enlarged ventricles out of proportion to cortical atrophy. The patient's symptoms have been present for approximately 6 months, and there is no H/O significant head trauma or other known causes of cognitive decline.
a. What is the diagnosis? *(2 marks)*
b. What is the characteristic triad of symptoms associated with this condition? *(3 marks)*
c. What is the term used to describe enlarged ventricles out of proportion to cortical atrophy? *(2 marks)*
d. Name some differential diagnosis for this condition. *(3 marks)*

Q28. Short-statured boy of 12 years having a mental impairment and presented with fever and tetany in emergency.

There was a shortening of the distal phalanx of the thumb (murderer thumb or porter thumb)

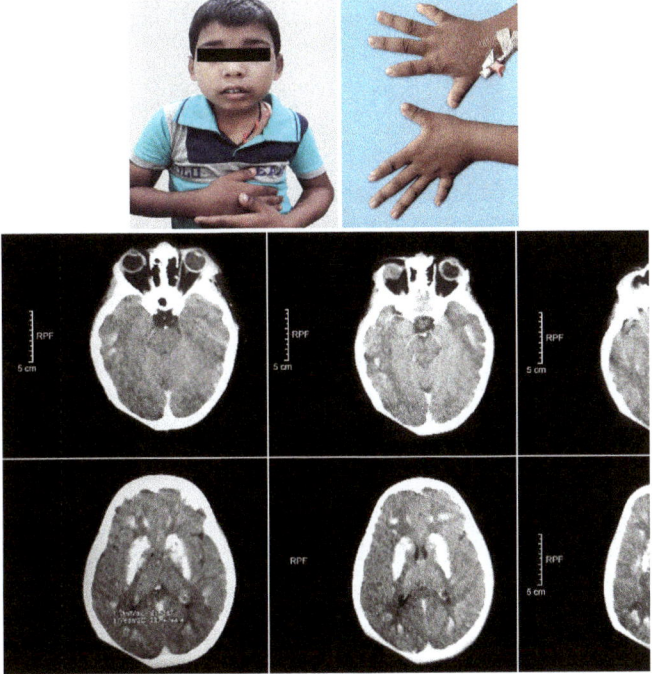

Calcium—6.1 mg/dL (8.4-10.4), Phosphate—5.6 mg/dL (2.6-4.5), and Mg—2.6 mEq/L

a. What is the CT scan finding? (2 marks)
b. What are the components of AHO? (5 marks)
c. What is your diagnosis? (3 marks)

Q29. A male subject of 29 years attended endocrinology clinic for infertility. On further questioning, he has preserved libibo with difficulty in releasing objects from handgrip.

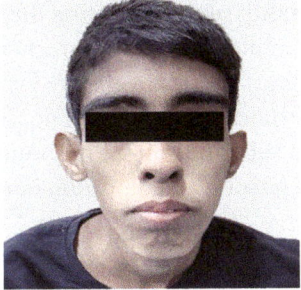

a. Describe the face. (2 marks)
b. What is your diagnosis? (2 marks)
c. Describe the neurological and EMG findings. (6 marks)

Q30.

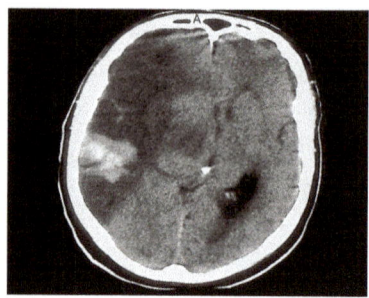

a. Describe the findings as seen. (3 marks)
b. What is the cause of the lesion? (3 marks)
c. Describe briefly the management of the patient. (4 marks)

Q31. A 17-year-old boy, a known c/o epilepsy since infancy, was on antiepileptic drugs and has now presented with oral mucositis, peeling of skin, and rashes with severe blackish discoloration.

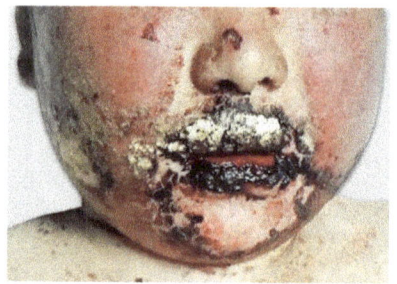

a. Identify the adverse drug reaction (ADR). (2 marks)
b. Mention antiepileptic drugs known to cause the ADR. (2 marks)
c. What other class of drugs are known to commonly cause the above ADR? (3 marks)
d. How will you manage the case? (3 marks)

Q32. 5 years ago, a 62-year-old Mrs M was diagnosed with a neurodegenerative disorder in which there was destruction of motor nerves affecting the control of movement. In routine course, people with this disorder could not survive for >4 years resulting in death due to the inability of the inspiratory muscles to contract leading to suffocation. Presently, M's condition is steadily deteriorating and it is expected that she will not be able to live through the month. She is anxious about the pain and suffering in her final hours. She requests her doctor to give her opioids in high doses for pain as soon as suffocation or choking starts to hasten her death and make it painless.

a. What is Mrs M requesting for? (1 mark)
b. Is it legally valid in India? (1 mark)
c. Is this request same as do-not-resuscitate (DNR)? (2 marks)
d. Name four geriatric giants. (4 marks)
e. Name two national programs concerned with the welfare of elderly population in India. (2 marks)

Q33. A 6-year-old child presented with imbalance in walking and had the abnormal eye movement—saccadic initiation problem.

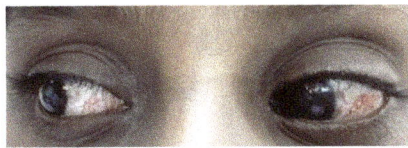

a. What is the ocular finding? (2 marks)
b. Mention three causes of this ocular finding. (2 marks)
c. What could be the probable diagnosis for this child? (2 marks)
d. Mention two non-neurological manifestations of the disease. (4 marks)

Q34. A 13-year-old college student presented with behavioral disturbances and involuntary movements of the hands for 6 months. His brother committed suicide 5 years ago with preceding psychiatric illness.

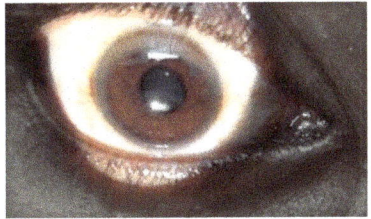

a. What is the ocular finding? (2 marks)
b. Mention four causes of this ocular finding. (2 marks)
c. What could be the probable diagnosis for this child? (2 marks)
d. Mention four non-neurological manifestations of the disease. (2 marks)
e. What is the scoring system used to diagnose this disease in this child? (2 marks)

Q35. A 23-year-old male came for evaluation of ataxia for 1 year. He had poor vision for the last 10 years and was operated for the same in both the eyes. On general examination, the below finding was noted.

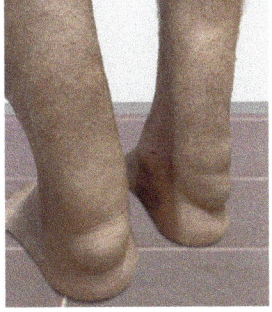

a. What is the clinical finding? (2 marks)
b. What are the causes of the above finding? (3 marks)
c. What could be the probable diagnosis for this boy? (2 marks)
d. Mention four non-neurological manifestations of the disease. (3 marks)

Neurology

Q36. This lady presented with 2 days H/O right sides lower motor neuron (LMN) facial palsy.

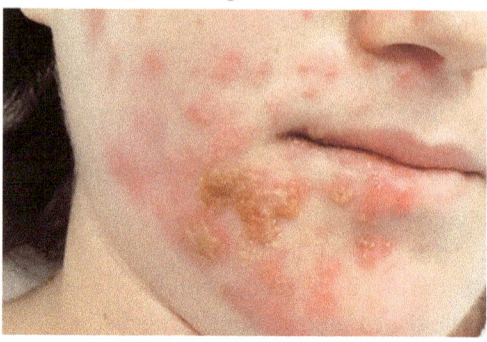

a. What is the skin lesion that you see? (2 marks)
b. What is the diagnosis for the patient? (2 marks)
c. What is the preventive measure for the above condition? (3 marks)
d. Where is the site of lesion for right LMN facial nerve palsy with restricted abduction of right eye? (3 marks)

Q37. A 25-year-old woman presented with weakness in bilateral LL till the level of hip. There were absent sensations below the level of hip. Reflexes were absent with normal bowel and bladder sensations.
a. What is the clinical diagnosis? (2 marks)
b. What is the most common subtype of this disease? (2 marks)
c. What is the treatment of choice for this disease? (2 marks)
d. What is the classical nerve conduction study results found in this disease? (2 marks)
e. Which bacterium is postulated in the occurrence of this disease? (2 marks)

Q38. You were called to the endocrine surgery unit to opine on a 32-year-old lady who had undergone total thyroidectomy developed a granular cell tumors (GCTs). The patient is now conscious and oriented but has complaints of vague symptoms.
a. Name two clinical signs of you will elicit in her to reach to your probable diagnosis. (3 marks)
b. What is your probable diagnosis? (4 marks)
c. What is Erb's sign? (3 marks)

Q39. A 45-year-old make presented with paraplegia. On examination, he is asked to raise the head from a supine position; you notice that there is *upward movement of the umbilicus.*
a. What is this sign? (3 marks)
b. Where is the anatomical localization of the lesion? (4 marks)
c. In which muscle disease, this sign was documented? (3 marks)

Q40. A 34-year-old male presented with H/O abnormal movement of his limbs for >2 years. On clinical examination, you noted that there is delayed relaxation of the quadriceps femoris after eliciting the patellar tendon reflex.
a. What sign is elicited in the above clinical vintage? (2 marks)
b. What is the most probable diagnosis? (2 marks)

c. What is the endocrine cause for the above sign? (2 marks)
d. What is the Mendelian pattern of inheritance of this disease? (2 marks)
e. Which anatomical structure in brain is affected? (2 marks)

Q41. A 48-year-old female presented with excruciating tick-like pain in the right side of her face for 3 years. Vascular imaging of her brain is given as below.

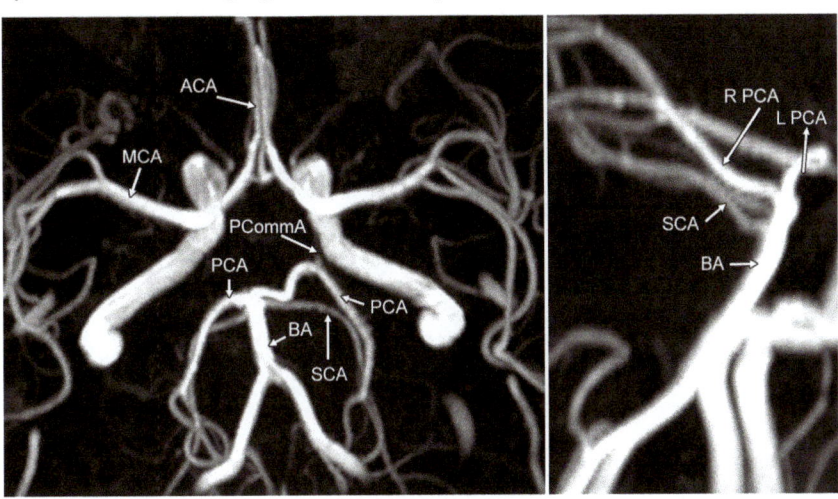

(ACA: anterior cerebral artery; BA: basilar artery; MCA: middle cerebral artery; PCA: posterior cerebral artery; SCA: superior cerebellar artery)

a. What is your probable diagnosis? (2 marks)
b. Which vessel is the most common culprit vessel for this condition? (3 marks)
c. What is the drug of choice for this condition? (2 marks)
d. What is surgical intervention done for refectory cases? (3 marks)

Q42. A 45-year-old lady complained of transient electric shock-like sensation extending down the spine upon flexion of the neck. She had a past H/O weakness of all four limbs which recovered after a month of treatment. The MRI—spine of the lady is shown below.

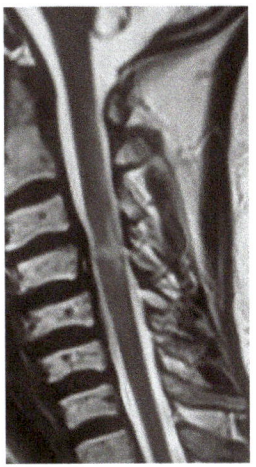

a. What is the name of the sign? (2 marks)
b. What is the motor equivalent of the sign? (3 marks)
c. What is the probable diagnosis for this lady? (3 marks)
d. What is the criterion used for the diagnosis of this disease? (2 marks)

Q43. A 55-year-old chronic smoker presented with pain in the right upper limb and chest. He complains of radiating pain from shoulders to tips of fingers. The below image shows his eye examination in dim light.

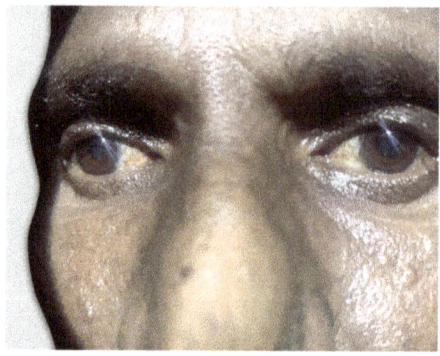

a. What is the sign in this image? (2 marks)
b. What is the probable diagnosis of this individual? (2 marks)
c. Name one other reason for the above clinical sign. (2 marks)
d. Which is the antibody most commonly associated with this individual disease, causing sensory-motor neuronopathy and encephalitis? (4 marks)

Q44. A 53-year-old male presented with inability to move his left eye, blurring of vision, and pain in left side of face. Clinical examination revealed external ophthalmoplegia with redness and swelling of left eye. Vision in left eye was 6/18.

There was numbness of left side of face present. There was black discoloration in the hard palate of the patient. His MRI image is given below.

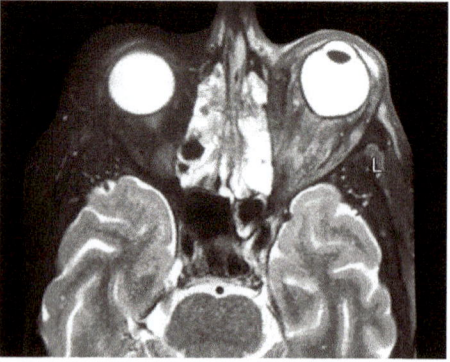

a. What is your diagnosis? (2 marks)
b. What is the probable ethology? (2 marks)

c. How do you differentiate between orbital apex syndrome and superior orbital fissure syndrome? *(3 marks)*
d. Which branch of trigeminal nerve passes through foramen rotundum? *(3 marks)*

Q45.

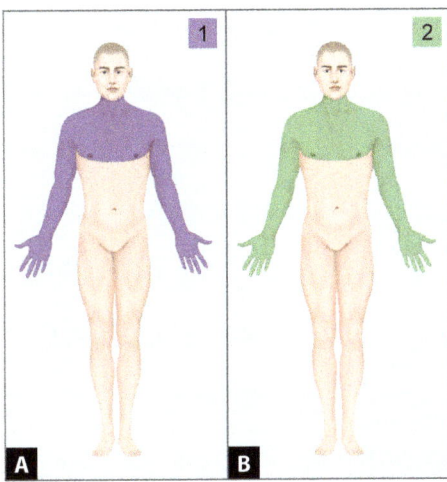

(A) Loss of pain and temperature sensation with preserved position and vibration sensations
(B) Loss of position and vibration sensations with preserved pain and temperature sensation
a. Which is the tract affected in patient No. 1? *(2 marks)*
b. Which are the tracts affected in patient No. 2? *(3 marks)*
c. Mention the site of lesion in patient No. 1. *(3 marks)*
d. Mention the site of lesion in patient No. 2. *(2 marks)*

Q46. A 45-year-old male with diabetes and HTN presented with involuntary rhythmic movement of his soft palate.
a. What is your probable diagnosis? *(2 marks)*
b. What is the triad associated with this condition? *(4 marks)*
c. Most common etiology for lesion in this anatomical location. *(4 marks)*

Q47. A 38-year-old male presented with H/O oscillopsia. Examination showed jerky nystagmus with fast phase downward in primary position which worsens on down gaze.
a. What is the eye movement described for him? *(5 marks)*
b. Where is the anatomical site of lesion for him? *(5 marks)*

Q48. A 38-year-old lady presented with giddiness and oscillopsia. Examination showed jerky nystagmus, which was slow and high amplitude on attempting to look to right side but was fast and low amplitude on attempting to look to left side.
a. What is the eye movement described for her? *(2 marks)*
b. Where is the anatomical site of lesion for her? *(2 marks)*
c. Which side is the localization of lesion for her? *(2 marks)*

d. Which other reflexes would be lost in this patient's eye? *(2 marks)*
e. What is the syndrome associated with central nervous system (CNS) tumors for this patient? *(2 marks)*

Q49. A 68-year-old male presented with right-sided headache, transient visual obscuration (TVO) for 6 months' time. His CT and MRI brain is normal.

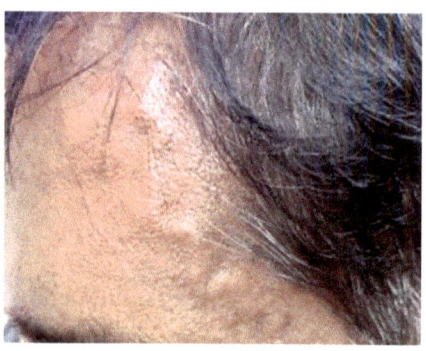

a. What is the probable diagnosis? *(2 marks)*
b. Name two important investigations. *(2 marks)*
c. What is the drug of choice? *(3 marks)*
d. What is the minimum size of biopsy to be taken? *(3 marks)*

Q50. A 50-year-old diabetic patient was brought to the emergency room (ER) with complete left-sided ophthalmoplegia. His oral cavity examination is as below.

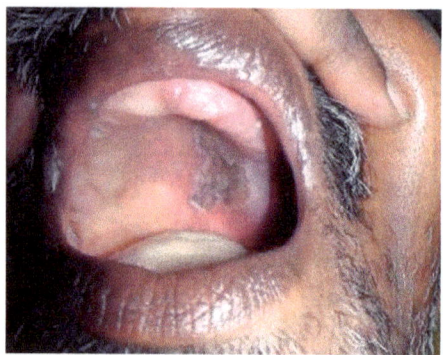

a. What is the finding? *(2 marks)*
b. What is the diagnosis? *(3 marks)*
c. What is the treatment of choice? *(3 marks)*
d. What is the drug of choice *(2 marks)*

Q51. An 18-year-old man presented to ER with H/O sudden jerks in the early morning hours. While on observation within next 1 hour had generalized tonic–clonic seizure (GTCS).
a. What is the likely diagnosis? *(2 marks)*
b. What is the drug of choice for him? *(2 marks)*

c. What is the drug of choice if the patient was an unmarried female? *(3 marks)*
d. Which is the drug that should be avoided in these patients? *(3 marks)*

Q52. A 65-year-old male presented to the ER with H/O inability to use his right upper and lower limb for 3 hours. CT brain is given below.

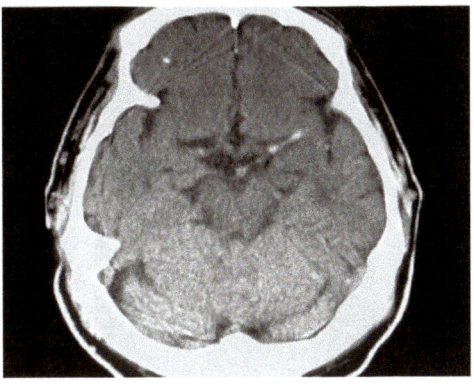

a. What is the interpretation of the CT brain? *(2 marks)*
b. What is the diagnosis? *(2 marks)*
c. What is the next best intervention for him? *(2 marks)*
d. What is Alberta stroke program early computed tomography score (ASPECTS) and its clinical implication? *(4 marks)*

Q53. A 26-year-old primigravida on her first trimester was admitted for imbalance in walking for the past 1 week. On examination, she had horizontal nystagmus. Optic disk was normal. Her MRI brain is shown below:

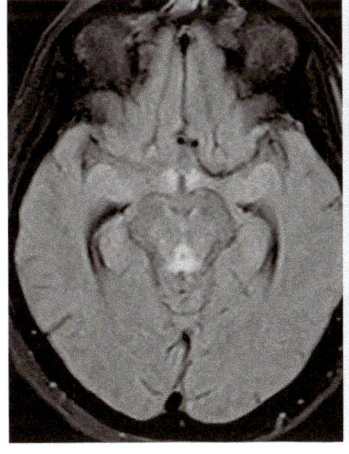 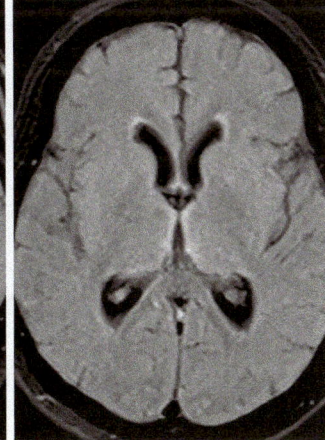

a. What is the probable diagnosis? *(2 marks)*
b. What is the specific history to be asked to her? *(2 marks)*
c. What are the other causes for this condition? *(3 marks)*
d. What is the treatment of choice? *(3 marks)*

Q54. A 30-year-old gentleman had quadriplegia in 2022. He was diagnosed with transverse myelitis. He was treated with steroids and had made a partial recovery. Now presented to ER with intractable hiccough and vomiting for the past 3 days.

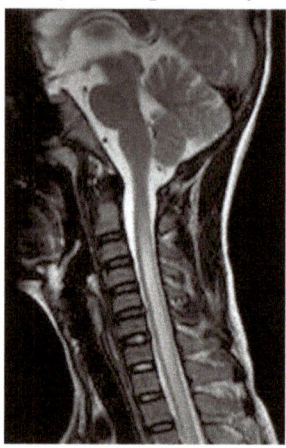

a. What is the abnormal finding in the MRI image? *(2 marks)*
b. What is the probable diagnosis? *(2 marks)*
c. Which area in his brain is responsible for the gastrointestinal tract (GIT) symptoms? *(2 marks)*
d. Which antibody will be positive blood of this patient? *(2 marks)*
e. What kind of molecular mimicry has been postulated in the genesis of this disease? *(2 marks)*

Q55. A 60-year-old man consulted general physician (GP) for his giddiness. He was diagnosed as high BP and sublingual nifedipine was given. Next day he presents to ER with right leg weakness and his BP had normalized. His MRI is given below.

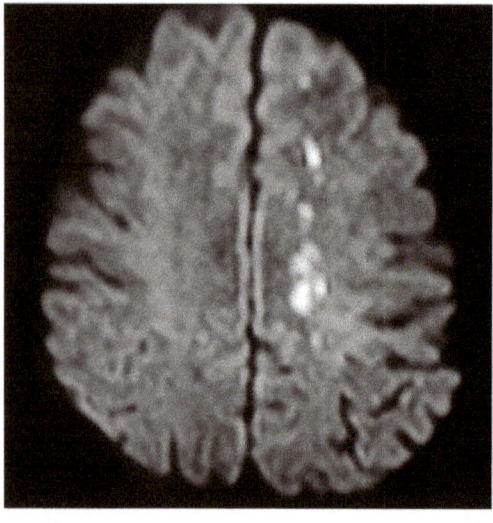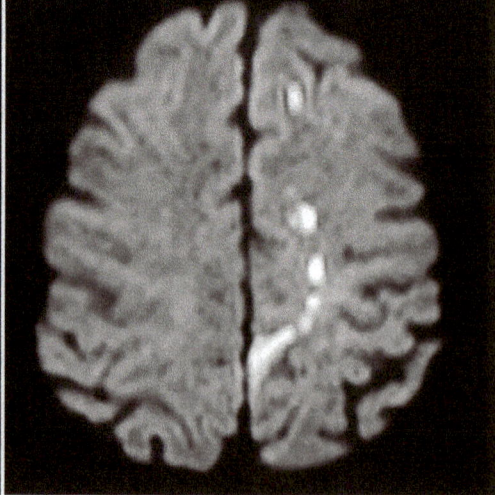

a. What MRI imaging sequence is shown above? *(3 marks)*
b. What is the diagnosis? *(3 marks)*
c. What is the next investigation you suggest? *(4 marks)*

Q56. Mrs Sharma, a 42-year-old software engineer, suddenly collapsed at home, unable to move or speak. She was conscious but could only communicate by blinking her eyes. Medical tests revealed a pontine stroke, leading to locked-in syndrome (LIS).
a. Name three important clinical features of locked-in syndrome? *(3 marks)*
b. What is the site of lesion in locked-in syndrome? *(3 marks)*
c. Name most common causes for locked in syndrome. *(4 marks)*

Q57. A 28-year-old woman presents to the ER with a H/O recurrent episodes of unusual movements. During these episodes, she experiences forceful rotation of her torso by at least 180° around the horizontal body axis. Sometimes, these episodes are accompanied by a preceding forced head version. The events last for a brief duration and are associated with altered awareness.

During the neurological examination, the patient's torso is observed to rotate forcefully, and there is a distinct semiology of gyratory seizures. The ictal focus is suspected to be in the frontal or temporal lobe, and further investigations, including imaging and electroencephalogram (EEG), are planned to localize the exact origin. It is noted that the rotation of the torso is contralateral to the direction of head version and ipsilateral when the body rotates "en bloc" without head version.

a. What is the semiology of gyratory seizures? *(3 marks)*
b. Where is the ictal focus in gyratory seizures? *(4 marks)*
c. Which antibody can be positive in this disease? *(3 marks)*

Q58. A 70-year-old man was referred for chronic progressive dorsal myelopathy. As his recent MRI showed longitudinally extensive transverse myelitis (LETM) from D6 extending up to conus, he was started on pulse intravenous methylprednisolone (IVMP). Following the steroid course, he had worsening of weakness. His MRI lumbar spine (LS) is shown below:

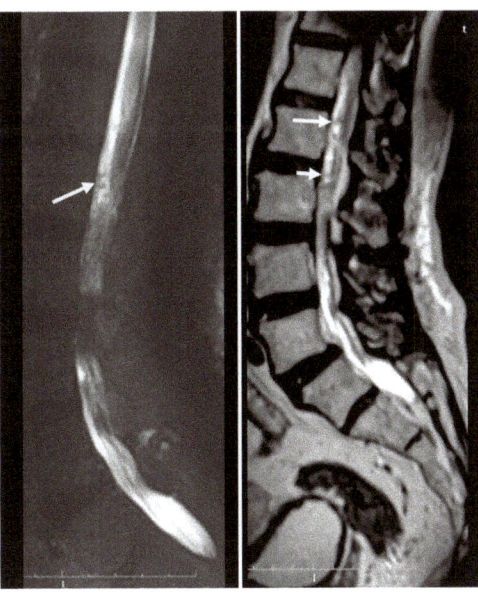

a. What is the likely diagnosis? (5 marks)
b. What is the next best investigation to confirm your diagnosis? (5 marks)

Q59. A 45-year-old woman presented with chief complaints of severe headache and vomiting followed by hemiparesis. She was attended to a neurologist and a CT scan of brain with contrast was done. Answer the following questions:

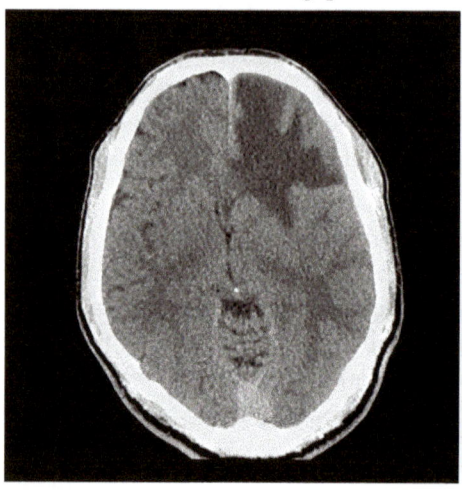
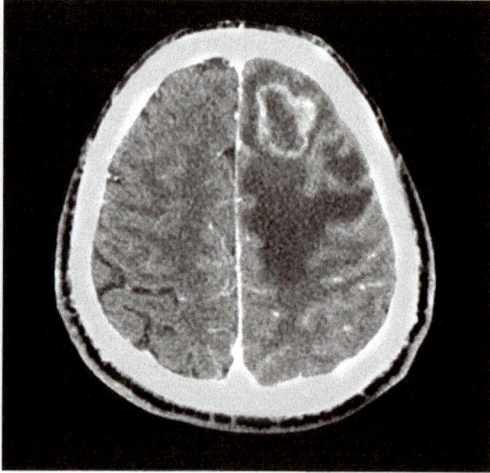

a. Describe three abnormalities in this CT scan. (3 marks)
b. Which of the following is the most likely cause? (3 marks)
c. Mention two differential diagnoses. (2 marks)
d. How can you manage the patient (two modalities)? (2 marks)

Q60. This 30-year-old patient has presented with H/O fever, headache, and vomiting for 3 days. He has H/O chronic sinusitis.

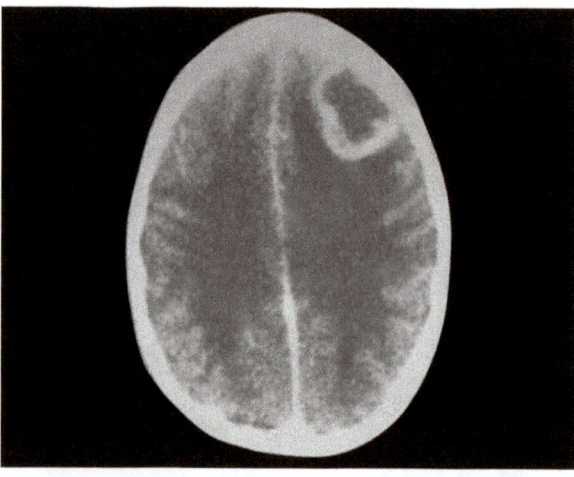

a. What investigation is shown and what is the diagnosis? (3 marks)

b. Name three most useful drugs for this problem. *(3 marks)*
c. What is the definitive treatment for this patient? *(4 marks)*

Q61. A 65-year-old male visited to the emergency department with H/O sudden onset of left-sided weakness. A CT scan of brain was done immediately.

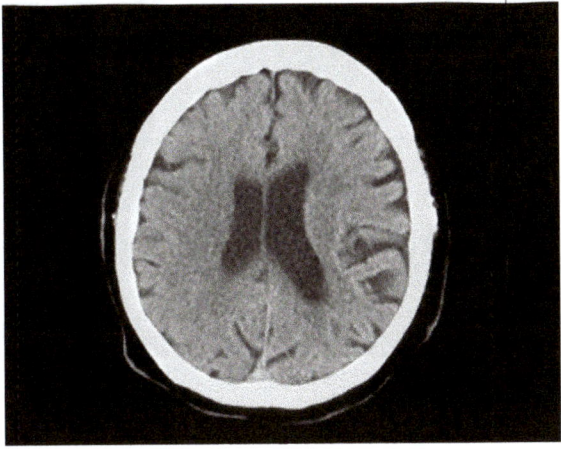

a. What does the CT scan show? *(3 marks)*
b. What is the diagnosis? *(2 marks)*
c. What are other signs for the diagnosis in CT scan? *(2 marks)*
d. What is the treatment? *(3 marks)*

Q62. A 43-year-old woman complained of headaches, nausea, and vomiting. Within 2 hours of being admitted to the hospital, she suddenly lost consciousness.

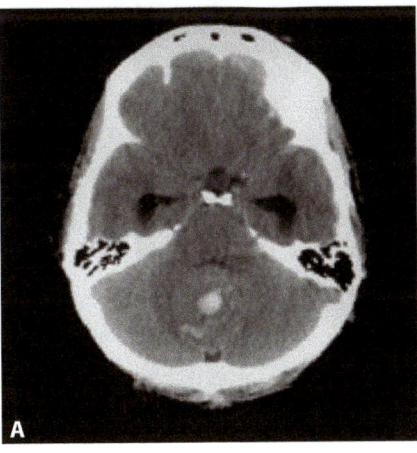 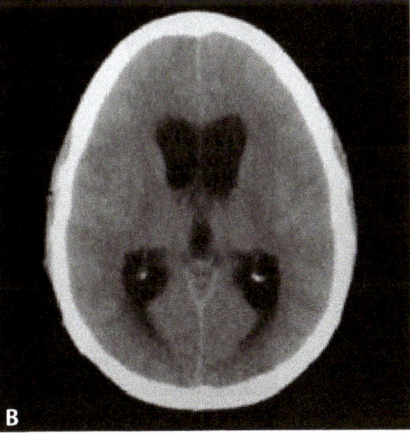

Look at the Images A and B. Answer the following questions:
a. Write down three important radiological features. *(3 marks)*
b. What is the diagnosis? *(4 marks)*
c. Write down the most probable cause of this lesion. *(3 marks)*

Neurology

Q63. This 45-year-old male presented to the emergency department after an unwitnessed fall with head strike. He underwent CT. A noncontrast axial reformat is shown below:

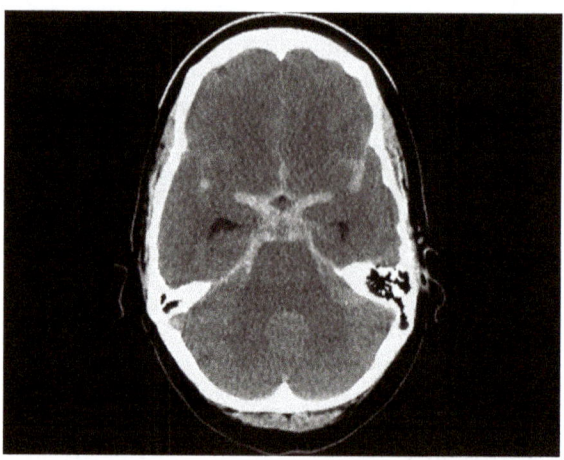

Answer the following questions:
a. What is the most likely diagnosis? (3 marks)
b. Mention three cardinal clinical presentations. (2 marks)
c. What may be the cause? (2 marks)
d. What is the definite treatment? (3 marks)

Q64. A 68-year-old male patient presented with severe headaches followed by loss of consciousness. A CT scan was done immediately. Answer the following questions:

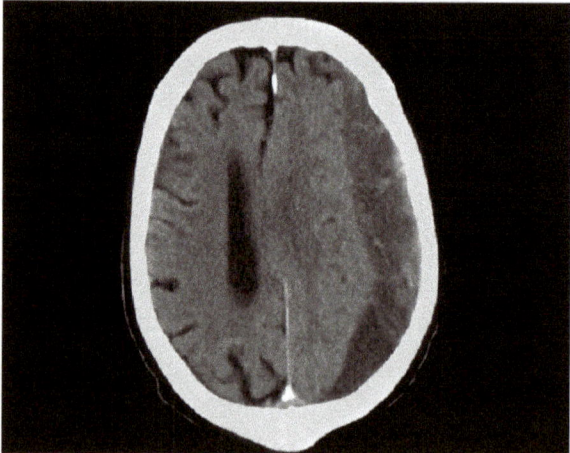

a. Describe two abnormalities in this CT scan. (3 marks)
b. Which of the following is the most likely cause? (2 marks)
c. Mention four clinical features of this patient. (2 marks)
d. What is the definite treatment? (3 marks)

Q65. A 62-year-old woman without any medical history reported headaches persisting for the past 3 months, unresponsive to typical pain relievers, accompanied by behavioral disturbances. The symptoms intensified, marked by vomiting, although there were no sensory-motor deficits or seizures. She underwent a contrast-enhanced MRI (A) and fluid-attenuated inversion recovery (FLAIR) (B). Answer the following questions:

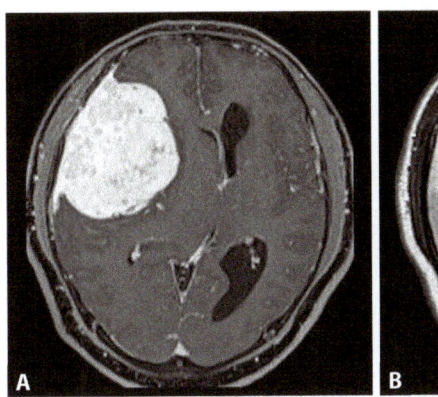
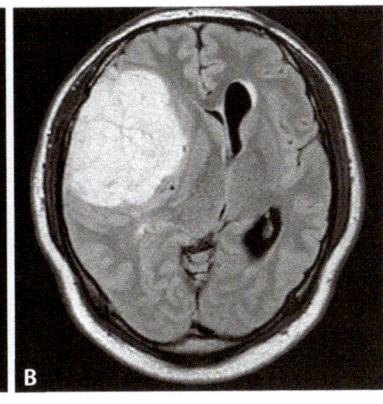

a. Describe the film (three important features). (3 marks)
b. What is the most likely diagnosis? (4 marks)
c. What are the treatment modalities? (3 marks)

Q66. A 58-year-old man was admitted to hospital having experienced pain in the lower back and left leg for 2 years and a sudden exacerbation of the symptoms for 5 days before admission. MRI of the LS has done and shown below.

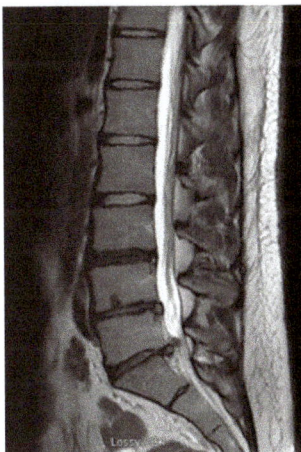
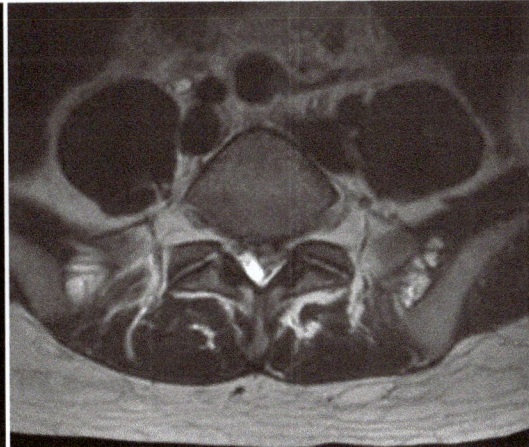

a. What are the findings of MRI (three findings)? (3 marks)
b. What is the diagnosis? (2 marks)
c. Enumerate three neurological signs for this patient. (2 marks)
d. What is the treatment? (3 marks)

Q67. A 45-year-old man presented with neck pain radiating to both shoulders along with a stiff and awkward gait. During the physical examination, increased reflexes were observed in both the arms and legs, and bilateral Babinski responses were noted. MRI of the cervical has done and shown below.

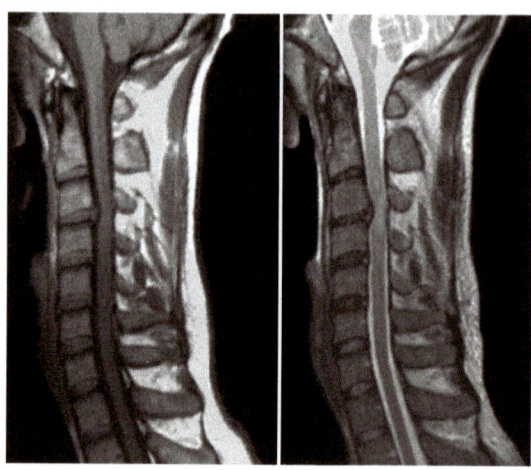

a. What are the findings of MRI (three findings)? (3 marks)
b. What is the diagnosis? (2 marks)
c. What is the most likely cause? (2 marks)
d. What is the treatment? (3 marks)

Q68. A 53-year-old housewife reported weakness and atrophy in her right forearm and hand persisting for 1 year. Additionally, she described severe and nearly debilitating paresthesias affecting all four limbs, including both hands and feet, for the past 6 months. MRI of cervical has done. Answer the following questions:

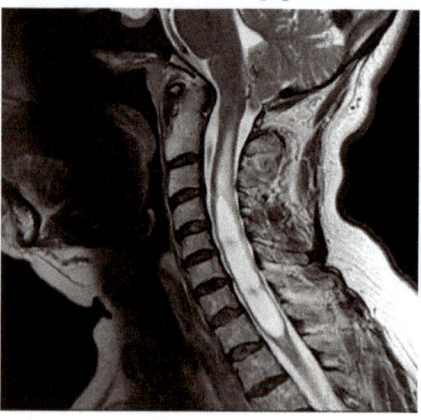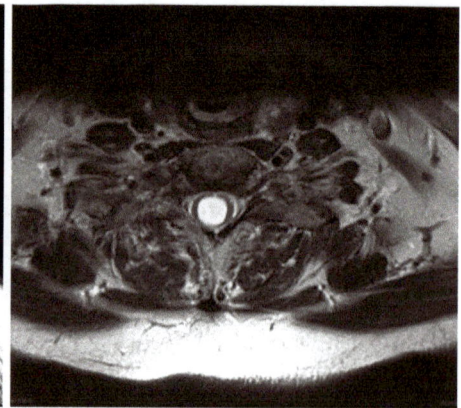

a. What are the findings of the MRI? (3 marks)
b. What is the diagnosis? (2 marks)
c. What is dissociated sensory loss? (2 marks)
d. What is the treatment? (3 marks)

Q69. A 13-year-old boy with an unremarkable medical history presented at our outpatient clinic due to fever and back pain. Approximately 4 months before seeking medical attention, he occasionally experienced high fever. The lower back pain had been ongoing for 3 months, initially attributed to his regular track and field training. However, 4 days before the clinic visit, he developed a high fever, and the back pain worsened. Despite taking acetaminophen, his symptoms did not improve. An MRI was performed (see Images A and B). Answer the following questions:

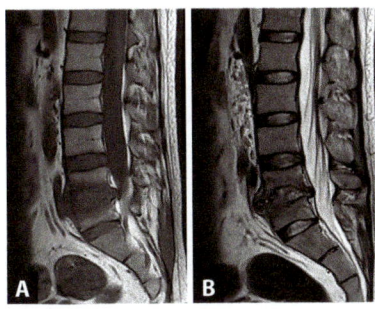

a. What are the findings of the MRI? (3 marks)
b. What is the diagnosis? (3 marks)
c. What is the treatment? (4 marks)

Q70. A 9-year-old girl was brought to the outpatient department (OPD) by her mother with complaints of brief episodes of complete unawareness lasting a few seconds to a minute for a period of 6 months. She further explains that her daughter does not have any convulsions, tongue bites, urinary incontinence, or falls. The child has multiple episodes (average of 10–15) of lapse of awareness in a day. The child does not respond during those episodes when called her name and is also amnestic for the event. Her EEG is given below.

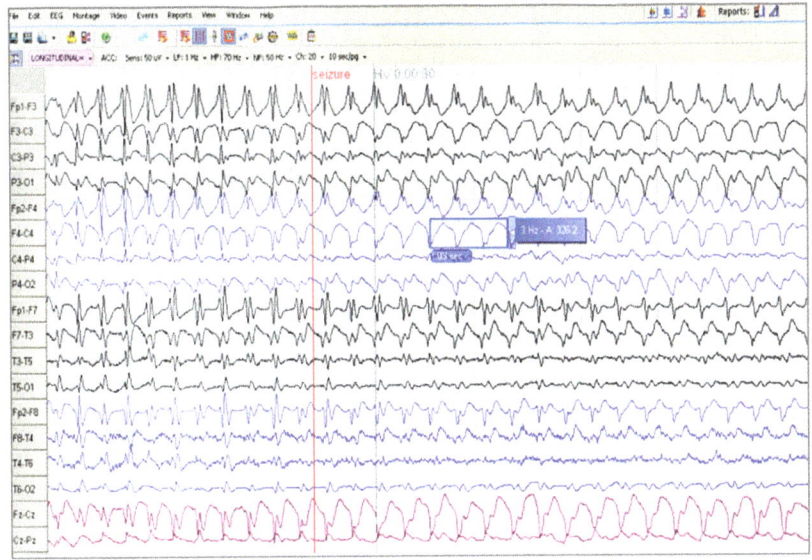

a. What is the diagnosis? (2 marks)
b. What is the EEG finding? (2 marks)
c. Is there any provocative test to bring out the event? (2 marks)
d. What is the specific drug for this type of epilepsy and discuss its mechanism of action? (2 marks)
e. Name any two alternative drugs that can be used. (2 marks)

Q71. A 25-year-old female presented with acute-onset right facial and left truncal numbness with blurred vision. She denied any febrile illness preceding her complaint. There was no H/O trauma or toxin ingestion. On examination, she had a normal higher function. Her left medial rectus was paralyzed on testing extraocular muscle movement and at the same time she had abducting nystagmus of the right eye. She had reduced sensation to touch, pain, and temperature on her face and the left trunk. She also had mild left appendicular ataxia. Her MRI FLAIR axial section is given below.

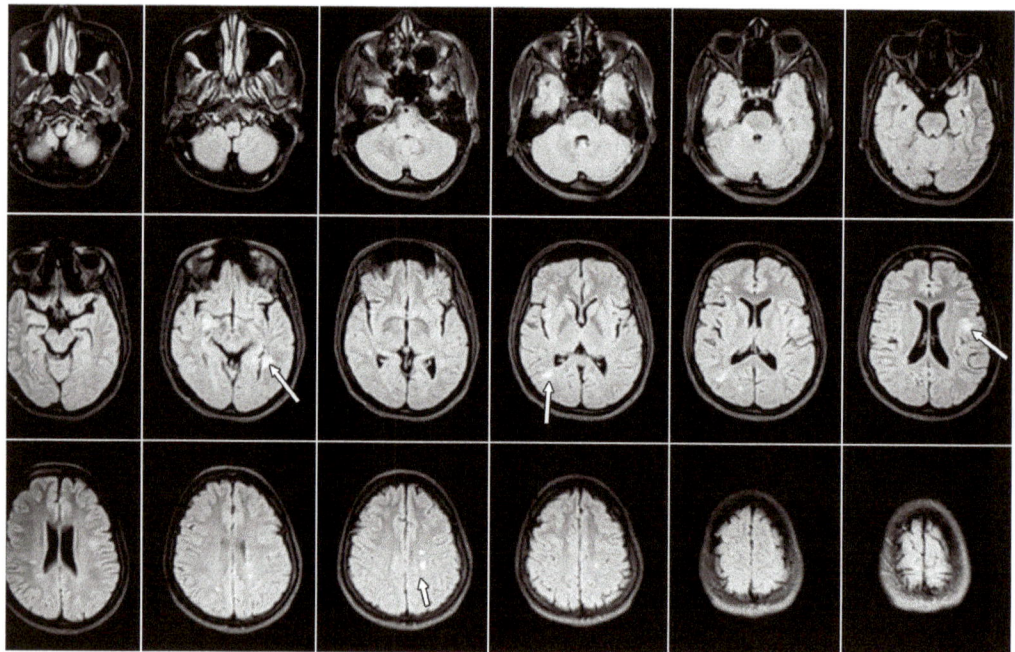

a. What is the ocular finding and what structure is responsible for the above described? (2 marks)
b. Name two conditions causing the above ocular phenomena. (2 marks)
c. What is the treatment for this acute attack? (2 marks)
d. Give two differential diagnoses for this MRI image. (2 marks)
e. Name the cerebrospinal fluid (CSF) investigation that may aid in diagnosis with this clinicoradiological presentation. (2 marks)

Q72. A 34-year-old male presented with rest tremors of the right upper and the lower limbs for the past 6 months. He also reported slowness of activities in his daily living. His elder sister also had such similar illness.

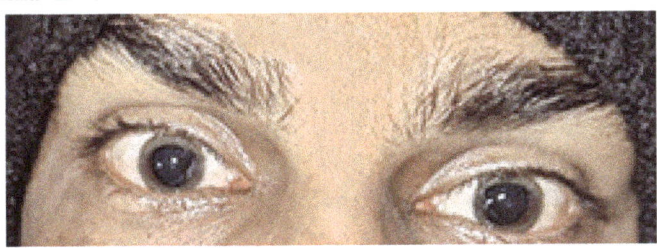

a. What is the eye sign in the patient's image? (1 mark)
b. What is the mode of inheritance of this disease? (1 mark)
c. What are the named signs described in the MRI of the brain of such patients? (2 marks)
d. Name two drugs used for the management of the above entity. (2 marks)
e. What is the curative treatment for this patient? (1 mark)
f. What drugs can be used to symptomatically treat this patient? (2 marks)
g. Name of the gene that is defective. (1 mark)

Q73. A 44-year-old male chronic alcoholic presented with acute confusional state and unsteadiness while walking for the past 1 week. On examination, he was disoriented and had vertical nystagmus. He had appendicular ataxia and gait ataxia in addition to bilateral upper limb postural tremor. His MRI diffusion-weighted imaging is shown below.

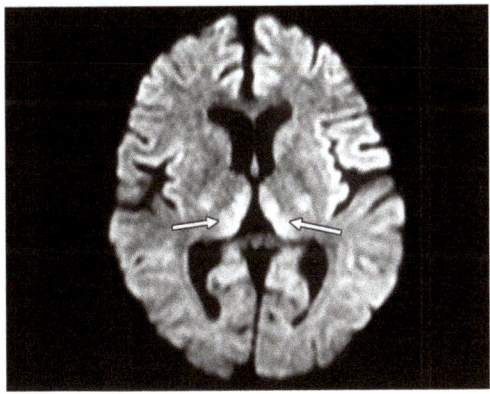

a. What is the diagnosis? (1 mark)
b. What is the acute management? (2 marks)
c. What is the sequela, if not treated promptly? (1 mark)
d. Name two other settings in which this disease entity can develop. (2 marks)
e. What is the classic triad of this disease entity? (3 marks)
f. What is the pathomechanism? (1 mark)

Q74. A 57-year-old diabetic patient presented with acute onset vertical diplopia along with unsteadiness while walking and reeling to the left. His MRI of the brain film is shown below.

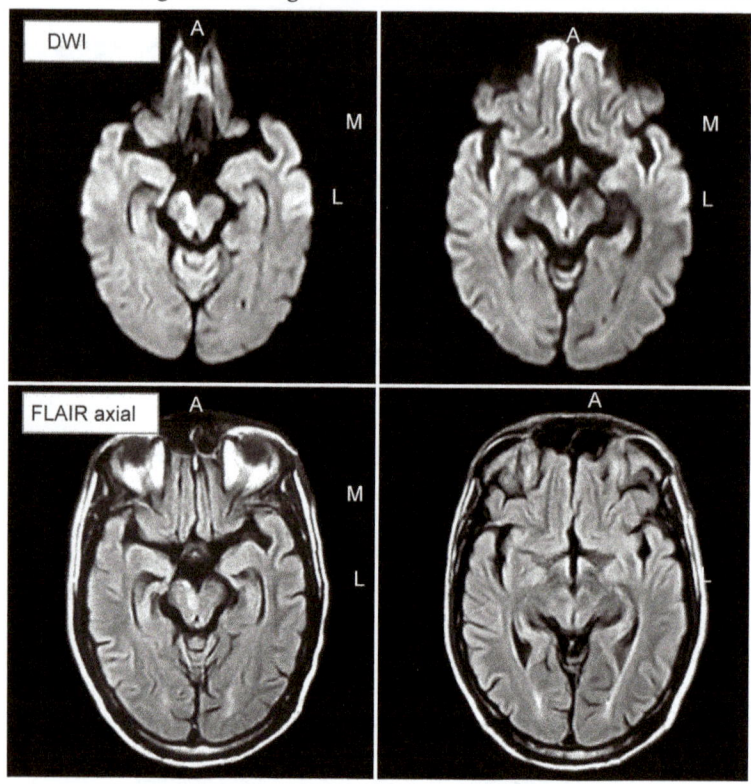

(DWI: diffusion-weighted imaging; FLAIR: fluid-attenuated inversion recovery)

a. Discuss the blood supply of the involved structure. *(3 marks)*
b. Name two eponymous syndromes associated with lesions of the involved structure. *(2 marks)*
c. Which structure controls vertical gaze? *(2 marks)*
d. What are the cranial nerves that originate from the involved structure? *(2 marks)*
e. All extraocular muscles are supplied by cranial nerves from the involved structure except. *(1 mark)*

Q75. A 70-year-old female presented with tremulousness of both hands (right more than left) at rest along with slowness of activities of daily living for a period of 2 years. She also has difficulty in traveling in the bike as she tends to fall while climbing. She does not have any memory impairment or myoclonus. She denies a H/O any chronic drug intake.

a. What is the probable diagnosis? *(1 mark)*
b. Mention three nonmotor symptoms. *(3 marks)*
c. Staging used for measuring severity. *(1 mark)*
d. Name the surgical option for advanced disease. *(1 mark)*
e. Name two drugs causing such similar conditions. *(2 marks)*
f. Name two drugs used to treat this condition. *(2 marks)*

Q76. A 33-year-old male alcoholic presented with acute-onset horizontal diplopia (binocular) with a headache for 2 days. The headache is holocranial with no response to analgesics. His MRI of the brain and venogram are shown below.

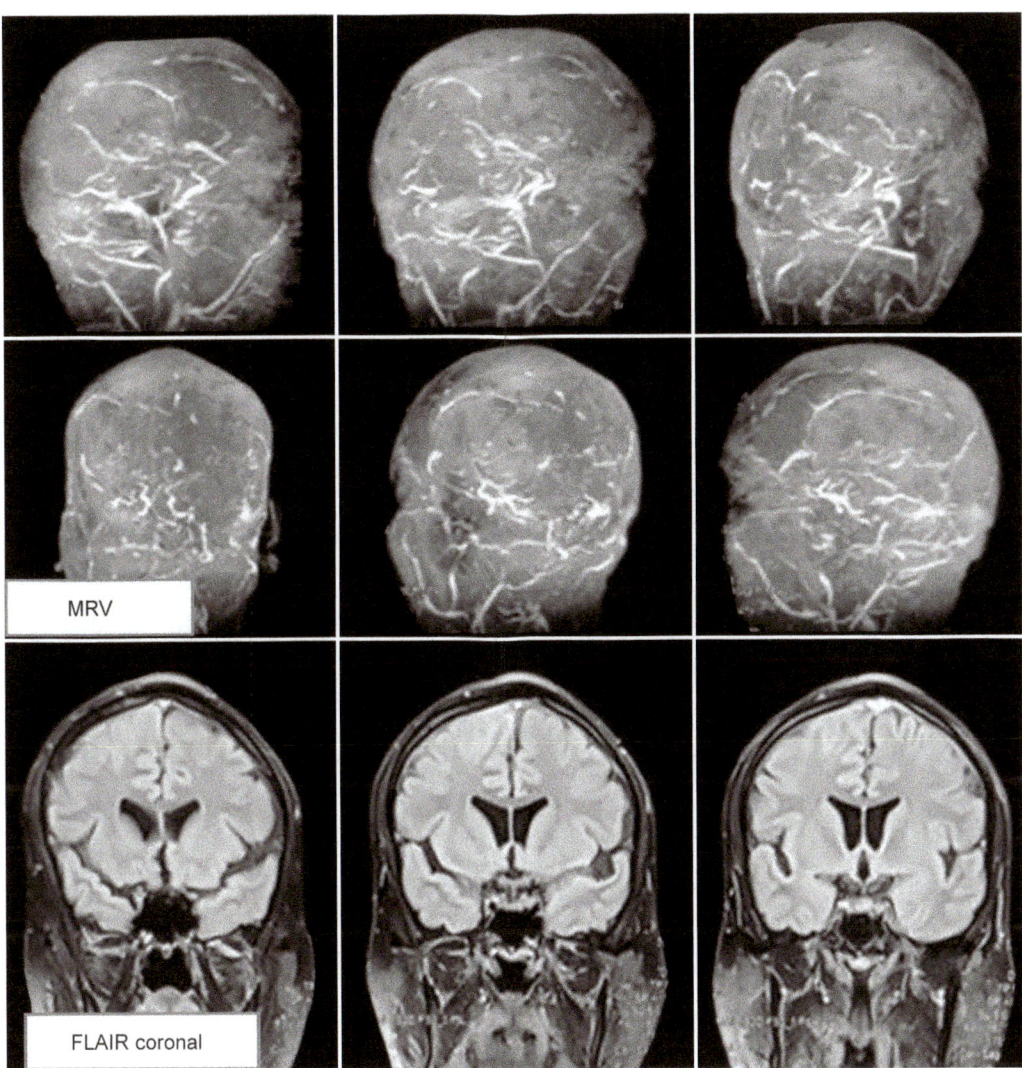

(FLAIR: fluid-attenuated inversion recovery; MRV: magnetic resonance venography)

a. What are the provoking factors for this condition? (2 marks)
b. What are the magnetic resonance (MR) venogram findings? (1 mark)
c. What is the acute management? (2 marks)
d. Name two hypercoagulable states associated with this condition. (2 marks)
e. Mention the duration of treatment. (1 mark)
f. Name the oral drug used after acute treatment. (1 mark)

Q77. A 36-year-old female with no family history presented with acute onset focal deficit in the form of right upper limb weakness, slurred speech, and right facial lag. Her past history revealed frequent migraine attacks. Her MRI of the brain showed a lacunar infarct in the left internal capsule. Her MRI also has other clues for the etiology of stroke.

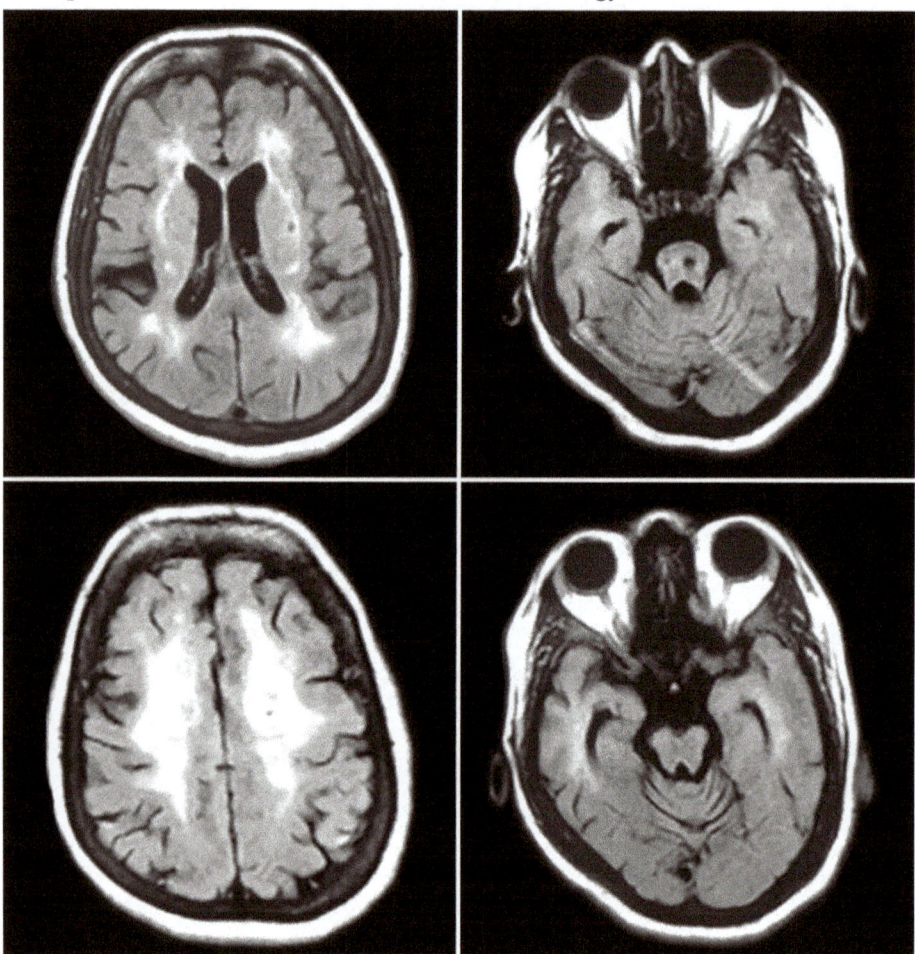

a. What is the etiology of stroke? (2 marks)
b. Is the condition familial and if yes mention the pattern of inheritance? (2 marks)
c. What radiological clue leads to the suspicion of this condition? (2 marks)
d. What is the pathology behind this entity? (2 marks)
e. Mention four lacunar syndromes. (2 marks)

Q78. A 57-year-old female presented with altered sensorium, acute onset for 2 days. H/O fever preceding the altered sensorium 10 days ago. Her MRI of the brain diffusion-weighted sequence is shown below. Her CSF analysis revealed high protein (124 mg/dL), CSF cells 280, predominantly lymphocytes, and low glucose (35 mg/dL).

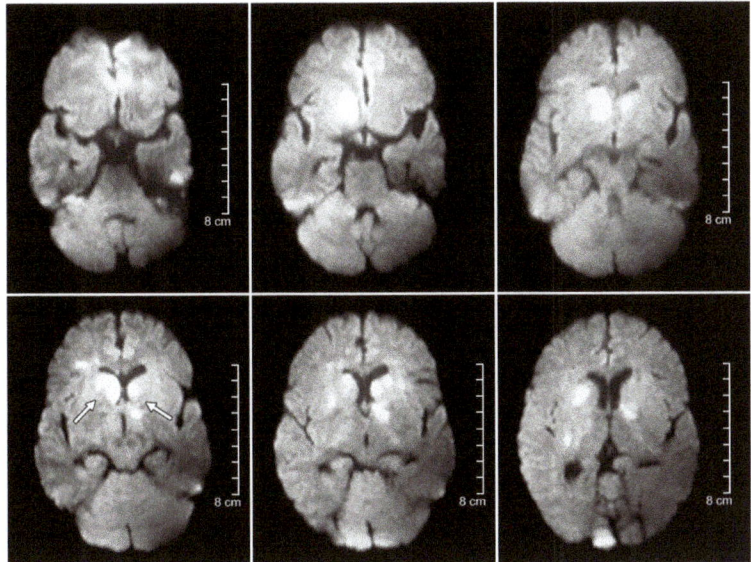

a. What is the MRI suggestive of? (2 marks)
b. What is the mechanism behind the MRI finding? (1 mark)
c. How long will you treat this patient? (1 mark)
d. What is the usual regimen of drugs used? (4 marks)
e. Is there a role for polymerase chain reaction test in this condition? (2 marks)

Q79. A 63-year-old man with chronic kidney disease was admitted with headache, acute and new onset for a week. H/O fall by self, 1 week ago. On examination, he is awake and irritable. Mild disorientation noted. His CT of the brain is shown below.

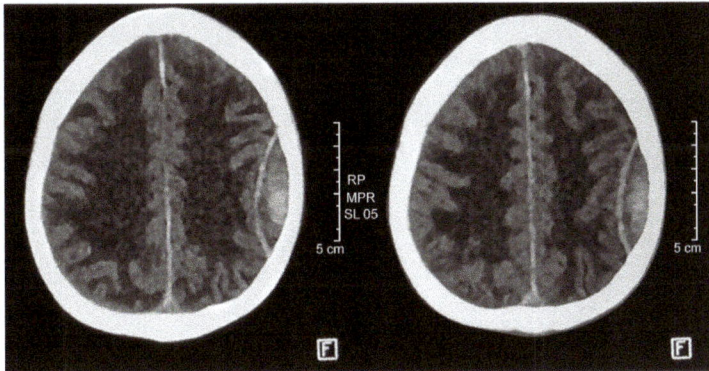

a. What is the CT finding? (2 marks)
b. Mention the mechanism of development of this finding. (2 marks)
c. How will you manage this condition? (2 marks)
d. Mention two etiologies leading to this condition. (2 marks)
e. Mention two complications if this condition is not treated. (2 marks)

Q80. This 10-year-old boy was brought by his mother with complaints of poor scholastic performance. His picture is shown below.

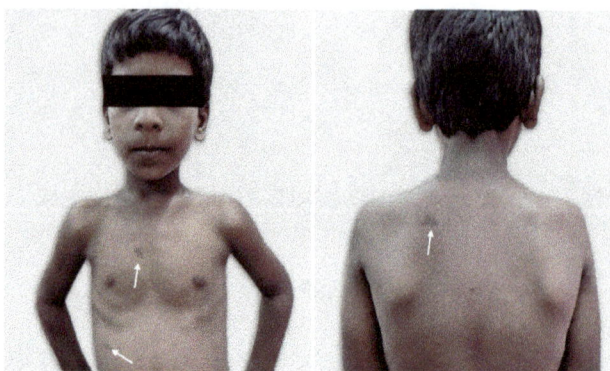

a. Name the neurocutaneous marker and the syndrome associated with it. (2 marks)
b. Mention the mode of inheritance. (2 marks)
c. When are the lesions shown above considered pathological? (2 marks)
d. What gene is mutated in this syndrome and where it is located? (2 marks)
e. Mention two ocular findings in this syndrome. (2 marks)

Q81. A 52-year-old female had urinary and fecal incontinence since childhood. Her MRI spine axial images are given below.

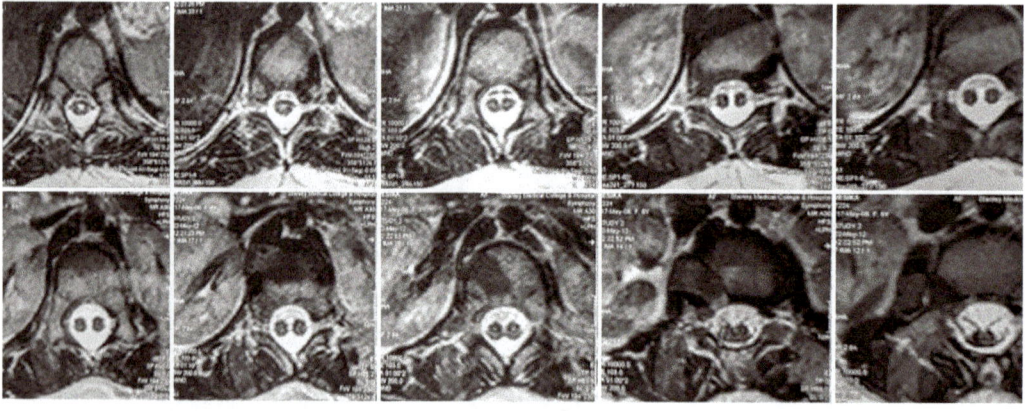

a. What is abnormal in this MRI? (2 marks)
b. Mention any four conditions related to this abnormality. (4 marks)
c. What is the preventive measure to avoid such abnormality? (2 marks)
d. What is the pathogenesis? (2 marks)

Q82. This 45-year-old female presented with frequent episodes of stereotyped repetitive movements in the form of lip-smacking, and repetitive left-hand movements in the form of picking with altered awareness lasting a few minutes. Her CT of the brain is shown next.

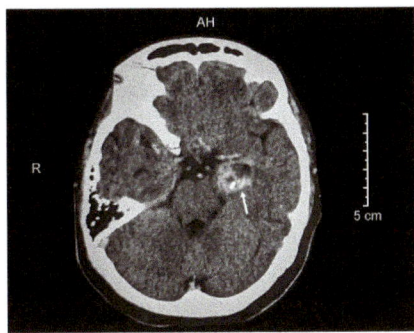

a. What is the CT finding? (3 marks)
b. What antiepileptics are preferred? (2 marks)
c. What are the side effects of surgically removing this lesion? (2 marks)
d. How would be the aura if the seizure arises from the above structural lesion? (3 marks)

Q83. A 22-year-old female in the immediate postpartum period complained of a holocranial headache followed by a generalized GTCS. Her antenatal period was uneventful. Her BP in the postpartum period never exceeded 120/80 mm Hg. Her MRI sequences are given below.

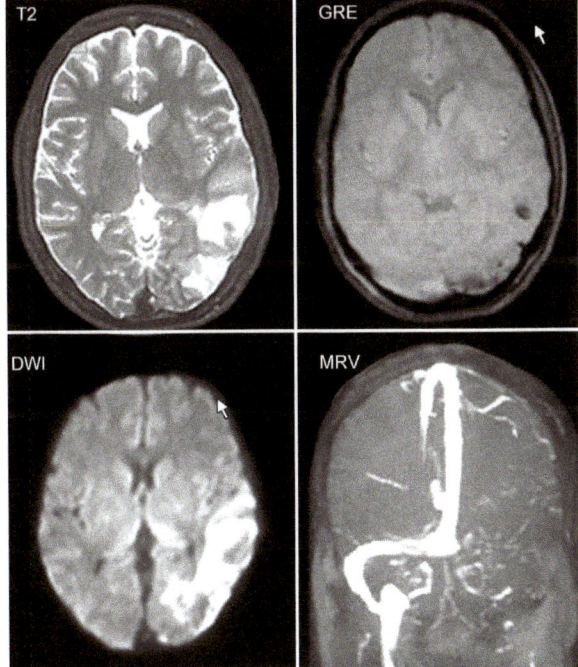

(DWI: diffusion-weighted imaging; GRE: gradient recalled echo; MRV: magnetic resonance venography)

a. Mention the MRI findings. (4 marks)
b. What is the management? (2 marks)
c. Mention the two causes of secondary headaches in pregnancy. (2 marks)
d. Name two complications of this condition if untreated. (2 marks)

Q84. A 48-year-old male with midbrain cavernoma presented with the left upper limb tremor for the past 3 years. His tremor is present at rest (mild in amplitude). On outstretched hands, the tremor becomes coarse and high in amplitude. Severe intention quality tremor noted on finger nose test.

a. Name the tremor. (2 marks)
b. Discuss the treatment options. (4 marks)
c. Mention any two causes of this tremor. (2 marks)
d. What structure in the midbrain is responsible for such tremors? (2 marks)

Q85. A 49-year-old hypertensive male, irregular on treatment, presented with sudden onset altered sensorium with a BP of 230/120 mm Hg and paucity of movements noticed in the right upper and lower limb. His CT of the brain image is shown below.

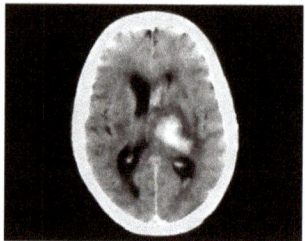

a. What is the CT finding suggestive of? (2 marks)
b. Mention two etiologies for this condition other than HTN. (2 marks)
c. What should be the target BP reduction in this patient? (2 marks)
d. Mention two poor prognostic factors for this condition. (2 marks)
e. What antihypertensives are preferred? (2 marks)

Q86. A 54-year-old male diabetic and hypertensive was admitted with sudden onset dizziness and unsteadiness while walking and reeling to the right. He also had vomiting, intractable hiccoughs, coughs up when drinking any liquid, and his voice became hoarse. His MRI is shown below.

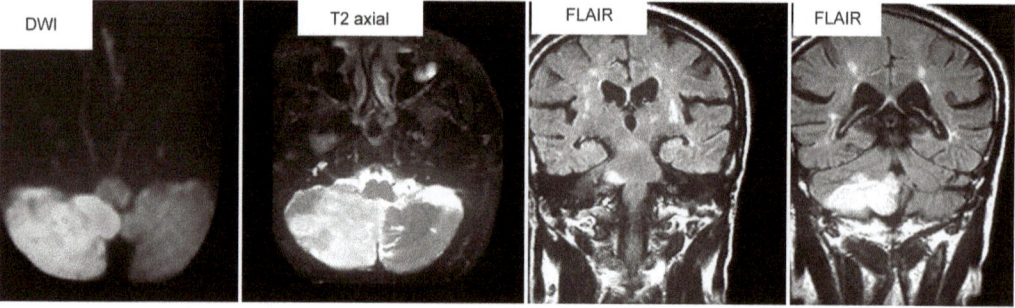

(DWI: diffusion-weighted imaging; FLAIR: fluid-attenuated inversion recovery)

a. Name the most common artery involved in this condition and mention the eponym for this condition. (2 marks)
b. Discuss the key MRI findings. (2 marks)
c. Discuss the blood supply of the involved structures. (6 marks)

Q87. A 62-year-old male who is a known coronary artery disease patient with heart failure, reduced ejection fraction, and dilated chambers, developed sudden onset quadriparesis with urinary incontinence. His LLs were weaker than his upper limbs. His MRI is shown below.

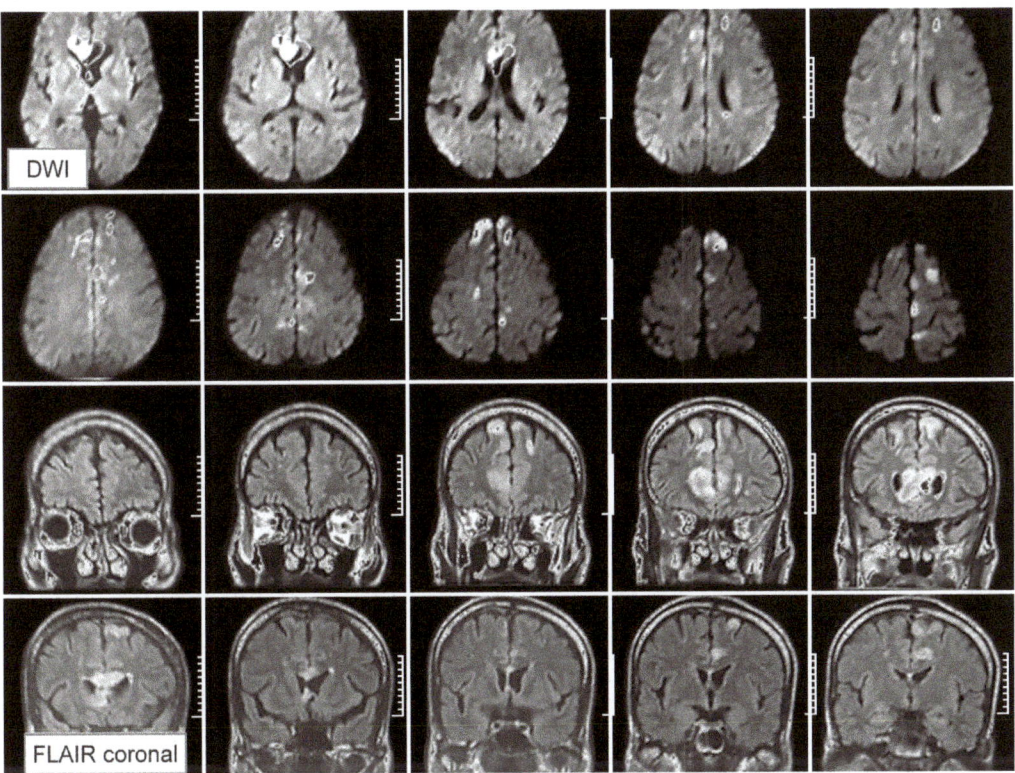

(DWI: diffusion-weighted imaging; FLAIR: fluid-attenuated inversion recovery)

a. Discuss the MRI findings. *(2 marks)*
b. Discuss the probable etiology for this condition in this patient. *(2 marks)*
c. Mention the brain areas supplied by the involved vessel. *(4 marks)*
d. Mention two branches of the involved vessel. *(2 marks)*

Q88. A 65-year-old diabetic for the past 3 years with high glycated hemoglobin (HbA1c) of 10.5% consulted a physician and he was started on insulin for a tight glycemic control. Three months later his HbA1c dropped to 8.0%. Soon after patient started noticing thinning of both thighs (asymmetric) along with neuropathic pain which was excruciating particularly, at night. All these symptoms developed subacutely and were progressive. He was started on pregabalin 75 mg by his physician and noted little improvement in pain. Subsequently, he had difficulty in getting up from squatting position and climbing stairs. The patient noticed his left LL was weaker than the right LL. Meanwhile, the patient lost a weight of 6 kg in the last 2 months. On examination, he had a bilateral, areflexic, proximal (right 3/5) (left 2/5) more than distal (right 4+/5) (left 4/5) weakness of both LLs.

a. What is the condition and other name for this? (2 marks)
b. Discuss the management options. (3 marks)
c. Mention the two risk factors. (2 marks)
d. Discuss its prognosis and the natural course of the illness. (3 marks)

Q89. A 62-year-old female presented with difficulty in chewing *rotis* for the past 1 month. She also complained of fatigability. She also noticed that her speech gets slurred after a prolonged conversation. She also mentioned that her eyelids become droopy toward the end of the day. All her symptoms worsen particularly at the evening time. Her repetitive nerve stimulation (RNS) of the trapezius muscle is given below.

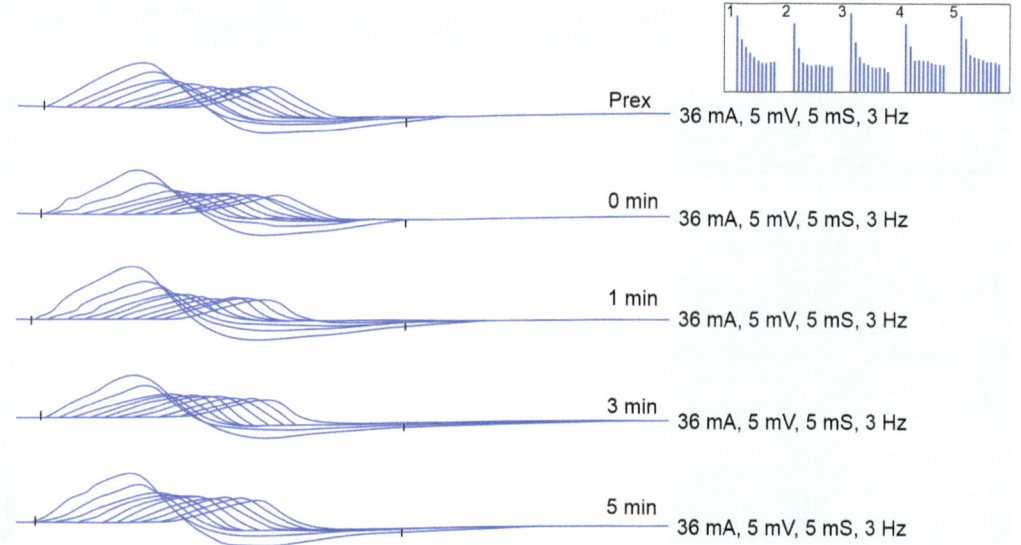

	Amplitude (mV)					Decrement (%)				
Tr	Prex	0 min	1 min	3 min	5 min	PREX	0 min	1 min	3 min	5 min
1	7.17	6.60	7.54	6.62	7.51	0.0	0.0	0.0	0.0	0.0
2	5.25	4.28	5.04	4.56	5.39	−26.7	−35.2	−33.2	−31.1	−28.3
3	4.23	3.10	3.71	3.31	3.97	−40.9	−53.0	−50.8	−50.0	−47.1
4	3.94	2.83	3.11	3.14	3.78	−45.1	−57.2	−58.8	−52.6	−49.6
5	3.64	2.70	2.94	3.26	3.52	−49.2	−59.2	−61.0	−50.7	−53.1
6	3.28	2.68	2.59	3.15	3.60	−54.2	−59.5	−65.7	−52.4	−52.2
7	2.88	2.78	2.40	3.13	3.28	−59.8	−57.9	−68.1	−52.8	−56.4
8	3.01	2.60	2.43	2.88	3.29	−58.0	−60.6	−67.8	−56.5	−56.2
9	3.14	2.49	2.47	2.86	3.29	−56.2	−62.4	−67.2	−56.9	−56.2
10	3.05	2.56	2.35	2.79	3.06	−57.4	−61.2	−68.9	−57.8	−59.2

Tr	Prex	Area (mV mS)				PREX	Decrement (%)			
		0 min	1 min	3 min	5 min		0 min	1 min	3 min	5 min
1	59.2	50.4	57.2	50.1	59.4	0.0	0.0	0.0	0.0	0.0
2	40.3	28.6	33.9	31.7	39.1	−31.8	−43.2	−40.7	−36.8	−34.1
3	33.3	18.9	26.3	22.2	28.8	−43.7	−62.6	−54.0	−55.7	−51.5
4	29.6	17.4	24.2	22.0	26.7	−50.0	−65.5	−57.7	−56.0	−55.0
5	26.5	16.0	25.0	21.1	22.9	−55.3	−68.4	−56.3	−57.8	−61.4
6	24.2	15.8	20.1	19.6	25.3	−59.1	−68.7	−64.9	−60.9	−57.3
7	19.9	16.5	18.7	19.1	22.9	−66.3	−67.3	−67.3	−61.8	−61.5
8	21.1	15.7	19.1	17.0	21.4	−64.4	−68.9	−66.5	−66.1	−63.9
9	21.7	14.6	19.2	16.9	20.9	−63.4	−71.1	−66.4	−66.2	−64.7
10	21.5	14.9	19.2	17.3	19.0	−63.6	−70.5	−66.5	−65.4	−67.9

a. What are the findings in the RNS? (1 mark)
b. What is the pathophysiology of the disease? (3 marks)
c. Discuss the symptomatic management of this patient. (2 marks)
d. What is the treatment of crisis in this patient? (2 marks)
e. Mention two drugs used for long-term immunotherapy. (2 marks)

Q90. A 64-year-old male with uncontrolled diabetes (random blood sugar of 600 mg/dL) presented with acute onset of involuntary, jerky, random, purposeless movement of all four limbs more on the left side. The movements disappear in sleep. His CT of the brain is shown below.

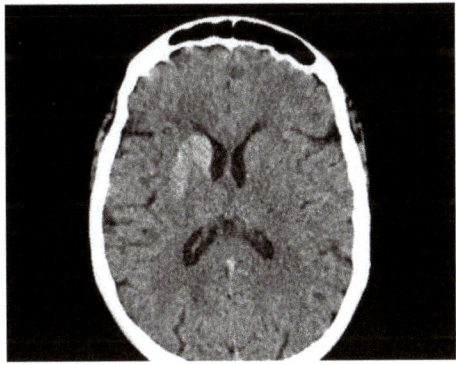

a. Mention the CT finding and the involuntary movements. (2 marks)
b. Mention other common causes of such involuntary movement in children and adults. (3 marks)
c. Explain the symptomatic management of these movements. (2 marks)
d. Mention three other involuntary movements associated with diabetes mellitus. (3 marks)

Q91. A 58-year-old married male, who studied up to 9th standard, working as EB officer-foreman was brought by his wife and son for developing a new habit of drinking alcohol for the past 3 years. Initially, he used to drink alcohol occasionally but now he drinks daily. He also exhibits disinhibitory activities, such as claiming that he is a senior section engineer and switching on the electric board connections inappropriately. Due to his cognitive decline, he was given medical leave at his workplace for a few months. He also could not do minor electrical repair work. He shows no interest in family members. He frequently exhibits anger outbursts and irritability. He also had difficulty in recognizing people and things by their names for the past 7 months. His CT of the brain is shown below.

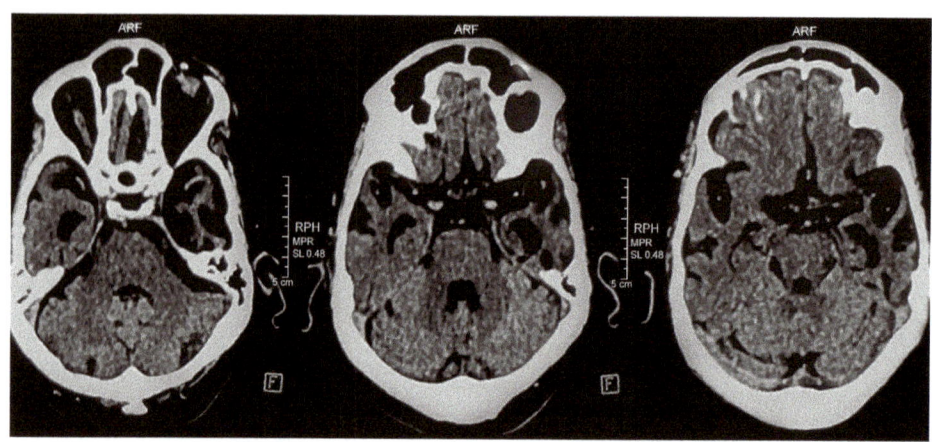

a. What type of dementia presents like this? (2 marks)
b. Mention the CT findings. (2 marks)
c. Is the above condition familial? (2 marks)
d. Discuss the variants of this dementia. (3 marks)
e. What is prosopagnosia? (1 mark)

Q92. A 73-year-old woman presented with forgetfulness for the past 3 years which was progressive. Her husband reported that she frequently misplaced personal items, forgot keys, repeated the same questions, and forgot to add salt to dishes often. She also could not pay the EB bills on time and forgot to collect the remaining money after purchase from shops. She had insight into her problem and feels frustrated often according to her husband. However, she could remember her family members and other personal information. She had trouble finding her way back to home and has been brought to home twice with the help of neighbors. She has no difficulty in naming, comprehends well, and speaks fluently. She had shown less interest in previous hobbies but did not report a low mood. Her husband did not notice any change in her behavior or personality. She was able to take care of her personal hygiene. She did not have any visual symptoms and could recognize familiar faces. There was neither slowness in her activities nor fluctuating level of consciousness. She did not feel her limbs as foreign and there were no involuntary jerks. Her past medical history was notable for long-standing HTN, diabetes mellitus, and hyperlipidemia. She did not sustain any head injury, seizures, or headaches in the past. Family history was notable for late-onset dementia in her mother. She had studied up to 8th standard, never drank alcohol, did not smoke tobacco, or use recreational drugs. She eats a mixed diet and had a regular bowel and bladder habits.

a. What could be the possible dementia? (1 mark)
b. Discuss the risk factors for developing this type of dementia. (2 marks)
c. Discuss the variants of this dementia. (3 marks)
d. Discuss the MRI findings of this type of dementia. (2 marks)
e. Mention any two preventive measures. (2 marks)

Q93. A 45-year-old male, a known c/o ethanol-related decompensated chronic liver disease (DCLD) was admitted for altered sensorium after an episode of hematemesis. His wife revealed that he did not pass stools for the last 2 days. He initially had an altered sleep pattern and later progressed to a lethargic and drowsy state. His MRI T1 sagittal section is shown below.

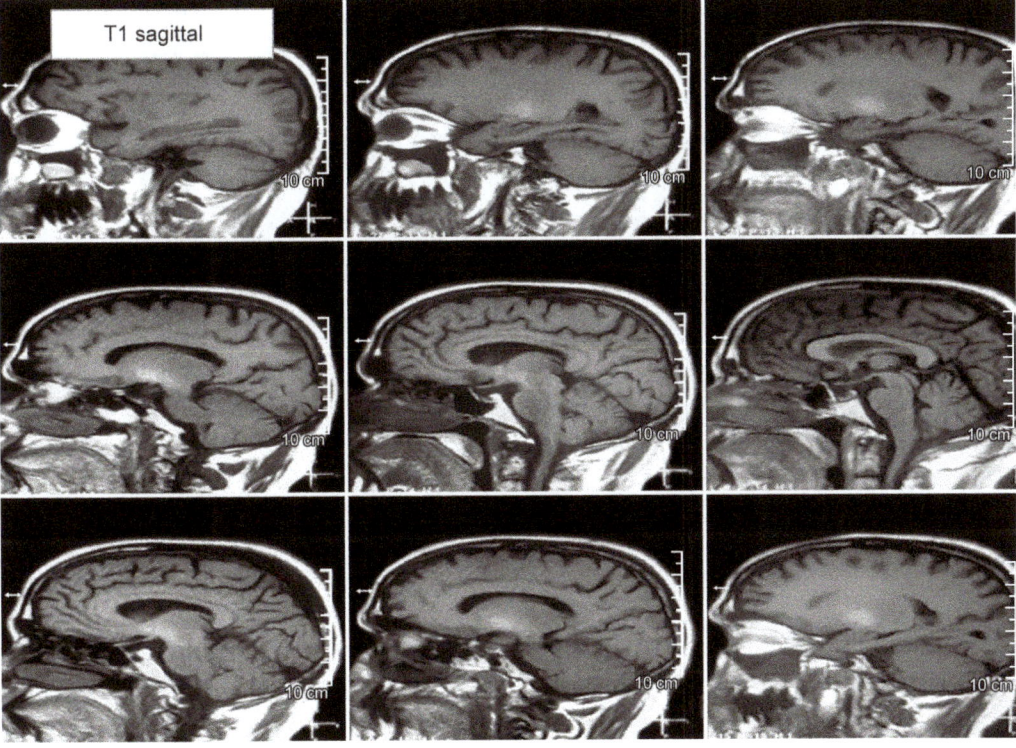

a. Mention the MRI findings. (2 marks)
b. What is the mechanism behind the MRI findings? (2 marks)
c. Discuss the management of this condition. (2 marks)
d. Discuss the EEG findings expected in this condition. (2 marks)
e. Describe the grading used to assess severity of this condition. (1 mark)
f. Describe the role of testing ammonia in this patient. (1 mark)

Neurology

Q94. A 45-year-old man with sudden onset thunderclap headache and drowsiness presented to the emergency ward. His CT of the brain is shown below.

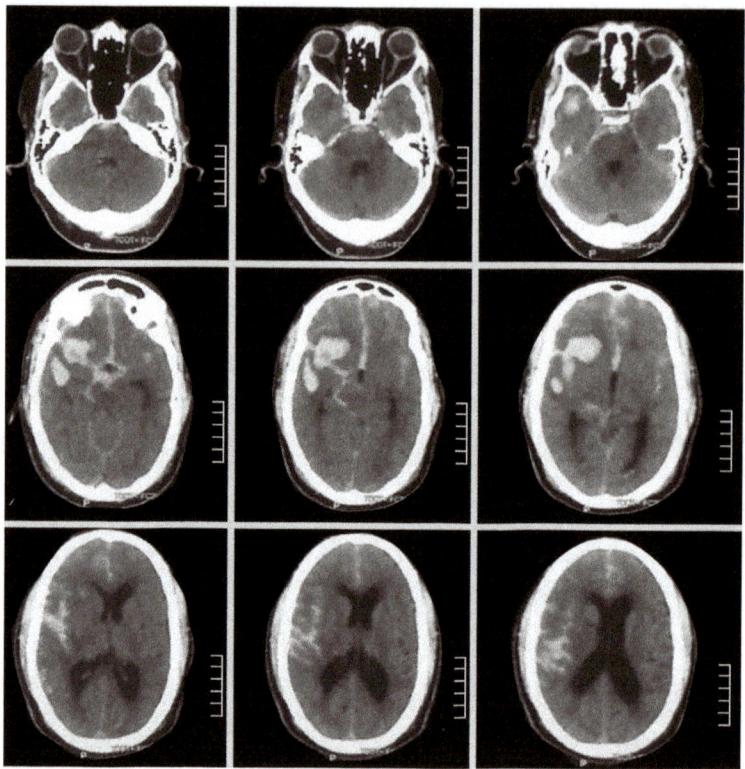

a. Mention the CT brain findings. *(1 mark)*
b. What drug is used to prevent cerebral vasospasm, mention dose and duration? *(3 marks)*
c. Discuss the risk factors for this condition. *(2 marks)*
d. Explain the surgical options for this patient. *(2 marks)*
e. Describe the grade used for assessing severity. *(2 marks)*

Q95. A 19-year-old female, was admitted with acute weakness of both LLs followed by upper limbs for 1 day. She had a H/O paresthesia in both feet prior to weakness. She had difficulty in swallowing with nasal regurgitation. Her weakness was preceded by acute gastroenteritis 1 week ago. On examination, she had bifacial and palatal weakness. Her gag reflex was sluggish and she had neck weakness too. Her single breath count was 14/min. She had symmetric, areflexic, hypotonic weakness in the upper limbs and two-fifths in the LLs. Her plantar reflexes were flexor and her sensory system examination was unremarkable.

a. What is the most probable clinical diagnosis? *(1 mark)*
b. What are CSF abnormalities in this condition? *(2 marks)*
c. Discuss the specific management. *(2 marks)*
d. Mention any two variants. *(2 marks)*
e. What are the nerve conduction abnormalities? *(3 marks)*

Q96. A 30-year-old male with fever, malaise, pain, and vesicular eruption for 5 days.

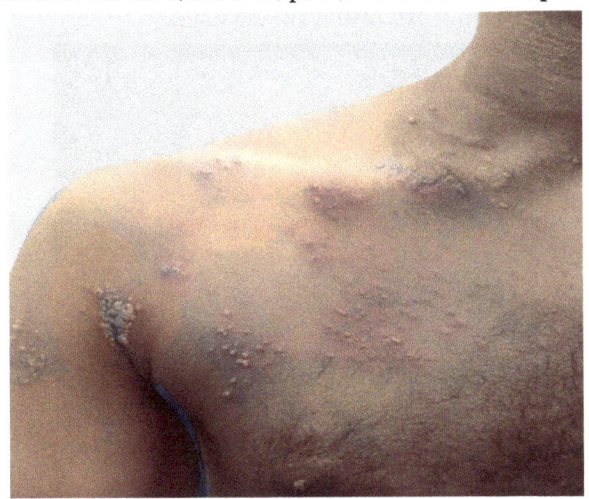

a. What is the diagnosis? (1 mark)
b. Discuss its pathophysiology. (2 marks)
c. Mention the drug used to treat with dose and duration. (3 marks)
d. The common complication and management. (2 marks)
e. Mention the preventive measures involved. (1 mark)
f. Discuss the risk factors for developing this condition. (2 marks)

Q97. An 83-year-old male with gait disturbance followed by urinary incontinence, and memory impairment for 2 years. His MRI of the brain is shown below.

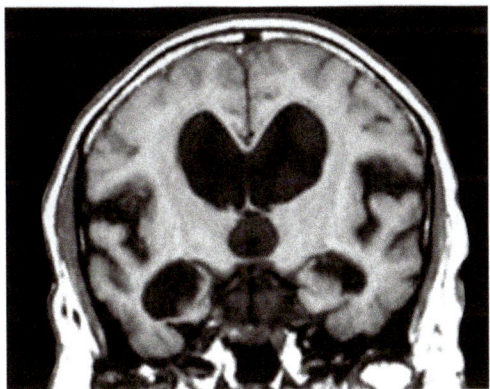

a. What is the diagnosis? (1 mark)
b. What type of gait disturbance is noticed in such patients? (2 marks)
c. What radiological findings help in diagnosis? (2 marks)
d. Discuss the management. (2 marks)
e. Discuss the factors suggesting unfavorable outcomes following shunt surgery. (2 marks)
f. Name of the triad seen in this condition. (1 mark)

Q98. A 45-year-old man with chronic progressive gait disturbance along with choreic movements and cognitive decline. His MRI is shown below.

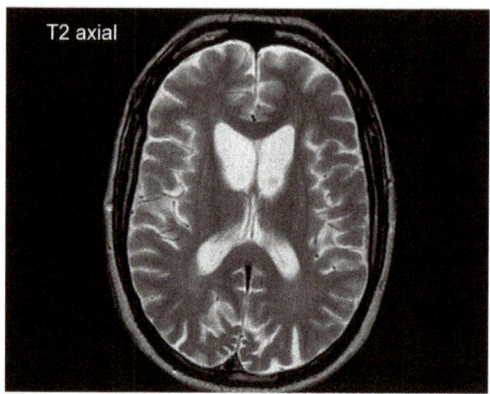

a. What is the probable diagnosis? (1 mark)
b. Is it genetic and if yes what is the mode of transmission? (2 marks)
c. Mention the MRI findings. (1 mark)
d. What is anticipation? (1 mark)
e. Discuss the pathophysiology. (2 marks)
f. Discuss the variant of this disease. (1 mark)
g. What is the management? (2 marks)

Q99. A 32-year-old female with subacute onset of behavioral disturbance with memory loss. Her FLAIR axial section MRI of the brain is shown below.

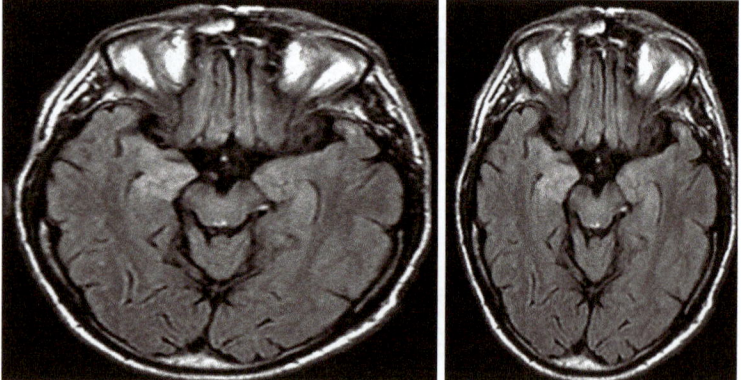

a. Mention the MRI findings. (1 mark)
b. Name two radiological differential diagnoses for this image. (2 marks)
c. What is the anatomical substrate behind episodic memory? (2 marks)
d. What semiology of seizure is expected if it arises from this involved structure? (3 marks)
e. What would be the EEG finding in case if the above patient is suffering from herpes simplex virus (HSV) encephalitis? (2 marks)

Neurology

Q100. A 27-year-old female was found in a comatose state in ER. She was on a poor diet plan with an intent to lose weight. She was found malnourished. Prior to developing this comatose state she had a fever for 10 days and drowsy sensorium which progressed to such a comatose state. Her MRI of the brain with contrast is shown below.

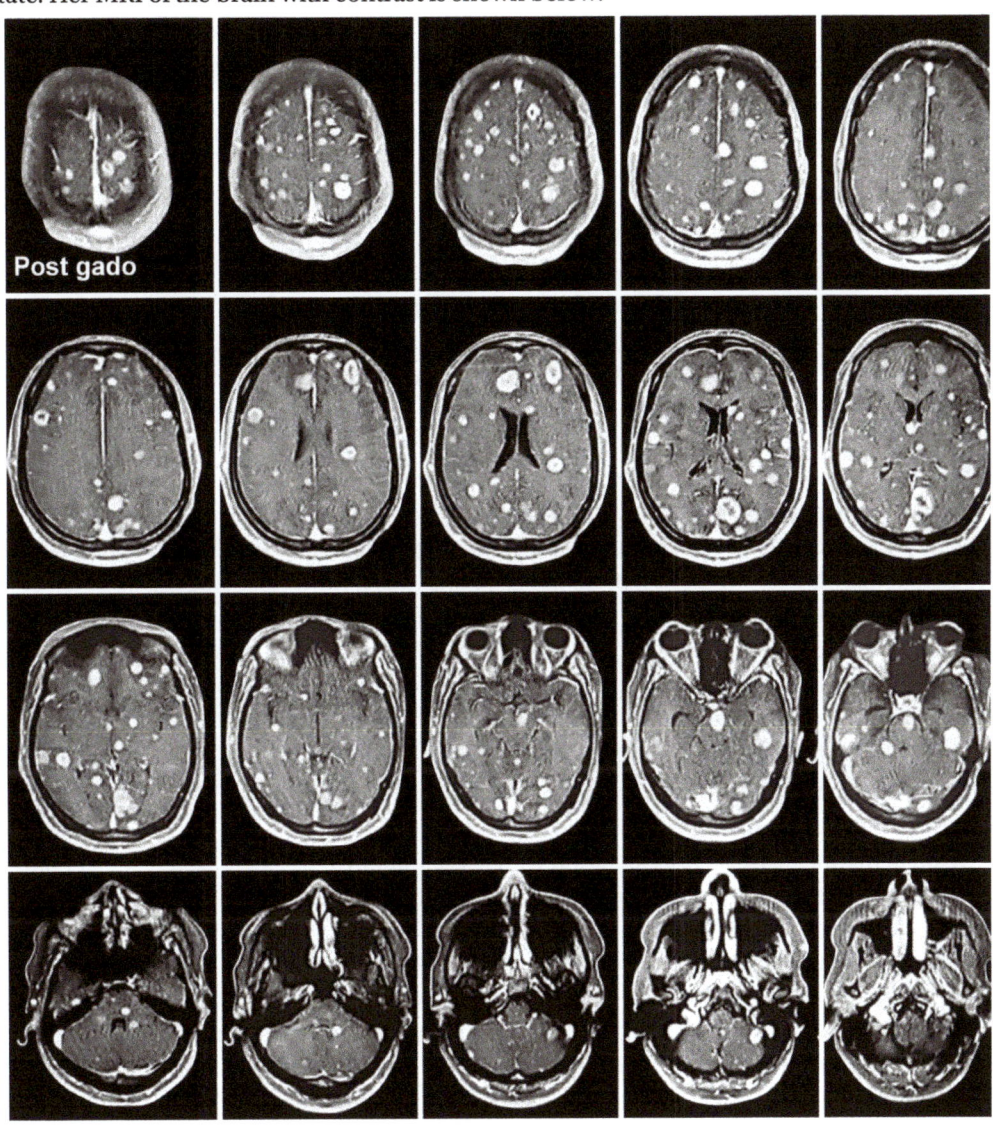

a. Name two radiological differential diagnoses for this patient. (2 marks)
b. What would be the duration of treatment in case of tuberculous etiology? (1 mark)
c. Mention three major clinical spectrums of CNS tuberculosis. (3 marks)
d. Mention the MR spectroscopy finding in tuberculoma. (2 marks)
e. Mention two major adverse effects of isoniazid. (2 marks)

Neurology

Q101. A 34-year-old male presented with unsteadiness while walking for 3 years, clumsiness of both upper limbs, and slurring of speech for 1 year. He is swaying to either side while walking akin to a drunkard and has difficulty in negotiating narrow pathways. It was not associated with worsening in the dark or walking on cotton wool sensation. He has difficulty in bringing a glass of water to the mouth, resulting in spillage of water, and smearing over the face with solid food particles. His speech is similar to that of a drunken person. Positive findings include bilateral gaze-evoked nystagmus, dysmetric saccades, broken pursuits, scanning dysarthria, and dysdiadochokinesia. Finger nose, finger-finger nose, and heel-shin tests were impaired bilaterally. He was not able to do tandem walking.

a. What is the involved neuroanatomical structure in this case? *(2 marks)*
b. Which part of the involved structure is predominantly affected by alcohol consumption? *(2 marks)*
c. Which part of the involved structure governs eye movements and body equilibrium during stance and gait? *(2 marks)*
d. Which part of the involved structure controls saccade and pursuit? *(2 marks)*
e. Name two drugs causing ataxia. *(2 marks)*

Q102. A 58-year-old man presented with weakness and thinning of both LLs for 3 years followed by weakness and thinning of both upper limbs for 2 years. He later developed difficulty in swallowing and started noticing twitches in his thighs and shoulders for 6 months. He was also emotionally labile. On examination, the gag reflex was diminished. Wasting and weakness of bilateral sternocleidomastoid and trapezius were noted. The tongue was atrophic, flaccid with fasciculations and movements were weak. Generalized wasting with hypotonia was observed. Asymmetric quadriparesis with hyperreflexia noted. The right plantar response was extensor.

a. What is the probable diagnosis? *(2 marks)*
b. What is pseudobulbar palsy? *(2 marks)*
c. Discuss its pathophysiology. *(2 marks)*
d. Describe the drugs used to treat this condition. *(2 marks)*
e. What dementia has a close association with this condition? *(1 mark)*
f. Name any one criteria used to diagnose this condition. *(1 mark)*

Q103. A 60-year-old farmer presented with a slowness of all activities of daily living for 1 year followed by difficulty in walking for 8 months in the form of problems in initiation of walking, sudden freezing while walking, and difficulty in turning while walking. The patient also experienced recurrent falls for the past 6 months. He falls backward especially while turning not associated with loss of consciousness. His speech became slow, low-volume, and monotonous. One of the key findings on examination is vertical gaze palsy with slowing of horizontal saccades. The patient had predominantly axial rigidity compared to appendicular rigidity.

a. What is the most probable diagnosis? *(2 marks)*
b. What are the red flag signs in this case that are suggestive of atypical parkinsonism? *(3 marks)*
c. Mention two named signs in this condition seen in an MRI of the brain. *(2 marks)*
d. What is the procerus sign? *(1 mark)*
e. Discuss its pathology. *(2 marks)*

Q104. A 67-year-old diabetic and hypertensive male who is a right-handed person presented with acute onset right homonymous hemianopia. His MRI (diffusion sequence) is shown below.

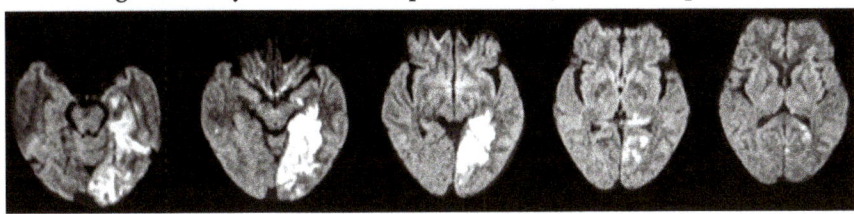

a. Discuss the MRI findings. (2 marks)
b. Which artery is involved? (2 marks)
c. Where is exner area located? Discuss its involvement. (2 marks)
d. Which site is involved in alexia with agraphia? (2 marks)
e. Which site is involved in alexia without agraphia? (2 marks)

Q105. A 23-year-old female in the immediate postpartum was brought to the intensive care unit (ICU) from the obstetrics and gynecology (OBG) ward with a H/O one episode of GTCS lasting 2 minutes with frothing and tongue bite. She gave birth to twin babies by lower segment cesarean section (LSCS) 14 hours earlier. Her vitals immediately after seizure pulse rate (PR)—84, respiratory rate (RR)—22, BP 140/90 mm Hg, S1 S2 heard, and lungs clear. The patient recovered from postictal confusion within 15 minutes and had transient blurred vision. Otherwise, no focal deficits. She already had received a loading dose of magnesium sulfate 4 g IV. She was on maintenance dose of MgSO$_4$ 1 g/h. She had a second episode of GTCS lasting <30 seconds 6 hours later. This time her BP was 150/90 mm Hg. Otherwise her vitals were within normal limits. She recovered within 10 minutes from postictal confusion. Labetalol 100 mg oral was started thrice daily along with an antiepileptic [levetiracetam 500 mg IV TDS]. MRI of the brain FLAIR sequence is shown below. There was no diffusion restriction.

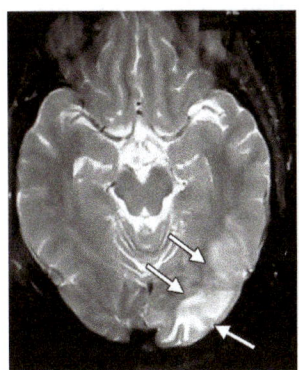 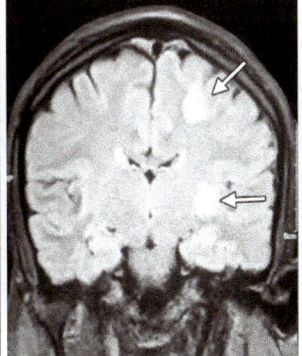 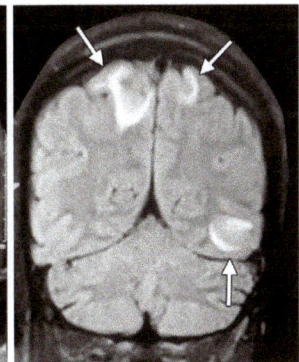

a. Discuss its diagnosis. (2 marks)
b. What is the management for it? (2 marks)
c. Enumerate the drugs causing this condition. (2 marks)
d. Is this condition reversible? (2 marks)
e. Discuss its pathophysiology. (2 marks)

Q106. A 19-year-old female presented with generalized body pain and swelling of all four extremities for 10 days. She had myalgia and fever for 3 days. She also had difficulty in getting up from the sitting position and difficulty in combing her hair. She had malar rash and flat red rash over the back of the fingers shown in the figures below. Uniform swelling of both upper and lower extremities that were tender on palpation was observed. Power was 2/5 in both R and L upper limbs (proximal > distal) whereas 4/5 in both R and L lower limbs (proximal > distal). Her CPK was 7026 U/L, LDH 2529 U/L, SGOT 1152 U/L and SGPT 439 U/L.

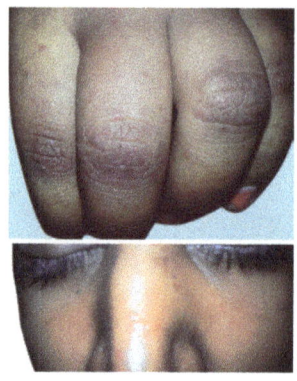

a. Name the skin lesions. *(2 marks)*
b. Describe its management. *(2 marks)*
c. Expalin the muscle biopsy findings. *(2 marks)*
d. Name the criteria used for the diagnosis. *(1 mark)*
e. Is cancer screening recommended in such patients? Explain. *(1 mark)*
f. Name two autoantibodies associated with this disease. *(2 marks)*

Q107. A 20-year-old college student presented with a change in personality for 4 months, followed by diminished vision and involuntary jerking of limbs periodically for the past 2 months. His sensorium progressively deteriorated and became bed-bound. He had a past H/O measles in childhood. His CSF showed lymphocytic pleocytosis without elevation of protein. His MRI and EEG are given below.

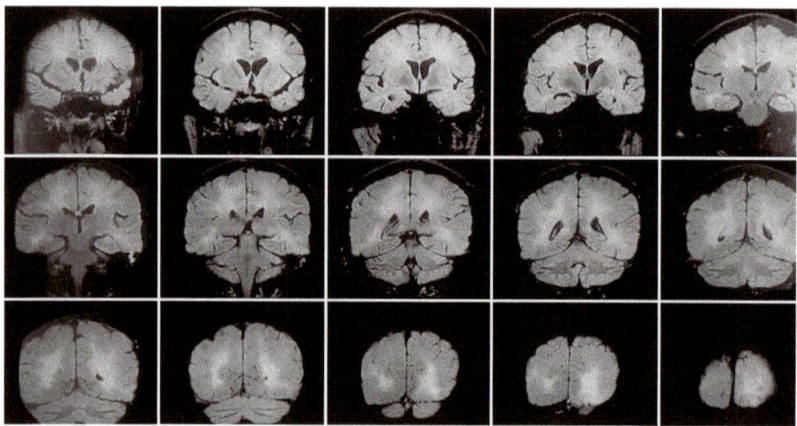

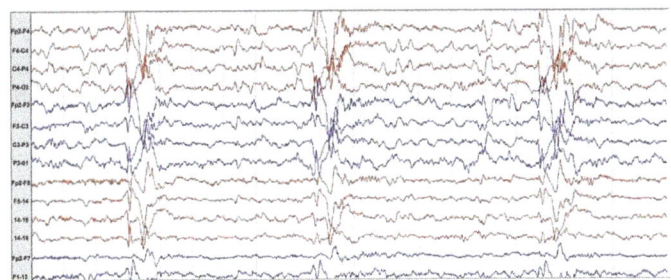

a. What is the most probable diagnosis? (2 marks)
b. Discuss the EEG finding. (2 marks)
c. What is the preventive measure? (1 mark)
d. Enumerate the management. (2 marks)
e. What is the name of the criteria used for the diagnosis? (1 mark)
f. Explain the stages of this disease. (2 marks)

Q108. A 60-year-old male patient with no other comorbid conditions presented with a sensation of tingling and numbness that began in the LLs around 1 year back, and gradually progressed to involve both the upper limbs as well. The patient experienced a cotton-wool sensation over his soles as he walked. The patient then developed a weakness in both his LLs 3 months back, with difficulty in using both his proximal and distal muscles, and was associated with stiffness of both LLs. Neurological examination revealed increased tone in both LLs, decreased power in both LLs, exaggerated knee jerks, and absent ankle jerks bilaterally, with bilateral extensor plantar reflexes. Additionally, abdominal, and cremasteric reflexes were absent. Sensory system examination revealed loss of fine touch, vibration and proprioception in both LLs and distal upper limbs, with decreased sensation in the abdomen and thorax as well. Pain and temperature sensations were relatively normal. Memory and other cognitive functions were normal. His peripheral smear and MRI spine are shown below.

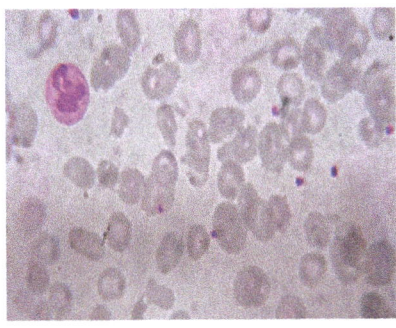
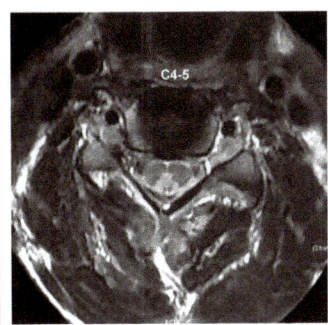

a. Discuss its diagnosis. (2 marks)
b. Explain the treatment for it. (2 marks)
c. Mention two settings to develop such a condition. (2 marks)
d. What is the peripheral smear finding? (2 marks)
e. Name the radiological sign in the MRI spine. (1 mark)

Q109. A 50-year-old male presented with sharp lancinating pain over his right face for the past 2 years. The pain lasts a few seconds and he could not tolerate the pain. The pain gets triggered whenever he is exposed to cold air, chewing or laughing. The painful episodes occur multiple times a day and no response to analgesics.
a. Discuss its diagnosis. (2 marks)
b. Explain the medical treatment for it. (2 marks)
c. What is its surgical treatment? (2 marks)
d. Discuss its pathophysiology. (2 marks)
e. What neurological examination abnormality is expected in these patients? (1 mark)
f. Out of the three subdivisions of trigeminal sensory nerves which of them is commonly affected by this condition? (1 mark)

Q110. A 50-year-old presented with new-onset seizures which were focal in nature; three to four episodes in 1 week each episode lasting <5 minutes with full recovery of sensorium. Her EEG and MRI with contrast were normal. She was started on carbamazepine and discharged. She developed behavioral changes and psychoses subsequently. 1 month later she had a GTCS episode lasting 15 minutes and landed in ER.
a. What would be the first step in managing this patient? (2 marks)
b. What is the first-line drug to be used? (2 marks)
c. Name any two second-line drugs for this patient. (2 marks)
d. What anesthetic agents can be used if seizures are refractory? (2 marks)
e. What is super refractory status epilepticus?

Q111. A 22-year-old female presented with high-grade fever for 5 days and drowsiness for 2 days. On examination, she was drowsy but was able to obey simple motor commands. She had no neck rigidity. She was treated empirically with acute encephalitis syndrome. Her MRI of the brain diffusion sequence is shown below. A CSF smear showed mononuclear cells. CSF protein was 50 mg/dL and glucose was 75 mg/dL.

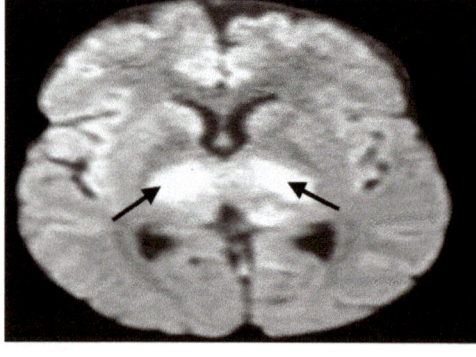
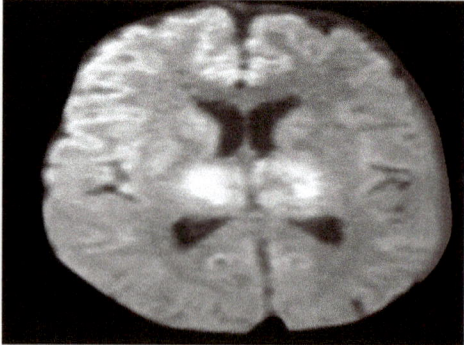

a. Mention two radiological differential diagnoses for this patient. (2 marks)
b. Mention two common viruses causing encephalitis in India. (2 marks)
c. Mention the blood supply for the involved structure. (3 marks)
d. What is the prevention of Japanese encephalitis? (3 marks)

Q112. A 50-year-old myasthenia gravis patient was admitted for respiratory distress and swallowing difficulty. He was diagnosed to have myasthenic crisis and planned for intravenous immunoglobulin (IVIG) therapy.
a. What is the usual dosage for an adult? *(2 marks)*
b. How to differentiate cholinergic crisis from myasthenic crisis? *(2 marks)*
c. What is the alternative treatment in patients with myasthenic crisis apart from IVIG? *(2 marks)*
d. Mention two complications of IVIG. *(2 marks)*
e. Mention two monoclonal antibodies that can be used in myasthenia gravis. *(2 marks)*

Q113. A 40-year-old male presented with unilateral headache, tearing, and redness of the eye. He becomes agitated during the headache due to severe pain. The headache has recurred daily at 5 PM for the past 4 weeks. He had a similar episode of headaches last year. The headache lasts on average for 40 minutes. There is a poor response to nonsteroidal anti-inflammatory drugs (NSAIDs) but the headache subsided after inhalation of oxygen 15 L/min.
a. What is the diagnosis? *(2 marks)*
b. In whom this headache is common; male or female? *(1 mark)*
c. Mention one secondary cause of this type of headache. *(2 marks)*
d. Mention prophylaxis to prevent such headaches. *(2 marks)*
e. Mention three to four other trigeminal autonomic cephalalgias. *(3 marks)*

Q114. A 70-year-old diabetic and hypertensive individual presented with quadriparesis and dysarthria. On examination, he had tongue weakness and flaccid quadriparesis with bilateral extensor plantar reflexes. He also had bilateral horizontal nystagmus. His MRI is shown below.

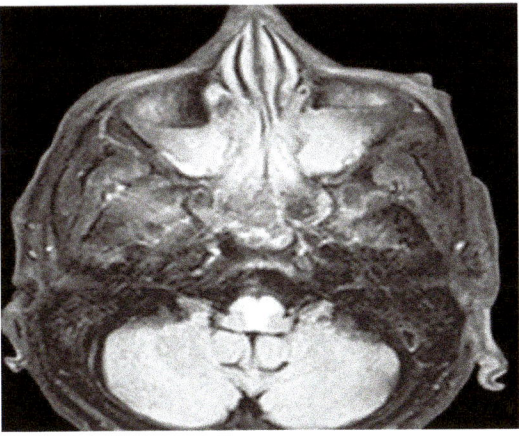
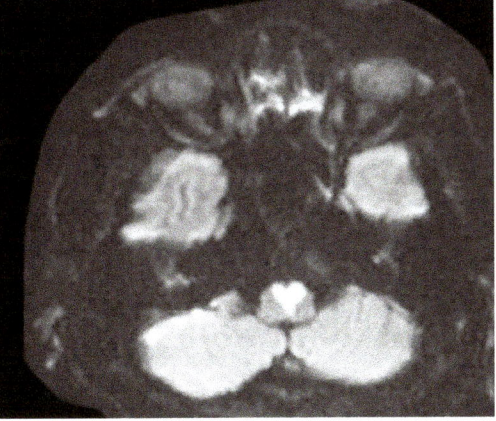

a. Discuss the MRI findings. *(2 marks)*
b. Mention four structures located in the involved structure. *(4 marks)*
c. What is area postrema syndrome (APS)? *(2 marks)*
d. Explain the function of the nucleus tractus solitaries. *(2 marks)*

Q115. A 27-year-old male presented to the OPD with insidious onset, progressive, difficulty in walking and climbing stairs from the age of 9 years. At present, he can walk only a few steps with support and cannot get up from a sitting position. He also had difficulty in raising his hands above the shoulder and in gripping objects for the past 1 year. He had no associated sensory or cranial nerve disturbances. He was the elder of two siblings born of second-degree consanguineous parents. A three-generation pedigree analysis showed no similar complaints. Motor system examination showed atrophic muscle groups, hypotonia, and hyporeflexia in the lower extremities. Gower's sign was present. Power in the proximal and mid groups of the LL was MRC grade 3 on both sides while it was MRC grade 2 in the distal groups in the LLs. His upper limb examination revealed atrophic muscle groups, hypotonia and hyporeflexia with power of MRC grade 4 in the proximal muscles and MRC grade 3 in the distal groups. The remaining neurological examination was within limits.

a. What group of muscle diseases would you classify this patient? (2 marks)
b. What test is to be done for this patient to confirm diagnosis? (2 marks)
c. Expalin the role of dystrophin protein in muscle. (2 marks)
d. What is Gower's sign? (2 marks)
e. What group of muscle diseases present with episodic weakness and rhabdomyolysis? (2 marks)

Q116. A 52-year-old male with comorbidities of HTN and diabetes on irregular treatment presented with acute onset of focal deficit in the form of right upper limb and LL weakness, slurred speech, and right facial droop since 10 AM today morning. He came to you within 3 hours of the onset of the deficit.

a. What are two investigations that are needed to thrombolyse this patient? (2 marks)
b. What is the current time window for thrombolysis? (2 marks)
c. What should be the BP and blood glucose levels prior to thrombolysis? (2 marks)
d. What scale is commonly used for measuring neurological deficits in stroke? (1 mark)
e. What was the symptomatic intracranial hemorrhage risk in thrombolysis using recombinant tissue plasminogen activator (rtPA) in the NINDS (National Institute of Neurological Disorders and Stroke) trial? (1 mark)
f. How will you treat large vessel occlusion (LVO)? (2 marks)

Q117. A 24-year-old female presents with new-onset headaches that have occured mostly at night or in the early morning for the past 2 months. These involve dull frontal and occipital pain with associated tinnitus. She also had brief periods of blacked-out vision lasting a few seconds whenever she changed her posture. Her physical examination demonstrates bilateral papilledema. MRI of her brain is normal. CSF protein, sugar, cell count, cytology, gram stain, and acid–fast bacteria (AFB) stain were unremarkable.

a. What is the most probable diagnosis? (2 marks)
b. What CSF abnormality is expected? (2 marks)
c. What are the management options? (2 marks)
d. What cranial nerve palsy can occur due to this condition? (2 marks)
e. Mention two side effects of acetazolamide. (2 marks)

Q118. A 14-year-old girl developed neck pain, radiating to her right hand, aggravated with the movement of head and shoulder, and relieved by taking rest for a month. She also had difficulty in walking because of a stiff type of proximal weakness of both LLs and occasional tripping. A general physical examination revealed gibbus at the cervical level with anterocollis; however, she had no spinal tenderness. On examination, of the nervous system, she had spastic quadriparesis in the MRC grade of four-fifths in all four limbs with exaggerated deep tendon reflexes and bilateral extensor plantar. CT of the thorax showed mediastinal and hilar lymphadenopathy. Her MRI of the spine is given below.

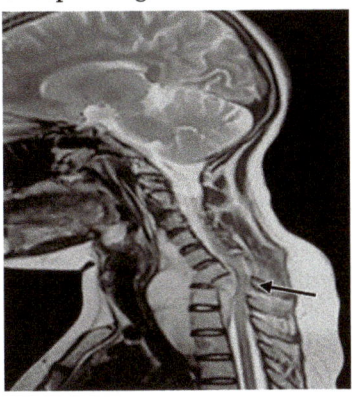

a. What are the MRI findings? (2 marks)
b. Which is the most common organism producing such a clinical condition? (1 mark)
c. What is a cold abscess? (2 marks)
d. Mention two radiological differential diagnoses. (2 marks)
e. What is the mechanism of gibbus? (3 marks)

Q119. A primigravida with severe postpartum hemorrhage went into shock, remained drowsy, and failed to produce breast milk in the puerperium. Her cortisol and prolactin levels were also low. After replacing corticosteroids her clinical condition improved. Her MRI FLAIR sequences are given below.

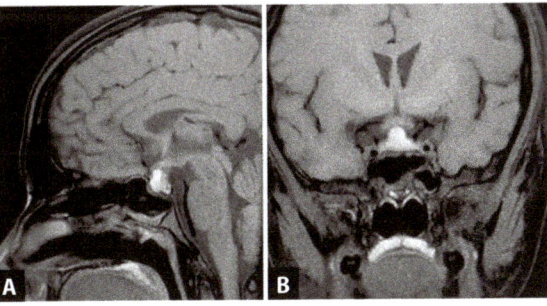

a. What are the MRI findings? (2 marks)
b. What is pathomechanism? (3 marks)
c. Explain its management. (3 marks)
d. Which is the most common initial symptom of this disease? (2 marks)

ANSWERS

Ans. 1

a. Myeloneuropathy
b. Vitamin B12 deficiency (subacute combined degeneration of cord), paraneoplastic syndrome, Sjögren's syndrome, and neurosyphilis
c. MRI spine, Vitamin B12 levels, antineuronal antibody 1, and venereal disease research laboratory (VDRL) test

Ans. 2

a. CT scan with contrast showing multiple rings enhancing lesions.
b. Cerebral toxoplasmosis (HIV, neurosymptoms, and multiple brain lesions with ring enhancement).
c. General imaging differential considerations include:
   - Primary CNS lymphoma
   - Cerebral metastases
   - Other infections:
     - CNS tuberculoma
     - CNS cryptococcosis
     - Bacterial abscesses
     - Neurocysticercosis
d. *Management:* Sulfadiazine and pyrimethamine

Ans. 3

a. There is edema of VII cranial (facial) nerve. Facial nerve changes are widespread but most severe in the narrow labyrinthine segment where edema causes compression and the tenuous blood supply worsens the damage.
b. Differential diagnosis: Herpes zoster infection, Lyme disease, otitis media, Guillain–Barré syndrome (GBS), HIV infection, sarcoidosis, and Sjögren's disease
c. (1) Oral prednisolone (within 3 days × 7 days), (2) Oral acyclovir or valacyclovir for severe symptoms, and (3) eye care

Ans. 4

Deviation of lips to right side suggesting Bell's palsy along with puffiness of eyes with conjunctival erythema.

Ans. 5

a. Hypertensive intracranial hemorrhage.
b. Putamen
c. For prognostication:

Score	Predicted mortality %
5+	100
4	97
3	72
2	27
1	13
0	0

d. BP control/mannitol/evacuation.

Ans. 6

a. Cerebral venous thrombosis (CVT)
b. Risk factors for thrombosis are prothrombotic conditions, obesity, oral contraceptives, and pregnancy or the puerperium along with malignancy, infection, head injury, and mechanical precipitants.
c. Anticoagulation—heparin/warfarin/management of raised intracranial temperature (ICT)

Ans. 7

a. Ice pack test—reversibility of ptosis
b. Myasthenia gravis
c. Anti-AchR/anti-MuSK/anti-LRP4
d. Osserman system:

Class	Symptoms
I	Only ocular involvement
IIa	Generalized muscle involvement without pulmonary involvement
IIb	Bulbar manifestation
III	Rapid progression of generalized bulbar disease and weakness in respiratory muscles
IV	Class 1 or 2 patients presenting progressive symptoms within 2 years

Ans. 8

a. CNS toxoplasmosis; *Toxoplasma gondii*
b. Cryptococcal meningitis, CNS lymphoma, and progressive multifocal leukoencephalopathy
c. Pyrimethamine, sulfadiazine, and spiramycin (in pregnancy)
d. Treatment failure refers to loss of antiviral efficacy to the current regimen criteria:
   - Plasma viral load >1,000 copies/mL at or after 6 months of art with >95% adherence
   - CD4 count at 250 cells/mm^3 following clinical failure or persistent CD4 count below 100 cells/mm^3
   - New or recurrent WHO stage 3 or 4 conditions while on treatment

Ans. 9

a. Subdural hematoma (SDH)
b. Rupture of cortical bridging veins

Ans. 10

a. Large vessel thrombosis, lacunar stroke, and hypercoagulable states
b. Todd's paresis and hemiplegic migraine
c. IV thrombolysis, rtPA
d. - *Indications:* Onset of symptoms to drug administration <4.5 hours and CT showing absence of hemorrhage
   - *Contraindications:* Sustained BP >185/110 mm Hg despite treatment, platelet count <100,000/μL, and HCT <25%

Ans. 11

a. Alzheimer's dementia
b. MRI brain or PET scan
c. Donepezil and memantine
d. Alzheimer's disease, Parkinson's disease, and multi-infarct dementia
e. Thiamine, B12, and niacin

Ans. 12

a. The best description of the pupillary abnormality observed in this 26-year-old woman is "Adie's tonic pupil".
b. Adie's tonic pupil is characterized by an enlarged pupil (usually unilateral) that reacts poorly or sluggishly to light but does constrict when the patient focuses on a near object (accommodation). This pupillary abnormality is often associated with a decreased or absent deep tendon reflex (hyporeflexia or areflexia), particularly in the Achilles tendon (known as Holmes-Adie syndrome when both features are present).
c. The underlying cause of Adie's tonic pupil is usually damage or dysfunction of the ciliary ganglion or the postganglionic fibers of the oculomotor nerve (cranial nerve III). This condition is typically benign and may be idiopathic or associated with viral infections or other neurological conditions.

Ans. 13

a. Reversible cerebral vasoconstriction syndrome (RCVS) is characterized by multifocal arterial constriction and dilation in the cerebral vasculature and may be linked to nonaneurysmal subarachnoid hemorrhage.
b. The diagnosis of RCVS relies on the radiological evidence of vasospasm seen on cerebral angiogram features.
c. In comparison to patients with primary angiitis of the central nervous system (PACNS), those with RCVS are typically younger and predominantly female, with a 2.6-fold higher percentage. Additionally, identifiable triggers, such as medications, illicit drugs, or physiological stress are commonly associated with RCVS, while triggers are rarely identified in PACNS patients.
d. Calcium channel blocker nimodipine

Ans. 14

a. Fahr syndrome
b. Basal ganglia, hippocampus, dentate nucleus (DN), cerebral cortex, and cerebellar subcortical white matter
c. No definite treatment but managed like other neurodegenerative disorder depending on clinical manifestations.
d. Hypo- and pseudohypoparathyroidism, mitochondrial myopathy [mitochondrial encephalomyopathy, lactic acidosis and stroke-like episodes (MELAS)], infection (intrauterine/perinatal), and infections [cytomegalovirus (CMV), rubella, herpes, toxoplasma, neurocysticercosis (NCC)].

Ans. 15

a. Muscle wasting of distal hand muscles
b. Weakness of abductors, extensors, external rotators of arm and extensors of wrist, spasticity of muscles, increased deep tendon reflexes, fasciculations present in upper limbs and weakness of internal rotators, and flexors of knee and hip
c. Motor neuron disease and cervical myelopathy

Ans. 16

a. Image A: In primary position of gaze, the eyes appear normal. Image B: Horizontal gaze to the left is intact. Image C: On attempted horizontal gaze to the right, the left eye fails to adduct.
b. Left internuclear ophthalmoplegia
c. Left medial longitudinal fasciculus

Ans. 17

a. Seizure disorder
b. EEG with stimulation will show epileptic spikes
c. MRI brain with contrast

Ans. 18

a. Parkinsonism
b. Shuffling/festinating gait
c. L-Dopa

Ans. 19

a. Flexion contracture of right middle finger with tread-like band seen on the palm extending proximally from the base of the middle finger
b. Dupuytren contracture
c. Familial, diabetes, smoking tobacco, alcohol, and occupational
d. There is no exact cure for Dupuytren contracture. Surgical interventions, such as fasciectomy, needle fasciectomy, or dermafasciectomy may be helpful. Treatments can relieve symptoms and slow the progression.

Ans. 20

a. Intracerebral bleed with interventricular extension
b. Contraindications to thrombolytic therapy include prior intracerebral hemorrhage and ischemic stroke <3 months
c. Indications for thrombolytic therapy include diagnosis of acute ischemic stroke causing significant neurodeficit and age >18 years and presenting within <4.5 hours from onset of symptoms.

Ans. 21

a. Horner syndrome
b. Ptosis, miosis, and facial anhidrosis

Ans. 22

a. This is a NCCT of brain showing bilateral multiple calcific foci involving both cerebral hemisphere and more importantly bilateral basal ganglia (caudate nucleus and lentiform nucleus).
b. With the provided clinical H/O seizures and cognitive impairment and a positive family history, the provisional diagnosis is *Fahr's disease/bilateral striopallidodentate calcinosis/ primary familial brain calcification/calcinosis nucleorum.*
c. In order to label the case as Fahr's disease, secondary cause of bilateral basal ganglia calcification should be evaluated and ruled out (Fahr's syndrome). Secondary cause includes evaluation for blood and urine heavy metal levels, endocrine cause of hypercalcemia, and CSF analysis for infections.
d. Genes involved—*SLC20A2, PDGFB, PDGFRB,* and *XPR1*

Ans. 23

a. This is a MRI of dorsal lumbar (DL) spine with screening of whole spine compression showing compression collapse of D10-D11 vertebrae with cord compression at that level.
b. From the history as patient was a known c/o prior PTB with recent onset paraparesis due to involvement of D10-D11 vertebrae leading to compression of the cord, so our provisional diagnosis is *Pott's paraplegia* (involves classically lower thoracic and upper lumbar vertebrae)
c. *Management:* ATD as per National Tuberculosis Elimination Program (NTEP) protocol, surgical decompression, and physiotherapy.

Ans. 24

a. This is MRI brain sagittal section showing the pathological finding of midbrain atrophy, whereas the other brain stem structures are preserved giving the appearance of a humming bird so known as Humming bird sign.
b. From the history, the patient is having more predominant sign of postural instability and dementia and with the given MRI finding this is a case of progressive supranuclear palsy (PSP). PSP classically presents as H/O repeated falls on attempted downgaze and dementia so hence a member of atypical Parkinsonism. Other diseases included in this group are Lewy body dementia, multiple system atrophy, and corticobasilar degeneration.

Ans. 25

a. The NCCT brain shows ill-defined hypodensities in bilateral occipital areas and with the given clinical history it is suggestive of (s/o) *posterior reversible encephalopathy syndrome (PRES)*.
b. This is a case of PRES as evidenced by headache, vomiting, and seizures with underlying elevated BP in a case of SLE with suspected nephritis. Causes leading to PRES are eclampsia/preeclampsia, sickle cell disease, autoimmune disease, post organ transplant, and hemolytic uremic syndrome. On controlling BP and the underlying disease, the process is reversible. (*NB*: This can also be confused with neuropsychiatric manifestation of SLE but that will not present with such CT brain changes). MRI changes of the above case:

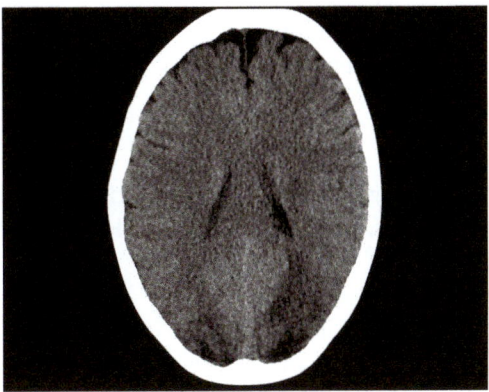

Ans. 26

a. This is a CECT scan of brain evidenced by blood vessels within the brain parenchyma showing contrast uptake with a hypodense lesion (triangular in shape) at the midpoint in the occipital region s/o cortical vein thrombus and the sign is known as "empty delta sign".
b. This is a case of *cortical venous sinus thrombosis* evidenced by H/O headache, with projectile vomiting and blurring of vision and prolonged H/O OCP intake and empty delta sign on CECT brain.
c. Management: Subcutaneous (S/C) low-molecular-weight heparin (LMWH) or IV heparin (anticoagulants should not be stopped even if venous bleed is present)

Ans. 27

a. Normal pressure hydrocephalus
b. Ataxia, dementia, and urinary incontinence (Adam's triad or Hakim's triad)
c. Boxcarring
d. Alzheimer's disease, Parkinson's disease with dementia, frontotemporal dementia, and Lewy body dementia.

Ans. 28

a. Bilateral basal ganglia calcification
b. Round face, obesity, short stature, brachydactyly, and mental impairment
c. Pseudohypoparathyroidism type 1A

Ans. 29

a. Face appeared hatchet shaped with bilateral ptosis along with visible atrophy of masseter and temporalis muscles
b. Myotonic dystrophy
c. EMG of distal extremity muscles revealed myotonic discharges with a waxing and waning frequency and a characteristic "engine revving" sound

Ans. 30

a. Hyperdense lesion spotted in right parietal cortex with penumbra, with hypodense lesion in the entire middle cerebral artery (MCA) territory of right hemisphere
b. Hemorrhagic conversion of right MCA territory infarct
c. Reverse anticoagulation, withhold antiplatelet agents, intracranial pressure (ICP) control measures, and supportive management

Ans. 31

a. Stevens-Johnson syndrome
b. Carbamazepine, phenytoin, phenobarbitone, and lamotrigine—most common antiepileptics
c. *Antimicrobials:* Sulfonamides, beta-lactams, quinolones; NSAIDs (paracetamol and oxicam), and allopurinol
d. Further management:
   - Cessation of the suspected causative drug(s)
   - Hospital admission: Preferably to an intensive care unit
   - Fluid replacement (crystalloid)
   - Nutritional assessment: May require nasogastric tube feeding
   - Temperature control: Warm environment
   - Pain relief
   - Sterile/aseptic handling
   - Use of topical anesthetics and nonadherent dressings

Ans. 32

a. Active euthanasia
b. No
c. No. DNR applies to only performing cardiopulmonary resuscitation (CPR) and other interventions to revive in case of cardiorespiratory arrest
d. Immobility, instability (falls), incontinence, and impaired intellect (memory)
e. National Programme for the Health Care for the Elderly: National Policy for Older Persons and Indira Gandhi National Old Age Pension Scheme

Ans. 33

a. Ocular telangiectasia
b. - Ataxia telangiectasia
   - Hereditary hemorrhagic telangiectasia/Osler-Weber-Rendu syndrome
   - Bloom syndrome
   - Generalized essential telangiectasia
c. Ataxia telangiectasia

d. • Abnormalities of the immune system—immunoglobulin A (IgA) deficiency
   • Increased sensitivity to radiation
   • Increased susceptibility to cancer
   • Ocular motor apraxia, strabismus, and nystagmus

Ans. 34

a. Kayser–Fleischer (KF) ring
b. • Wilson disease
   • Primary biliary cholangitis
   • Children with neonatal cholestasis
c. Wilson disease
d. • Hepatitis and cirrhosis
   • Hemolytic anemia and thrombocytopenia
   • Cataract
   • Arthralgia, arthritis, osteomalacia
   • Psychosis
e. Leipzig score

Ans. 35

a. Tendon xanthoma
b. • Familial hypercholesterolemia
   • Cerebrotendinous xanthomatosis
   • Drug induced-isotretinoin, estrogens, cyclosporine, and antiretroviral therapy.
   • Hyper-β-sitosterolemia
c. Cerebrotendinous xanthomatosis
d. • Childhood-onset cataract
   • Intractable diarrhea
   • Severe premature atherosclerosis
   • Total body bone mineral density will be low and intestinal calcium absorption will be decreased.

Ans. 36

a. Shingles or herpetic vesicles of herpes zoster
b. Ramsay Hunt syndrome
c. • Shingrix—recombinant zoster vaccine
   • Given as two doses 2–6 months apart
   • For individuals of age >50 years who have had past H/O varicella zoster.
d. Right pons

Ans. 37

a. Guillain–Barré syndrome
b. Acute inflammatory demyelinating polyneuropathy (AIDP)
c. IV immunoglobulin 0.4 g/kg/day for 5 days
d. Prolonged or absent F wave latency
e. *Campylobacter jejuni*

Ans. 38

a.
- Chvostek sign
- Trousseau sign

b. Post-thyroidectomy hypocalcemia—probably due to transient damage to parathyroid gland or permanent devascularization to parathyroid gland.

c. Hyperexcitability of the muscle by subthreshold electrical stimulus

Ans. 39

a. Beevor sign is an *abnormal upward (cephalad) umbilicus movement upon truncal flexion* while the patient is in a supine position

b. T10 spinal level lesion

c. Facioscapulohumeral muscular dystrophy (FSHD)

Ans. 40

a. Hung-up knee reflex
b. Huntington's chorea
c. Hypothyroidism
d. Autosomal dominant
e. Caudate nucleus

Ans. 41

a. Trigeminal neuralgia
b. Superior cerebellar artery
c. Carbamazepine
d. Microvascular decompression by suboccipital craniotomy

Ans. 42

a. Lhermitte's sign
b. McArdle sign—greater than 10% neck flexion-induced reduction in strength of muscles of limbs.
c. Multiple sclerosis
d. Mcdonald criteria

Ans. 43

a. Anisocoria
b. Pancoast tumor of right side
c. Cranial nerve three palsy
d. Anti-Hu antibody—causes paraneoplastic sensory-motor neuronopathy and encephalitis. Most common malignancy causing anti-Hu antibody is small-cell lung cancer

Ans. 44

a. *Cavernous sinus thrombosis:* Pain and redness of lest eye. External ophthalmoplegia suggestive of involvement of cranial nerve III, IV, and VI. Numbness of left side of face present suggestive of involvement of maxillary division of trigeminal nerve. Visual acuity was not lost suggestive of sparing of optic nerve.

b. Probably invading fungal sinusitis—mucormycosis (feature of orbital cellulitis with black discoloration in hard palate)
c. In orbital apex syndrome, optic nerve is affected causing relative afferent pupillary defect (RAPD) or blindness. While in superior orbital fissure and cavernous sinus syndrome optic nerve is spared.
d. • *Ophthalmic nerve (V1):* Superior orbital fissure
   • *Maxillary nerve (V2):* Foramen rotundum
   • *Mandibular nerve (V3):* Foramen ovale

Ans. 45
a. Crossing fibers of lateral spinothalamic tract is affected with sparing of dorsal column tracts.
b. Position and vibration sensations being carried by dorsal column tract is affected here.
c. The localization is intramedullary, probably due to the expansion of central canal causing damage of the crossing lateral spinothalamic tracts, at the level of C3 to T2. Probably syringomyelia.
d. Loss of position and vibration sensations bilaterally involving the upper limbs and neck, the site of lesion in the dorsal column tract could be crossing of medial meniscus at the cardiovascular (CV) junction

Ans. 46
a. Palatal myoclonus/palatal tremor
b. Dentato-rubro-olivary pathway (aka Guillain-Mollaret triangle consists of three nuclei)
   • *Ipsilateral* red nucleus (RN)
   • Ipsilateral inferior olivary nucleus (ION)
   • Contralateral cerebellar DN
c. Most common lesion is cerebrovascular accidents (CVAs)

Ans. 47
a. Downbeating nystagmus
b. CV junction/pontomedullary junction

Ans. 48
a. Bruns nystagmus
b. Right cerebellopontine angle (Bruns nystagmus is seen in cerebellopontine angle tumors)
c. Right cerebellopontine angle (the slow and high-amplitude component of Bruns nystagmus suggests the side of lesion)
d. Absent corneal reflex/absent conjunctival reflex due to involvement of spinal nucleus of trigeminal nerve
e. Vestibular schwannomas are associated with neurofibromatosis type 2

Ans. 49
a. Temporal arteritis/cranial arteritis/giant cell arteritis
b. • Erythrocyte sedimentation rate/C-reactive protein (ESR/CRP)
   • Biopsy of temporal artery

c. *Steroids:* Prednisolone 1 mg/kg/day. To be started at the earliest if you suspect clinically. Do not wait for the biopsy report.
d. Since temporal arteritis is patchy granulomatous depositions, there are high chances of missing the lesion. Therefore, at least 4–7 cm of arterial biopsy should be taken to avoid false-negative results.

Ans. 50

a. Left palatal lesion which does not cross the midline—probably infarct
b. In the back ground of diabetes mellitus and palatal lesion, it could be mucormycosis
c. All invasive mucormycosis should be surgically debrided whenever possible to improve the penetration of the antifungal given
d. Liposomal amphotericin B 5–10 mg/kg/day IV

Ans. 51

a. Juvenile myoclonic epilepsy (JME) (characterized by myoclonic jerks in teenage)
b. Sodium valproic acid
c. Avoid sodium valproic acid due to the teratogenic potential of the drug. We use levetiracetam/zonisamide/lamotrigine in child-bearing age group.
d. Sodium channel blockers like carbamazepine/oxcarbamazepine/phenytoin are avoided as they exacerbate myoclonic and absence seizures (but, they can be useful for the treatment of GTCSs in JME)

Ans. 52

a. The hyperdense MCA sign, also called Gács sign, is characterized by focal hyperdensity in the MCA on noncontrast brain CT. This sign directly visualizes thromboembolic material within the MCA lumen, making it the earliest visible indication of MCA infarction, typically observed within 90 minutes after the event. It is the longitudinal counterpart to the MCA dot sign and hyperdense basilar tip sign.
b. Acute CVA involving left MCA territory
c. Emergency IV thrombolysis
d.
   - ASPECTS. 1 point is deducted from the initial score of 10 for every region involved in MCA territory.
   - It is a CT score used for MCA territory infarct to predict the outcome following IV thrombolysis.
   - An ASPECTS ≤7 predicts a worse functional outcome at 3 months and high incidence of intracranial hemorrhage

Ans. 53

a. Wernicke encephalopathy—ataxia and ophthalmoplegia. MRI showing symmetric T2/FLAIR increased signal intensity in the mammillary body
b. History of hyperemesis
c.
   - Chronic alcoholism
   - Malnutrition
   - Any other causes of vitamin B1 deficiency
d. IV thiamine

Ans. 54

a. There is long segment T2 hyperintensity involving the cervical spine suggestive of LETM
b. Neuromyelitis optica spectrum disorder (NMOSD)
c. Area postrema
d. Anti-aquaporin-4 immunoglobulin G (AQP4 IgG) antibody will be positive in serum.
e. Cross reactivity between the astrocyte water channel aquaporin-4 in human brain and ABC transporter permease protein in bacteria *Clostridium perfringens*

Ans. 55

a. Diffusion-weighted image
b. Watershed infarct left anterior cerebral artery (ACA) territory
c. CT angiogram of carotid/Doppler of carotid

Ans. 56

a. Quadriplegia, lower cranial nerve palsy, mutism with preservation of consciousness, presence of only vertical gaze, and upper eye lid movement
b. Pons
c.

Cause	Mechanism
Ischemic	Basilar artery occlusion, hypotensive, or hypoxic events
Hemorrhage	Hemorrhage originating within or infiltrating into the pons
Traumatic	Direct brain stem contusion or vertebrobasilar axis dissection
Tumor	Primary or secondary infiltration of the ventral pons
Metabolic	Central pontine myelinolysis following rapid correction of hyponatremia
Demyelination	Multiple sclerosis affecting the ventral pons
Infectious	Abscess infiltrating the ventral pons and brain stem encephalitis

Ans. 57

a. Gyratory seizures are identified by the rotation of the torso by a minimum of 180° around the horizontal body axis with or without a preceding forced head version.
b. The ictal focus in gyratory seizures is usually in the frontal or temporal lobe, contralateral to head version and ipsilateral to "en bloc" body rotation without head version.
c. Anti-N-methyl-d-aspartate receptor (anti-NMDAR) antibody can be positive if the cause if autoimmune encephalitis.

Ans. 58

a. Spinal Dural arteriovenous (AV) fistula
b. Spinal digital subtraction angiography (DSA)

Ans. 59

a.
- Hypodense lesion present in the left frontal lobe
- Contrast enhancement with irregular thick wall of the lesion
- Marked surrounding vasogenic edema

b. Glioblastoma

c. • Brain abscess
   • Solitary brain metastasis
d. • Surgery
   • Radiotherapy

Ans. 60

a. CT scan brain with contrast shows brain abscess
b. • IV antibiotics for 6–8 weeks
   • Antiepileptic drugs
   • Mannitol
c. • Surgical evacuation
   • Treatment of sinusitis

Ans. 61

a. Cortical hypodensity/hypoattenuated area/loss of gray-white matter differentiation
b. Hyperacute ischemic stroke
c. (1) Hyperdense MCA sign and (2) insular ribbon sign
d. IV rTPA/mechanical thrombectomy

Ans. 62

a. • Hyperdense lesion in the cerebellum
   • Compression of the 4th ventricle
   • Dilatation of the lateral and third ventricles
b. Hematoma in the cerebellum with noncommunication hydrocephalus
c. Hypertension

Ans. 63

a. Subarachnoid hemorrhage.
b. • Thunderclap/severe headache
   • Vomiting
   • Loss of consciousness
c. Rupture left MCA aneurysm
d. Coiling/clipping

Ans. 64

a. • Concavo-convex hyperdense area with few hypodense shadows on the left parietal region
   • Compression of left lateral ventricle with midline shifting
b. Acute on chronic SDH
c. • Headache
   • Vomiting

- Loss of consciousness
- Right-sided weakness/hemiparesis

d. Burr hole/craniotomy

Ans. 65

a.
- Homogeneously enhanced mass within the right frontoparietal lobe
- A dural tail sign
- Compression of the left lateral ventricle and midline shift to the left

b. Meningioma in the right frontoparietal lobe

c. Surgical resection of the tumor

Ans. 66

a.
- Sagittal and axial MRI sections showing left paracentral L5-S1 disk herniation
- The extruded (free-floating) fragment compressing the nerve

b. Left-sided L5-S1 disk herniation with extruded fragment

c.
- Positive left Lasegue sign
- Weakness of the left extensor hallucis longus
- Decreased left ankle reflex

d. Surgery—minimally invasive surgery (MIS) microdiscectomy

Ans. 67

a.
- Sagittal MRI scans of the cervical spine reveal a substantial disk herniation between the C3 and C4 vertebral bodies, causing deformation of the spinal cord at that level.
- Thecal indentation is noted.
- Myelopathic changes/hyperintensity is noted at the level C3 and C4.

b. Cervical disk herniation at the level C3 and C4

c. Trauma

d. Surgery

Ans. 68

a. T2 hyperintense, nonenhancing ovoid region is seen within the spinal cord spanning from C2 to T1 level.

b. Syringomyelia at C2-T1

c. Dissociated sensory loss (sensory loss to pain and temperature while light touch, vibration, and position senses are preserved)

d. Laminectomy and syringotomy/shunt

Ans. 69

a.
- MRI sagittal T1-weighted image (T1WI) (A) shows destruction of L5-S1 intervertebral disk space and endplates of the adjacent vertebral bodies is marked, vertebral body alignment is normal.
- MRI sagittal T2WI (B) shows diskitis and destruction of the endplates of the adjacent vertebral bodies

b. Tuberculous spondylitis
c. Anti-TB drug [isoniazid (INH), rifampicin, pyrazinamide (PZA), and ethambutol]

Ans. 70

a. Absence epilepsy (typical).
b. 3 Hz spike and wave generalized discharge
c. Hyperventilation
d. Ethosuximide—antagonizes postsynaptic T-type calcium channel
e. Lamotrigine, valproate, levetiracetam, clobazam, and zonisamide (any two)

Ans. 71

a. Internuclear ophthalmoplegia and medial longitudinal fasciculus is responsible.
b. Multiple sclerosis and stroke.
c. Injection of methylprednisolone 1 g IV once daily for 5 days.
d. Multiple sclerosis and acute disseminated encephalomyelitis.
e. CSF oligoclonal bands

Ans. 72

a. Kayser–Fleischer ring
b. Autosomal recessive
c. The face of the giant panda sign and double panda sign.
   - The term "face of the giant panda sign" describes how the midbrain appears when the substantia nigra and RN are encircled by a high T2 signal in the tegmentum.
   - The combination of the giant panda's face and the miniature panda's face (the giant panda's cub) on T2-weighted images of the midbrain and pons, respectively, in Wilson disease is known as the "double panda sign".
   - The central tegmental tracts or the panda's eyes are relatively hypointense on the pons in contrast with the hyperintensity of the aqueduct opening into the fourth ventricle.
d. Copper chelation therapy with penicillamine and trientine is the cornerstone treatment for Wilson.
e. Liver transplant
f. Levodopa–carbidopa and trihexyphenidyl
g. *ATP7B* gene

Ans. 73

a. Wernicke encephalopathy
b. Injection of thiamine 500 mg IV three times a day for 3 days.
c. Korsakoff psychosis
d. Hyperemesis gravidarum and bariatric surgery
e. Ophthalmoplegia, ataxia, and confusion.
f. Thiamine is a cofactor for many metabolic processes including the Krebs cycle, pentose phosphate pathway, and deficiency results in neuronal cell death.

Ans. 74

a. Superior cerebellar artery, paramedian branches of a posterior cerebral artery (PCA), and quadrigeminal artery of a PCA.
b. Weber, Claude, Benedikt, and Nothnagel
c. Rostral interstitial medial longitudinal fasciculus
d. Third and fourth cranial nerves
e. Lateral rectus

Ans. 75

a. Idiopathic Parkinson's disease
b. Constipation, depression, insomnia, and nocturia
c. Hoehn and Yahr staging
d. Deep brain stimulation
e. Typical antipsychotics, such as chlorpromazine and calcium channel blockers like cinnarizine.
f. Levodopa–carbidopa, trihexyphenidyl, amantadine, selegiline, and pramipexole.

Ans. 76

a. Oral contraceptive pills, malignancy, alcoholism, trauma, and anemia.
b. Nonvisualization of major venous sinuses.
c. Injectable heparin or low molecular weight heparin.
d. Antiphospholipid antibody syndrome, hyperhomocysteinemia, and varicella zoster infection.
e. 3–12 months
f. Warfarin, nonvitamin K antagonist oral anticoagulants (NOAC) like dabigatran, and apixaban can be used though guidelines yet to recommend.

Ans. 77

a. Cerebral autosomal dominant arteriopathy with subcortical infarcts and leukoencephalopathy (CADASIL)
b. Yes and autosomal dominant.
c. Symmetric and progressive white matter hyperintensities particularly involving the external capsules and anterior temporal lobes.
d. *NOTCH3* gene is mutated in CADASIL. White matter blood vessels of the brain are affected by this mutation.
e. Pure motor stroke, ataxic hemiparesis, dysarthria-clumsy hand syndrome, and pure sensory stroke.

Ans. 78

a. MRI suggestive of bilateral caudate and genu infarct.
b. Vasculitis
c. 9–12 months
d. Isoniazid, rifampicin, streptomycin, ethambutol and pyrazinamide

e. Yes, GeneXpert in the CSF sample is a rapid diagnostic test for tuberculosis detection and rifampicin resistance.

Ans. 79

a. Left frontoparietal extradural hematoma
b. Tearing of branches of middle meningeal artery
c. Burr hole evacuation
d. Trauma and coagulopathy
e. Seizures and brain herniation

Ans. 80

a. Café au lait spot and neurofibromatosis type 1
b. Autosomal dominant
c. Six or more cafe-au-lait spots >5 mm prepubertal and >15 mm postpubertal.
d. The neurofibromin 1 *(NF1)* gene is located on band 17q11.2 and codes for neurofibromin.
e. Lisch nodules in the iris and optic nerve glioma sphenoid wing dysplasia.

Ans. 81

a. Diastematomyelia or split cord
b. Arnold–Chiari malformation, tethered cord syndrome, spina bifida occulta, and spina bifida with myelomeningocele.
c. Folic acid supplementation 0.4 mg/kg during antenatal time.
d. A persistent or abnormal adhesion between the ectoderm and endoderm creates an additional neuroenteric canal which in turn leads to the notochord developing into two hemicords

Ans. 82

a. CT of the brain plane shows a left medial temporal lobe mixed-density lesion (both hyperdense and hypodense). The hyperdensity is not homogenous and varies in signal density. The lesion could be a cavernoma.
b. Drugs effective for focal seizure such as phenytoin, carbamazepine, lamotrigine, and brivaracetam are preferred.
c. Quadrantanopia and memory loss
d. De Ja Vu, sense of fear, rising epigastric sensation, nausea, olfactory and/or gustatory hallucination, and depersonalization.

Ans. 83

a. T2 shows left temporooccipital hyperintensity with diffusion restriction and blooming suggestive hemorrhagic infarct. MRV shows the absence of flow in the left sigmoid and transverse sinus suggestive of CVT.
b. Anticoagulation parenteral in acute phase followed by oral anticoagulant
c. Reversible cerebral vasoconstriction syndrome and eclampsia
d. Cerebral edema, vision loss, status epilepticus, and brain herniation.

Ans. 84

a. Holmes tremor (rubral tremor, midbrain tremor, and thalamic tremor)
b. Treatment options:
   - *Surgical:* Stereotactic lesions at the thalamus may result in partial improvement. Nucleus deep brain stimulation of the ventral intermediate (VIM) nucleus can also be tried.
   - *Medical:* The most commonly used drugs are dopamine agonists, anticholinergics, trihexyphenidyl, levodopa, and topiramate.
c. The etiology of Holmes tremor commonly includes trauma, stroke (ischemic and hemorrhagic), infections, neurodegenerative (multiple sclerosis), tumors, and vascular lesions (cavernoma and AV malformations).
d. Red nucleus

Ans. 85

a. Hyperdensity noted in left gangliocapsular region with mild mass effect suggestive of intracranial hemorrhage
b. Trauma, oral anticoagulation overdose, and tumors.
c. BP target ≤140/90
d. Hyperglycemia, chronic kidney disease, coma, large hematoma with volume >30 mL, old age >80 years, intraventricular hemorrhage, and posterior fossa hemorrhage.
e. Nicardipine and labetalol

Ans. 86

a. Vertebral artery and Wallenberg syndrome (lateral medullary syndrome).
b. T2 FLAIR hyperintensity with diffusion restriction noted in the right lateral medulla and right cerebellum suggestive of the acute infarct.
c. The paramedian bulbar and lateral bulbar arteries comprise the two groups of blood vessels that supply the medulla. The medial aspect of the medulla is supplied by the paramedian bulbar arteries, which emerge from the vertebral arteries. The anterior spinal artery may also give rise to the paramedian bulbar arteries at the farthest caudal region of the medulla. The posterior inferior cerebellar artery (PICA) or the vertebral artery gives rise to the lateral bulbar branches, which supply the lateral region of the medulla.

   The anterior inferior cerebellar artery (AICA), PICA, and SCA are the three primary arteries that supply the cerebellum with blood. They are all part of the vertebrobasilar anterior system.

Ans. 87

a. FLAIR hyperintensity with diffusion restriction noted in bilateral parasagittal areas, corpus callosum, and centrum semiovale suggestive of acute infarct
b. Cardioembolism (since the infarct is bilateral, multiple, and the patient already has dilated cardiomyopathy)

c.

Anterior cerebral Artery	Sub-branches	Territories supplied
Central artery	Many small arterial branches	• Corpus callosum (rostrum) • Septum pellucidum • Caudate nucleus (head) • Anterior putamen (of lentiform or lenticular nucleus)
Cortical branches	• Orbital branches	• Frontal lobe (orbital surface): – Olfactory lobe – Medial orbital gyrus – Straight rectus
	• Frontal branches	• Medial frontal gyrus • Cingulate gyrus • Paracentral lobule • Superior frontal gyrus • Middle frontal gyrus • Precentral gyrus
	• Parietal branches	• Precuneus (superior parietal lobule) and nearby lateral surface

d. Heubner's, orbitofrontal, frontopolar, anterior internal frontal, middle internal frontal, posterior internal frontal, paracentral, superior parietal, inferior parietal, pericallosal, and callosomarginal arteries.

Ans. 88

a. Diabetic amyotrophy, better known as diabetic lumbosacral radiculoplexus neuropathy (DLRPN).
b. The management of pain symptoms, control of hyperglycemia, and increased mobility (physical therapy) comprise the treatment for diabetic lumbosacral radiculoplexus neuropathy (DLRPN). NSAIDs and paracetamol can be used to manage pain. Anticonvulsant medications, selective serotonin receptor inhibitors (SSRIs) for anxiety and depression, and amitriptyline for sleeplessness are other options. Steroids or opioids (oxycodone and tramadol) may be worth considering in cases of severe illness.
c. Trauma, infections, rapid glycemic control, and tight glycemic control.
d. The prognosis is good overall. The illness usually worsens over time before stabilizing and eventually recovering fully; however, some patients may still have some residual motor deficiency.

Ans. 89

a. Decremental response
b. The IgG1 and IgG3 subtypes of antibodies are present in antiacetylcholine receptor antibody-positive MG (AChR MG). They attach to the n-ACh receptor found in the skeletal muscles' postsynaptic membrane, activating the complement system and causing the membrane attack complex (MAC) to develop. The last stage of receptor degradation is

brought about by MAC. They could alternatively work by improving the endocytosis of the n-ACh receptor that is coupled to an antibody or by functionally inhibiting ACh's ability to bind to its receptor.
c. Pyridostigmine
d. IVIG or plasma exchange.
e. Azathioprine, mycophenolate mofetil, and corticosteroids.

Ans. 90

a. Right striatal hyperdensity seen in diabetic striatopathy manifesting as chorea
b. Adults—Huntington's disease (HD), thalamic infarct, SLE, and drugs like levodopa. Children—rheumatic fever
c. Haloperidol, tetrabenazine, and clonazepam.
d. Focal seizures, myoclonus, tremor, and restless legs syndrome.

Ans. 91

a. Frontotemporal dementia.
b. Bilateral severe temporal lobe atrophy (left more than right).
c. Yes, 20–50% could be familial.
d. Behavioral variants (bv-FTD), semantic dementia (SD), and progressive nonfluent aphasia (PNFA) are the three main variants.
e. Prosopagnosia is a form of visual agnosia characterized by an inability to recognize faces.

Ans. 92

a. Alzheimer's disease.
b. Hypertension, diabetes mellitus, head injury, aging, family history, smoking, and alcoholism.
c. Logopenic variant primary progressive aphasia, posterior cortical atrophy, behavioral/dysexecutive, acalculia, and corticobasal syndrome are some of the variants.
d. Brain MRI reveals moderate to severe atrophy of the hippocampus and medial temporal lobes bilaterally, and mild to moderate atrophy of the lateral temporal and parietal lobes.
e. Physical activity, HTN and diabetes management, cognitive training, and Mediterranean diet.

Ans. 93

a. T1 basal ganglia hyperintensity suggestive of hepatic encephalopathy in this case.
b. A rise in manganese concentration (a paramagnetic substance) in the CNS.
c. Ammonia lowering strategies, such are lactulose enema and rifaximin. Supplementation with branched-chain amino acids.
d. The initial EEG alterations often involve a slowing of the posterior dominant rhythm, succeeded by a progressive slowing of the background as theta and delta activity emerge. The triphasic waves have three separate phases and are nonspecific, sharp contoured waves with high amplitude. Surface positive and high amplitude (>70 µV) wave is preceded by a negative deflection, followed by a broad negative deflection that rises slowly.
e. The West Haven criteria
f. Normal ammonia levels in such patients question the diagnosis of hepatic encephalopathy.

Ans. 94

a. Right perisylvian fissure and hemispherical sulci hyperdensity, and right frontotemporal parenchymal hyperdensity suggestive of right frontotemporal hemorrhage with subarachnoid hemorrhage.
b. Nimodipine 60 mg every 4 hours for 21 days.
c. Hypertension, cigarette smoking, and family history.
d. The only effective treatment for an aneurysmal subarachnoid hemorrhage (aSAH) or a burst aneurysm is repair with surgical clipping or endovascular coiling, which should be carried out as soon as is practical, ideally within 24 hours of the diagnosis.
e. World Federation of Neurological Surgeons scale or Hunt–Hess scale.

Ans. 95

a. Guillain–Barré syndrome
b. Aalbumin-cytological dissociation in CSF.
c. IVIG and plasma exchange.
d. Acute motor axonal neuropathy (AMAN), acute motor sensory axonal neuropathy (AMSAN), acute AIDP, and Miller Fisher variant.
e. Distal latency prolongation, nerve conduction velocity slowing, temporal dispersion, conduction block, and sural sparing are seen in AIDP. Motor and sensory amplitudes are reduced in AMAN and AMSAN variants.

Ans. 96

a. Herpes zoster (shingles).
b. Herpes zoster is an infection caused by the varicella-zoster virus reactivating in a posterior dorsal root ganglion from its latent stage.
c. The antiviral medications used to treat herpes zoster include acyclovir 800 mg, taken five times a day for 5 days, valacyclovir 1 g, taken three times a day for five days, and famciclovir 500 mg, taken three times a day for 7 days. Creams containing topical antibiotics, such as soframycin and mupirocin, aid in preventing subsequent bacterial infections.
d. Postherpetic neuralgia. Pregabalin, gabapentin, and capsaicin patches are used to treat postherpetic neuralgia.
e. *Shingles vaccine:* Two injections given separately 2–6 months apart 0.5 mL vial for intramuscular injection.
f. Human immunodeficiency virus (HIV)/acquired immunodeficiency syndrome (AIDS), immunosuppression, family history, and older.

Ans. 97

a. Normal pressure hydrocephalus (NPH)
b. The most common description of NPH gait is "shuffling", "magnetic", and "wide-based".
c. Callosal angle is between 40 and 90° in patients with NPH.
A type of communicating hydrocephalus known as disproportionately enlarged subarachnoid space hydrocephalus (DESH) is marked by sulci crowding superiorly at the vertex and CSF spaces expanding more inferiorly, especially in the Sylvian fissures.

d. Ventriculoperitoneal shunt surgery
e. Risk factors for poor response after shunt surgery
   - Severe dementia
   - Dementia as a presenting symptom
   - MRI abnormalities, cerebral atrophy, and multiple white matter lesions misdiagnosis and delayed recognition
f. Hakims–Adams triad: NPH is a disorder of the elderly that characteristically presents with progressive gait impairment, cognitive deficits, and urinary urgency and/or incontinence.

Ans. 98

a. Huntington's disease
b. Yes and autosomal dominant
c. Bilateral caudate atrophy
d. Genetic anticipation is a phenomenon where the symptoms of a genetic condition become more severe and/or appear at an earlier age as they are passed from one generation to the next.
e. The main characteristic is the degradation of neurons in the cerebral cortex, caudate, and putamen. Chorea is caused by the selective degeneration of the medium spiny neurons in the basal ganglia that contain enkephalin through the indirect pathway.
f. Westphal variant (parkinsonism as a symptom of juvenile HD)
g. For the treatment of chorea, the American Academy of Neurology guidelines suggest using riluzole, amantadine, or tetrabenazine (TBZ). By preferentially depleting dopamine rather than norepinephrine, TBZ reversibly inhibits the central monoamine transporter type 2.

   In HD, tricyclic antidepressants and SSRIs are frequently used to treat anxiety, depression, and obsessive-compulsive disorders.

Ans. 99

a. Bilateral medial temporal lobe hyperintensity.
b. Autoimmune encephalitis and herpes encephalitis.
c. Hippocampus
d. Typical auras, such as rising epigastric sensations, déjà vu, affective phenomena (fear or sadness), and experiential phenomena, are included in the semiology of the medial temporal lobe. These auras are often followed by unilateral motor signs, such as head deviation or ipsilateral face or mouth contraction, and bilateral motor phenomena in the face or axial muscles. Oral automatisms and behavioral arrest are frequent, and bitemporal spread is a sign of altered consciousness, forgetfulness, autonomic abnormalities (such as changes in heart rate and breathing), and noticeable motor automatisms (such as dystonic and tonic posture).
e. The following abnormalities are noted in HSV encephalitis EEG:
   - Nonspecific diffuse high amplitude slow waves.
   - Temporal lobe spike-and-wave activity.
   - Periodic lateralized epileptiform discharges (PLEDs).
   - Uni- or bilateral periodic sharp waves.

Ans. 100

a. Any two differential diagnosis
   - Cerebral abscess
   - Tuberculoma
   - Neurocysticercosis
   - Metastasis
   - Glioblastoma
   - Demyelination
b. Three months intensive phase [HRZE(S)] and 9 months continuation phase (HRZ or HRE)
c. Tuberculoma, tuberculous meningitis, and arachnoiditis.
d. Tuberculomas usually demonstrate large lipid peaks on MRS with increased choline levels and decreased levels of NAA and creatinine.
e. *Isoniazid's major adverse effects:* Peripheral neuropathy, drug-induced lupus, psychoses, and seizures.

Ans. 101

a. Cerebellum
b. Anterior superior vermis
c. Vestibulocerebellum
d. Dorsal oculomotor vermis
e. Anticonvulsants such as phenytoin and anticancer drugs; such as 5-FU, cytarabine, and paclitaxel.

Ans. 102

a. Amyotrophic lateral sclerosis
b. A bilateral disruption of the corticobulbar pathways results in an upper motor lesion that causes pseudobulbar palsy. It is characterized by emotional instability, face and tongue weakness, dysphagia, and dysarthria.
c. Axon gliosis and degeneration in the lateral and anterior spinal cord columns are hallmarks of the pathogenesis of amyotrophic lateral sclerosis. Additionally gone are Betz cells in the motor cortex and motor neurons in the spinal cord's anterior horns.
d. Riluzole (50 mg BID) is the only medication that has demonstrated increased overall survival and is believed to lessen glutamate-induced excitotoxicity.
e. Frontotemporal dementia
f. El Escorial criteria and Awaji criteria.

Ans. 103

a. Progressive supranuclear palsy
b. Vertical gaze palsy, axial rigidity more than appendicular rigidity, and falls within a year.
c. Hummingbird sign and morning glory sign.
d. Dystonic contraction of the procerus muscle resulting in vertical wrinkles on the glabella and nose bridge may be a clinical indicator of early PSP.

e. Intracerebral accumulation of the microtubule-associated protein tau, with pallidum, striatum, RN, substantia nigra, pontine tegmentum, oculomotor nucleus, medulla, and DN being the areas that are preferentially involved.

Ans. 104

a. Left posterior occipitotemporal region and splenium of corpus callosum acute infarct.
b. Left PCA.
c. Exner's area is located in the left middle frontal gyrus and is involved in reading and writing.
d. Dominant angular gyrus
e. Dominant occipitotemporal area and splenium of the corpus callosum.

Ans. 105

a. Posterior reversible encephalopathy syndrome
b. BP control and antiepileptics
c. Tacrolimus and ciclosporin
d. Yes, reversible.
e. Dysregulation of cerebral autoregulation and sudden rise in BP leads to increased hydrostatic pressure. There is a breakdown of the blood-brain barrier, causing intravascular fluid to extravasate to the surrounding brain tissue, leading to edema.

Ans. 106

a. Gottron papules on fingers and heliotrope rash on face.
b. Corticosteroids and other immunosuppressants, such as azathioprine and rituximab.
c. Perivascular and perimysial inflammatory infiltrate and perifascicular atrophy.
d. Peter and Bohan
e. Yes cancer screening is recommended.
f. Anti-Jo and anti-Mi-2

Ans. 107

a. Subacute sclerosing panencephalitis (SSPE)
b. One of the characteristics of SSPE is the presence of quasiperiodic, high-voltage, repeated polyspike and sharp and slow wave complexes (Radermecker complexes), which last for one second and repeat every five seconds with slow background activity.
c. Vaccination for measles
d. Symptomatic management includes sodium valproate and clonazepam for myoclonus. The combination of intraventricular interferon-alpha plus oral isoprinosine has been the best regimen tried so far.
e. Dyken's criteria
f.

Stage	Change due to SSPE
Stage I	Behavioral decline (lethargy, inattention, or temper tantrums) and cognitive decline
Stage II	Myoclonic jerks, seizures, and dementia
Stage III	Rigidity, extrapyramidal symptoms, and progressive unresponsiveness
Stage IV	Coma, vegetative state, autonomic instability, and akinetic mutism

Ans. 108

a. Subacute combined cord degeneration due to vitamin B_{12} deficiency.
b. For individuals with neurological symptoms, a recommended dosage schedule is 1,000 µg every other day for two weeks, after which cyanocobalamin should be administered once a month.
c. Nutritional deficiency, fish tapeworm infestation, pernicious anemia, and gastric surgeries.
d. Macroovalocytes with hypersegmented neutrophils.
e. An inverted "V"-shaped high-intensity T2 signal is present on both sides of the posterior funiculus.

Ans. 109

a. Right trigeminal neuralgia
b. Oxcarbazepine, carbamazepine, pregabalin, and gabapentin.
c. Radiofrequency ablation and microvascular decompression.
d. Neurovascular compression in the trigeminal root entry zone is linked to classic trigeminal neuralgia. This compression can cause demyelination and a dysregulation of voltage-gated sodium channel expression in the membrane.
e. Normal neuroexamination
f. V2 or maxillary division

Ans. 110

a. Airway, breathing, and circulation assessment.
b. Midazolam (0.2 mg/kg, maximum 10 mg) intramuscular or lorazepam (0.1 mg/kg, maximum 4 mg) IV or diazepam (0.15 mg/kg, maximum 10 mg).
c. Phenytoin, sodium valproate, or levetiracetam
d. Propofol, thiopentone or midazolam infusion, and ketamine.
e. Status epilepticus that continues or recurs 24 hours or more after the initiation of anesthetic therapy.

Ans. 111

a. Deep CVT and artery of Percheron infarct.
b. Japanese encephalitis (JE) virus and *Enterovirus*.
c. The basilar communicating artery, PCA, and posterior communicating artery.
d. *Mosquito control measures:* As per the Government of India Guidelines, two doses of JE vaccines have been approved in routine immunization for endemic districts—one along with measles at the age of 9 months and the second with diphtheria–pertussis–tetanus (DPT) booster at the age of 16–24 months with effect from April 2013.

Ans. 112

a. 400 mg/kg/day for a total of 5 days.
b. The edrophonium test should be used to distinguish between a myasthenic crisis and a cholinergic crisis. The clinical signs of cholinergic crisis will get worse if 2 mg of edrophonium is administered. When there is a myasthenic crisis symptoms improve.
c. Large volume plasma exchange

d. Allergic reactions, myocardial infarction with high doses, fever, chills, headache, and thromboembolic events.
e. Eculizumab and rituximab

Ans. 113

a. Cluster headache
b. Male
c. Pituitary tumors
d. Verapamil and lithium
e. Paroxysmal hemicrania (PH), hemicrania continua (HC), short-lasting unilateral neuralgiform headache attacks (SUNAs) with conjunctival injection and tearing (SUNCT), and SUNA.

Ans. 114

a. FLAIR hyperintensity in both medial medulla with diffusion restriction suggestive of bilateral medial medullary acute infarct.
b. Hypoglossal nucleus, medial longitudinal fasciculus, pyramidal tract, and medial lemniscus.
c. Area postrema syndrome, which is characterized by otherwise intractable episodes of vomiting, hiccups, and nausea, is typically linked to neuromyelitis optica.
d. It is necessary for organizing and evaluating visceral afferent data. They are involved in breathing regulation. Taste-sensing neurons also form synapses in the nucleus tractus solitarius (NTS) prior to traveling to the thalamus and then the cortex.

ns. 115

a. Limb girdle muscle dystrophy
b. Genetic testing
c. Dystrophin is a protein that stabilizes the muscle membrane during muscle contraction. It connects the cytoskeleton to the plasma membrane, allowing for effective muscle contractions. Dystrophin also protects cells against contraction-induced damage.
d. Children with myopathies climb up their thighs with the aid of their hands to overcome the weakness of their pelvic and proximal LL muscles.
e. McArdle disease, carnitine palmitoyltransferase deficiency, drugs, and toxins.

ns. 116

a. Blood glucose levels and plain CT brain and CT angiogram.
b. Up to 4.5 hours.
c. Before administering alteplase in the setting of thrombolysis in arterial ischemic stroke (AIS), BP must be <185/110 mm Hg and it must remain <180/105 mm Hg for the next 24 hours. The ideal range for blood glucose is 50–400 mg/dL.
d. National Institutes of Health Stroke Scale (NIHSS)
e. 6%
f. Patients with LVOs should be offered mechanical thrombectomy, with or without IV thrombolysis, in an extended window of up to 24 hours of the last known well.

ns. 117

a. Idiopathic intracranial HTN.
b. An opening pressure >25 cmH$_2$O in adults is expected.
c. Weight loss, topiramate, and acetazolamide
d. Sixth nerve palsy (abducens).
e. Paresthesias of extremities, drowsiness, hypokalemia, and acidosis.

ns. 118

a. MRI of the cervical spine showed disc destruction of C6 to C7, posterior subluxation of C6 vertebral body over C7, and pre- and paravertebral collection from C6 to D2 suggestive of spondylodiscitis with the paravertebral collection.
b. *Mycobacterium tuberculosis (M. tuberculosis)*
c. Tuberculous abscesses typically lack all the inflammatory signs obvious in abscesses.
d. Pyogenic or fungal infections and neoplastic etiology.
e. In cases of paradiscal involvement, the most prevalent kind of lesion, *M. tuberculosis* lodges in the vertebra's subchondral marrow, causing disc degeneration. Because of this disc degeneration, an anterior wedge of the affected vertebrae forms, giving Pott's disease its distinctive kyphosis.

Ans. 119

a. Enlarged and hyperintense anterior pituitary suggestive of anterior pituitary infarct.
b. Pregnancy-related pituitary hyperplasia increases the anterior pituitary gland's overall nutritional and metabolic needs, but the blood flow does not increase.
c. The lifelong replacement of hormones that are lacking is the cornerstone of treatment for Sheehan syndrome. Levothyroxine replacement therapy is for hypothyroidism.
Prednisone or hydrocortisone can be used to replace cortisol in patients with insufficiency. If the uterus is present, gonadotropin insufficiency should be treated with a combination of progesterone and estrogen. Perhaps the most frequently depleted hormone is growth hormone, and each patient's needs must be taken into account while determining the appropriate dosage. The recommended course of treatment for individuals who develop diabetic insipidus is desmopressin (DDAVP).
d. The lack of lactation, or agalactorrhea, is the initial and most typical sign of Sheehan syndrome.

SECTION 13

Respiratory

QUESTIONS

Q1. A 32-year-old male presented with sudden-onset cough with profuse foul-smelling sputum, breathlessness, and fatigue. His chest X-ray (CXR) posteroanterior (PA) view was suggestive of hydropneumothorax left side.
a. Enumerate four physical signs on respiratory system examination. *(4 marks)*
b. Which complication has occurred in this situation? *(2 marks)*
c. How would you manage? *(4 marks)*

Q2. A 53-year-old lady presented with low-grade fever and weight loss and polyuria. On routine investigations her serum calcium was found to be elevated. (corrected serum calcium 14.3 mg%) CXR was suggestive of lower zone fibrosis.
a. Enumerate four further tests to decipher the cause of hypercalcemia. *(4 marks)*
b. What is the likely diagnosis? What is the mechanism of hypercalcemia in this case? *(4 marks)*
c. Enumerate two ways to treat acute hypercalcemia. *(2 marks)*

Q3. A 52-year-old man presented with cough for 4 weeks. He has lost 3 kg of his weight in last month. His CXR is shown below.

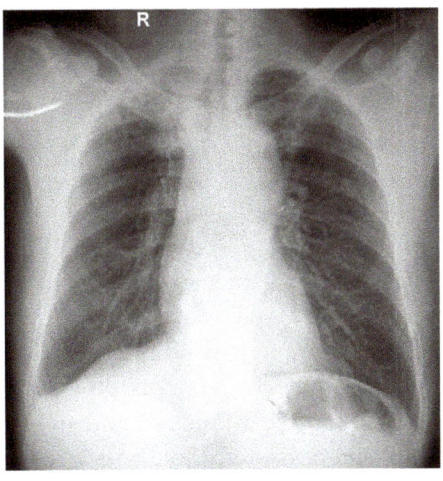

a. List the radiological abnormalities of his CXR. *(3 marks)*
b. What is the most probable diagnosis for the above abnormalities? *(3 marks)*
c. List two important questions you ask in the history to support the diagnosis? *(2 marks)*
d. List two investigations to confirm your diagnosis? *(2 marks)*

Q4. A 49-year-old woman was hospitalized due to pneumonia, experiencing three episodes of cough, fever, and purulent sputum in the last 6 months, one of which was accompanied by right-sided pleuritic chest pain. These episodes were managed at home by her family physician. Concurrently, she has been grappling with swallowing difficulties for the past 5 years, initially mild but progressively worsening. The sensation of food sticking in the low retrosternal area, affecting all types of solid food, has led to a weight loss of 5 kg over the last 2 months. Despite occasional improvement during meals, she now faces issues with regurgitation and vomiting of recognizable food. Three years ago, she underwent upper gastrointestinal endoscopy, which yielded normal results, providing temporary reassurance; however, the problem has since intensified. There is no pertinent medical or family history.

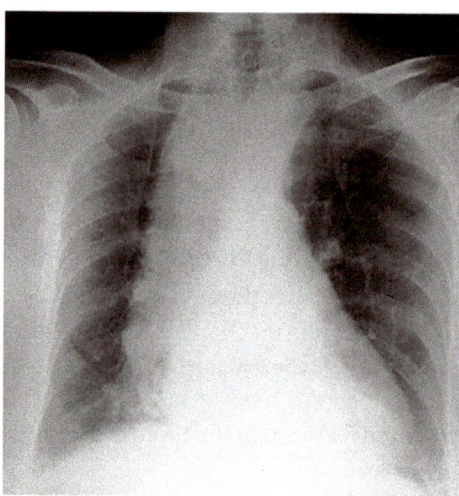

Examination: She looks thin. Respiratory system examination reveals some crackles at the right base. There are no evident abnormalities in the cardiovascular system, abdomen, or other systems on examination.

a. Which is the most likely cause of this patient's current condition? *(2 marks)*
b. How would you diagnose this? *(4 marks)*
c. How would you manage? *(4 marks)*

Q5. A 58-year-old woman visited the emergency department, reporting a 3-month history of general malaise, loss of appetite, and a weight loss of 4 kg. She also presented with sinusitis, purulent nasal discharge, nosebleeds, and new symptoms of (s/o) exertional dyspnea and hemoptysis. Painful joint symptoms began in the wrists, progressing to the ankles and knees.

On examination, the woman appeared fatigued and unwell, with swelling, warmth, tenderness, and restricted movement in the wrists and ankles. A palpable purpuric rash was observed on her shins. The cardiovascular, respiratory, abdominal, and neurological examinations revealed no remarkable findings. A CXR was conducted:

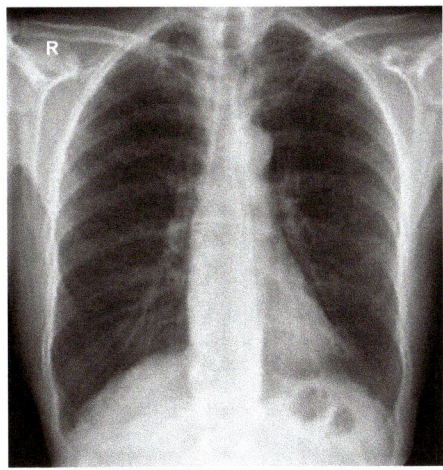

Observations: Temperature—37.9°C, heart rate—101 beats/min, respiratory rate (RR)—28 breaths/min, arterial oxygen saturation (SaO_2)—90% on room air

		Normal range
White cells	16.0	4–11 × 10^9/L
Neutrophils	14.5	2–7 × 10^9/L
Hemoglobin	9.8	13–18 g/dL
Platelets	580	150–400 × 10^9/L
Sodium	135	135–145 mmol/L
Potassium	6.8	3.5–5.0 mmol/L
Urea	39.2	3.0–7.0 mmol/L
Creatinine	745	60–110 µmol/L
Arterial gas sample on room air:		
pH	7.21	7.35–7.45
pO_2	7.4	9.3–13.3 kPa
pCO_2	4.8	4.7–6.0 kPa
Lactate	3.6	<2 mmol/L
HCO_3	14	22–26 mmol/L
Base excess	−6	−3 to +3 mmol/L
Urine dipstick:		
Protein	2+	
Blood	3+	
Urine microscopy	>100 red blood cells, red cell casts	

(HCO_3: bicarbonate; pO_2: partial pressure of oxygen; pCO_2: partial pressure of carbon dioxide)

a. What is the likely diagnosis? (2 marks)
b. How would you confirm this? (4 marks)
c. How would you manage this patient? (4 marks)

Q6. On the basis of electrocardiography (ECG) image answer the following questions.

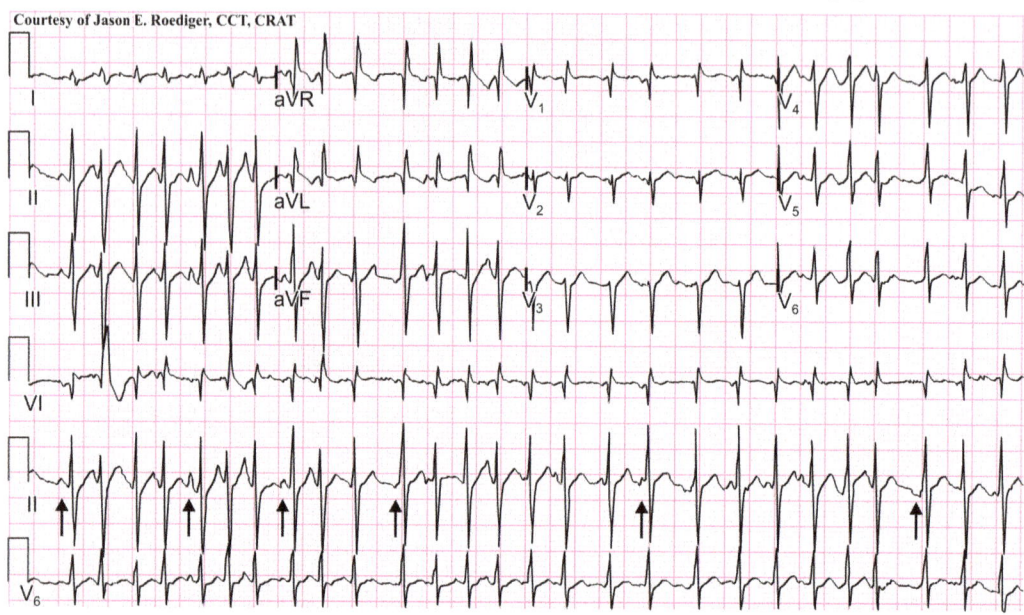

a. What does the ECG depict? (5 marks)
b. Which condition is associated with the given ECG. (5 marks)

Q7.

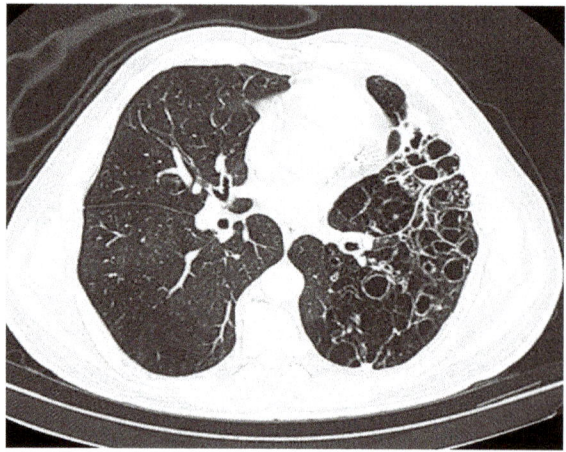

a. What is your most common provisional diagnosis? (5 marks)
b. Name one genetic syndrome associated with the given condition. (5 marks)

Q8. A 55-year-old male presented in emergency with acute-onset breathlessness. He was a smoker with 30 pack-year history. Examination revealed clubbing. His CXR is shown as follows:

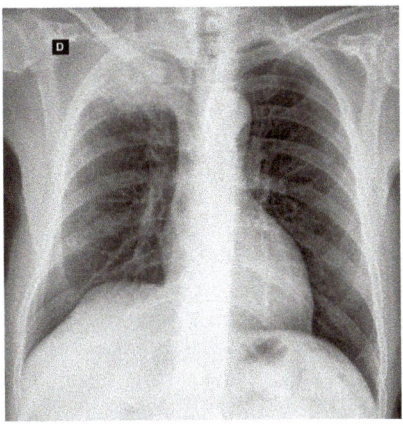

a. Name the condition. (2 marks)
b. Enumerate the components. (4 marks)
c. How will you confirm the diagnosis and which histopathology is commonly associated with it. (2 marks)
d. Give the full name of the scientist who first described it. (2 marks)

Q9. A 55-year-old female presented with lethargy and features of sleep apnea syndrome for 9 months. Her thyroid-stimulating hormone (TSH) was found to be 37 mIU/L. Her CXR suggested cardiomegaly.

a. Name four specific physical findings in her. (4 marks)
b. What is the cause of cardiomegaly? (2 marks)
c. Name three neurological complications. (3 marks)
d. Name one feature differentiating primary versus secondary cause (1 mark)

Q10. A 62-year-old lady with history of (H/O) chronic obstructive pulmonary disease (COPD) presented with acute onset shortness of breath (SOB) without any H/O fever.

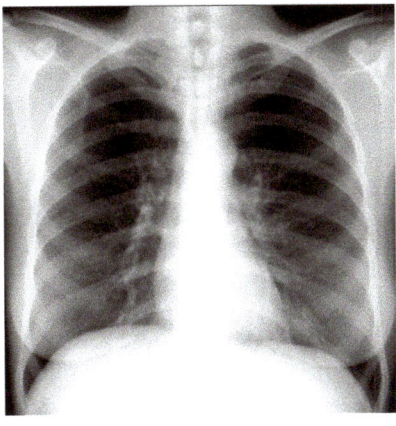

a. What is the abnormality in CXR? *(5 marks)*
b. How will you manage? *(5 marks)*

Q11. While being asked to perform percussion on a patient with sudden-onset dyspnea and chest pain, the resident observed stony dullness on the infrascapular area of right chest posteriorly which changed to hyperresonant in the scapular region.
a. What further signs is he expected to demonstrate on percussion and auscultation? *(4 marks)*
b. What additional auscultatory sign will appear if there is a communication with bronchus? *(2 marks)*
c. Name three disorders that can produce this condition. *(4 marks)*

Q12. While presenting the inspection finding on respiratory examination, the medical student mentioned that "trail sign is positive on left side".
a. Describe four conditions producing this sign. *(4 marks)*
b. In which condition can the trachea be on the same side of massive pleural effusion? *(3 marks)*
c. What is Oliver's sign? *(3 marks)*

Q13. A third-year medical student was fascinated to hear a "bronchial breathing" for the first time.
a. Draw the diagram of bronchial breathing. *(2 marks)*
b. Enumerate its types with one condition producing them. *(6 marks)*
c. Name two places where we can hear bronchial breathing in a normal person. *(2 marks)*

Q14. On the basis of CXR answer the following questions.

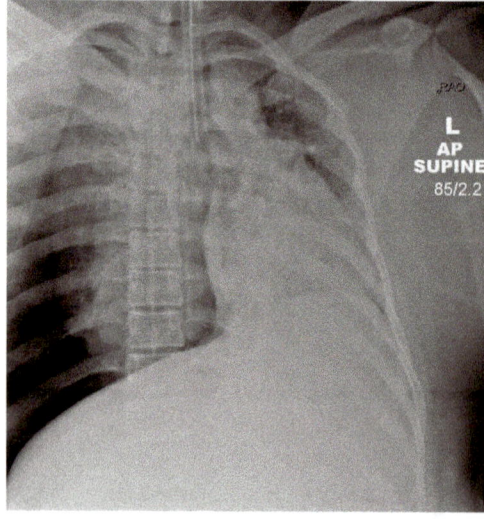

(AP: anteroposterior)

a. Identify the condition seen on the X-ray. *(5 marks)*
b. Emergency treatment of the condition. *(5 marks)*

Q15. A young obese male with body mass index (BMI) of 40 kg/m² came with complaints of (c/o) frequent road traffic accidents. He says he is feeling sleepy all the time and unable to concentrate to work. His wife c/o his snoring.
a. What is the likely cause of the given condition? (5 marks)
b. What is the best diagnostic modality in this patient and the complications of the above condition? (5 marks)

Q16. A 46-year-old male presented with chronic fatigue, cough, and dyspnea since past few days. On examination he had maculopapular lesion over skin. Serum ACE levels were elevated. High-resolution CT (HRCT) chest is given below.

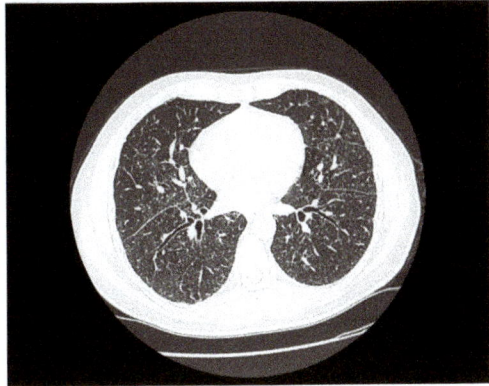

a. What is the most likely diagnosis? (5 marks)
b. How would you confirm the diagnosis? (5 marks)

Q17.

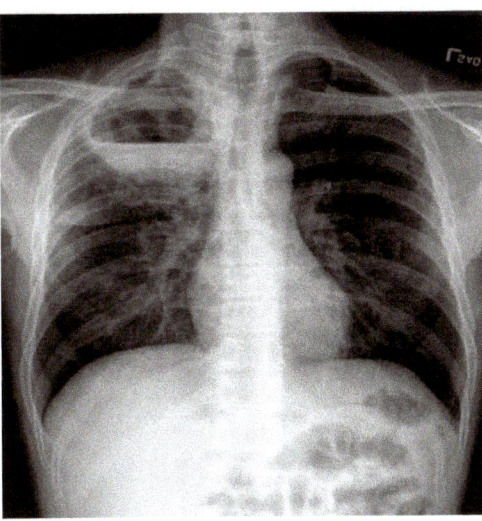

A 34-year-old alcoholic male presented with fever for 1 month, weight loss, night sweats, cough with halitosis, and SOB for 20 days associated with chest pain.

a. Read the X-ray findings. (3 marks)
b. What is your diagnosis? (2 marks)
c. What will be your treatment strategy? (2 marks)
d. What are its complications? (3 marks)

Q18. A 50-year-old male gives H/O dry cough since last 2 months with low-grade fever and weight loss. Suddenly since last 1 day he gives H/O painful nodular lesion over anterior aspect of shin. CXR was done for chronic cough which revealed the following:

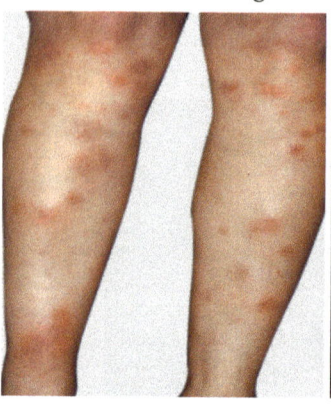
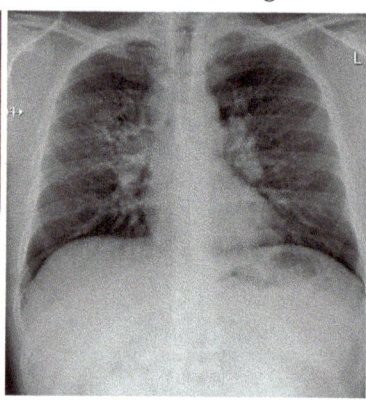

a. What are the skin manifestations? (3 marks)
b. What are the investigations needed to confirm the diagnosis? (4 marks)
c. What is the name of the staging system to stage this particular disease? (3 marks)

Q19. A patient who suffered from major road traffic acid (RTA) was given 3 units of whole blood one after another. At the end of third transfusion patient c/o SOB. Immediately the patient was shifted to intensive care unit (ICU) and monitors were connected. Patient was tachypneic, RR—36 breaths/min, peripheral oxygen saturation (SpO_2)—84% in right atrium (RA), pulse rate (PR)—110 beats/min, blood pressure (BP)—80/40 mm Hg and on auscultation bilateral (B/L) lung field revealed crepitations. Bedside CXR was ordered:

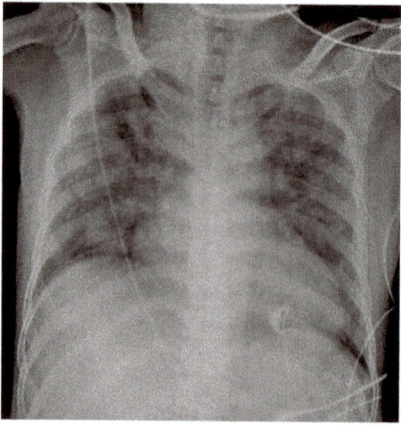

a. What is the diagnosis and treatment of the above condition? (5+5 marks)

Q20. A 25-year-old male patient presented to SCBMCH casualty with H/O SOB since last 1 hour which was sudden in onset and associated with severe left-sided chest pain which was sharp stabbing in nature and worsens with deep inspiration without any radiation. Patient has H/O loss of appetite and weight loss with yellowish discoloration of eyes and skin intermittently since last 1 year.

On examination:
Patient is in respiratory distress pallor +nt, icterus +nt
PR—120 beats/min, regular, thready BP—80/50 mm Hg
RR—36 breaths/min
On percussion: Hyperresonant note on left hemithorax on auscultation—breath sounds (BS) absent on left side of the chest
S1, S2 reduced in intensity
An urgent bedside ultrasonography (USG) was done which showed:

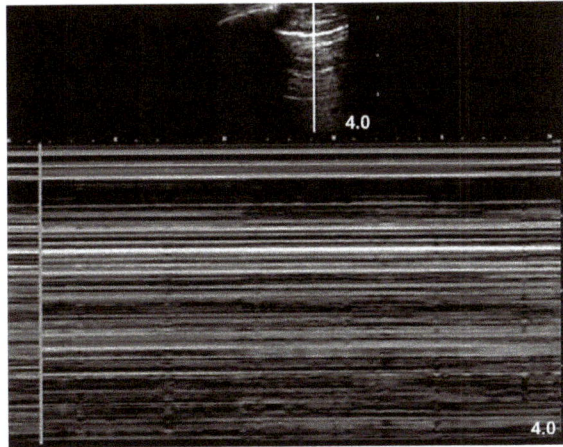

Immediately a chest drain was placed and the patient was stabilized hemodynamically. On further evaluation HRCT revealed:

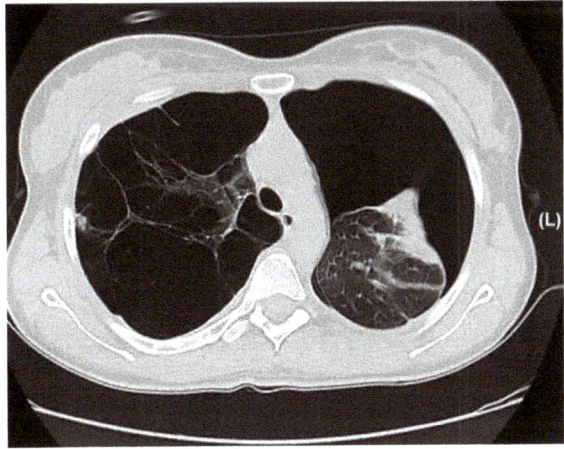

Liver biopsy (Bx) was done which revealed:

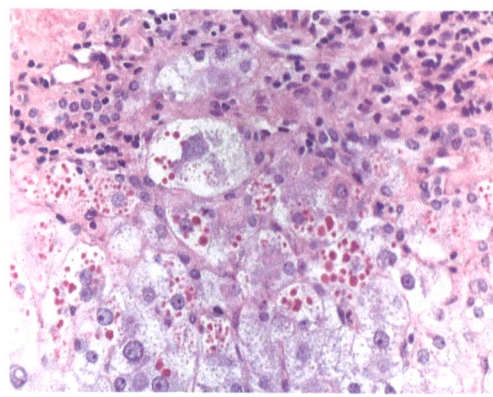

a. Read the USG of thorax. (3 marks)
b. Read the HRCT of thorax. (3 marks)
c. What is your diagnosis and the gene involved? (4 marks)

Q21. A 65-year-old male, who is a chronic smoker presented with c/o SOB and cough. Examination shows a B/L wheezing on chest auscultation and a blood oxygen saturation of 92%. A pulmonary function test (PFT) showed FEV_1/FVC (forced expiratory volume in 1 second/forced vital capacity) <0.7, an eosinophil count of 550 cells/µL and chest roentgenogram as shown below.

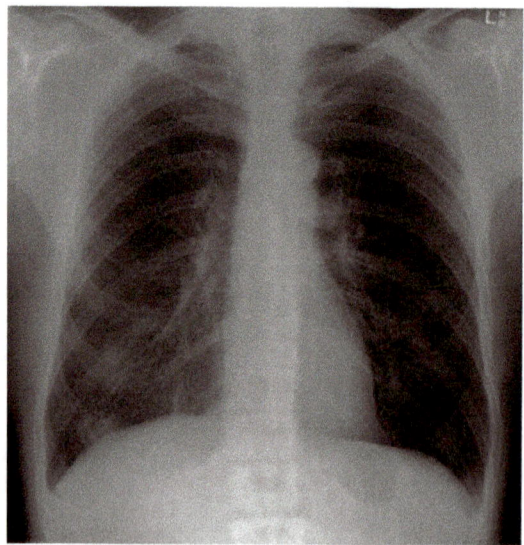

a. What is the diagnosis? (2 marks)
b. What are the clinical signs to look for in this condition? (3 marks)
c. What medications are used for managing the condition? (3 marks)
d. What is the role of measuring the eosinophil count in this condition? (2 marks)

Q22.

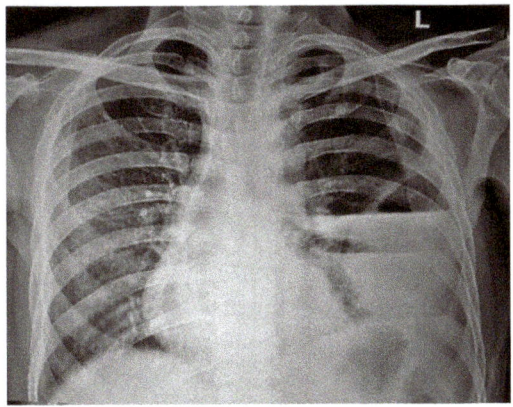

a. What is the diagnosis? (2 marks)
b. What are the differentials? (3 marks)
c. How do you treat the patient? (5 marks)

Q23. With regard to CXR shown below answer the following questions.

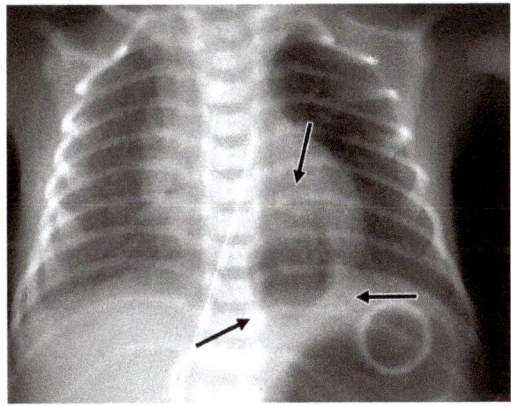

a. Identify the lesion marked by the arrows. (1 mark)
b. Name two common infectious causes, one noninfectious cause, and a drug abuse for the above. (2 + 1 + 1 = 4 marks)

Q24.

a. Define pulsus paradoxus. (1 mark)
b. Name two cardiac causes for pulsus paradoxus. (2 marks)
c. Name two respiratory causes for pulsus paradoxus. (2 marks)

Q25. A 66-year-old man presents with high-grade fever, night sweats, worsening cough with yellowish sputum and loss of weight for 3 weeks.

The CT chest is showed as below.

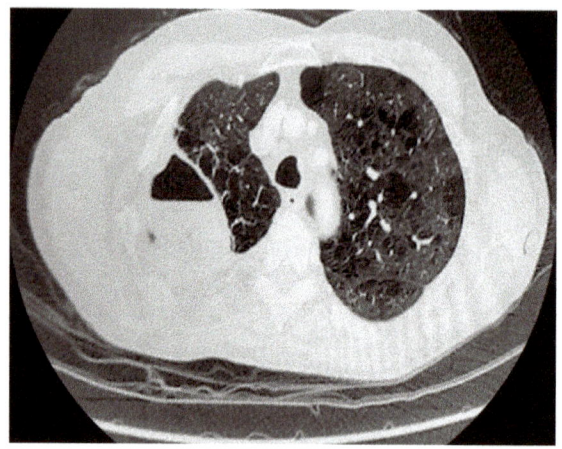

a. How do you describe the CT findings? (3 marks)
b. What is the diagnosis? (2 marks)
c. How do you treat this? (2 marks)
d. List two complications with delaying treatment. (3 marks)

Q26. A 33-year-old female, c/o lethargy, SOB since 6 months also has developed a rash over both shins.

Laboratory investigations are S/P (status post) raised erythrocyte sedimentation rate (ESR), serum calcium—12 mg/dL, CXR (image).

a. Identify the disease. (3 marks)
b. What is the cause of raised calcium in this case scenario? (7 marks)

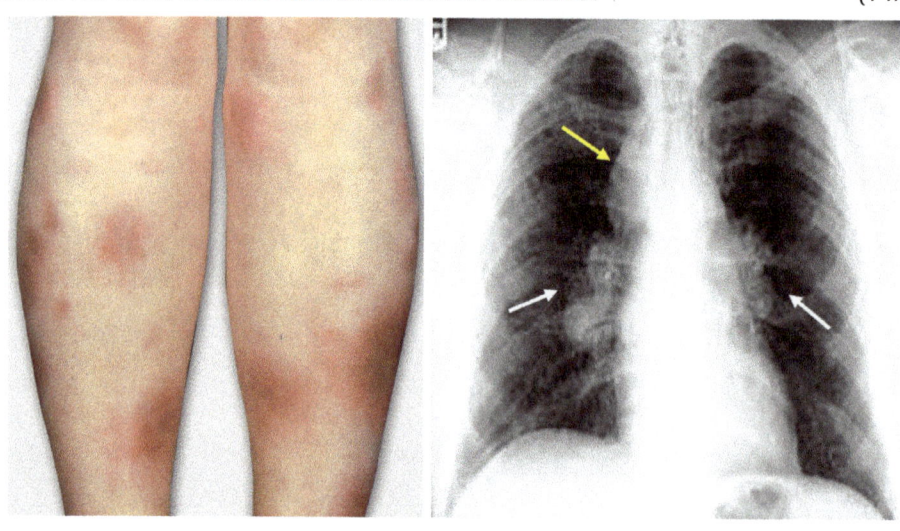

Q27.

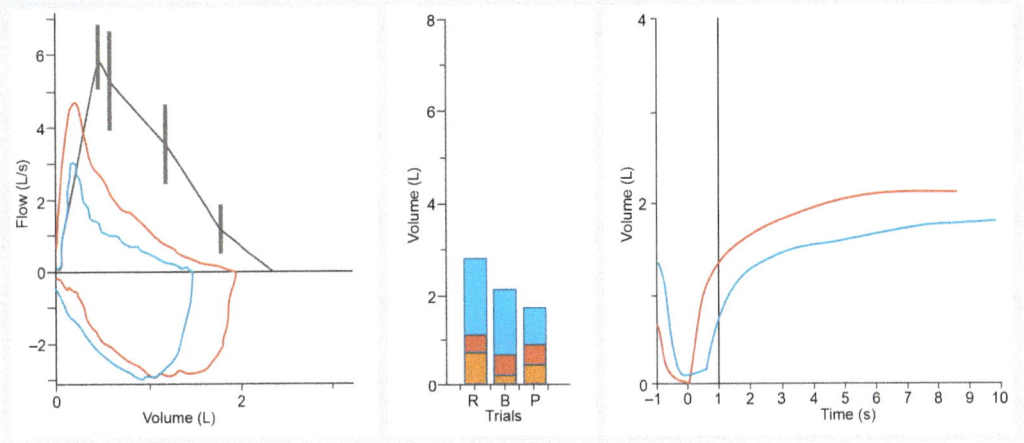

		Pred	Pre	Pre % Pred	Post	% Pred	% Change
FVC	(L)	2.39	1.73	72%	2.12	89%	23%
FEV$_1$	(L)	2.01	1.05	52%	1.40	70%	34%
FEV$_1$ % FVC	(%)	76.75	60.75	79%	66.10	86%	9%
PEF	(L/s)	5.96	3.05	51%	4.67	78%	53%
FEF 25	(L/s)	5.26	1.43	27%	2.49	47%	73%
FEF 50	(L/s)	3.55	0.69	20%	1.05	29%	51%
FEF 75	(L/s)	1.21	0.20	17%	0.25	21%	25%
FEF 25–75	(L/s)	2.76	0.54	19%	0.76	27%	41%
PIF	(L/s)	–	2.96	–	2.91	–	−2%
FET	(seconds)	–	9.72	–	8.36	–	−14%

(FEF: forced expiratory flow; FET: forced expiratory time; L/s: liter/second; PEF: peak expiratory flow; PIF: peak inspiratory flow; Pred: predicted)

a. Interpretation. (5 marks)
b. Global Initiative for Chronic Obstructive Lung Disease (GOLD) classification of airflow limitation severity in COPD. (5 marks)

ANSWERS

Ans. 1

a. Shifting dullness, succussion splash, coin test, cavernous bronchial breathing
b. Bronchopleural fistula
c. Chest tube drainage, video-assisted thoracoscopy (VATS), open window thoracostomy

Ans. 2

a. Parathyroid hormone (PTH), PTH-related protein (PTHrP), angiotensin-converting enzyme (ACE) levels, 1,25-dihydroxyvitamin D
b. Sarcoidosis
   In conditions such as sarcoidosis and other granulomatous diseases, activated mononuclear cells, notably macrophages, generate calcitriol from calcidiol independently of PTH.
c. Hydration and corticosteroids

Ans. 3

a. Right apical opacity due to pleuroparenchymal changes with a cavity and small right basal effusion
b. Old pulmonary tuberculosis (TB) with possible reactivation
c. Past history of TB, contact history of TB
d. Sputum for acid-fast bacilli (AFB), sputum for GeneXpert, sputum for TB culture and antibody sensitivity test (ABST)

Ans. 4

a. Achlasia cardia
b. The diagnosis can be confirmed by conducting a barium swallow, revealing the dilated esophagus. In earlier stages, precise cineradiology may be necessary, involving a barium-impregnated food bolus, or esophageal motility studies using a catheter equipped with multiple pressure sensors to identify abnormal motility in the esophageal muscles.
c. Achalasia can be addressed with muscle relaxants in milder cases but frequently necessitates interventions like endoscopic dilation or surgical procedures to disrupt the lower esophageal muscle.

Ans. 5

a. The woman's symptoms suggest pulmonary–renal syndrome with a purpuric rash, indicating active vasculitis, likely Wegener's granulomatosis.
b. Diagnosis involves detecting antineutrophil cytoplasmic antibody (ANCA) and Bx, with negative ANCA in 50% of renal cases. Wegener's granulomatosis is a systemic vasculitis affecting small-to-medium vessels. Tests include chest computed tomography (CT), lung function, and biopsies from affected areas. Management involves oxygen for hypoxia and intensive care for acute renal failure. Early specialist involvement is crucial.
c. Untreated Wegener's granulomatosis has a poor prognosis (median survival of 5 months). Treatment includes methylprednisolone, cyclophosphamide, and plasmapheresis for severe cases. Second-line agents are mycophenolate mofetil, rituximab, or leflunomide.

Ans. 6
a. Multifocal atrial tachycardia
b. COPD

Ans. 7
a. Bronchiectasis
b. Cystic fibrosis (CF), primary ciliary dyskinesia (PCD), alpha-1 antitrypsin (AAT) deficiency

Ans. 8
a. Pancoast syndrome
b. A superior sulcus tumor presents with ipsilateral shoulder and arm pain, along with paresthesias, paresis, and atrophy of the thenar muscles of the hand, accompanied by Horner's syndrome (ptosis, miosis, and anhidrosis).
c. Bronchoscopy and Bx/CT-guided Bx; squamous cell/adenocarcinoma
d. Professor Henry Pancoast in 1932

Ans. 9
a. Bradycardia, hung-up ankle jerk, thick coarsened skin, hypertension, hypothermia
b. Pericardial effusion, cardiomyopathy
c. Cerebellar signs manifesting with ataxia, tremor, and dysmetria; polyneuropathy; cranial nerve deficits; entrapment neuropathy (e.g., carpal tunnel syndrome)
d. *Heart:* Normal size, no hypertension, and low TSH in secondary cause

Ans. 10
a. Left-sided pneumothorax without mediastinal shift (see the left lung apex); always look for noninfective causes of COPD exacerbation if there is no H/O fever
b. Intercostal drainage (ICD) placement for pneumothorax, supportive management of COPD exacerbation

Ans. 11
a. Shifting dullness, coin test and succussion splash
b. Cavernous bronchial breathing and increase vocal resonance
c. Rupture of lung cavity in the pleura, gas-producing empyema, chest trauma

Ans. 12
a. Left upper lobe lung collapse or fibrosis, massive right-sided pleural effusion or pneumothorax, mediastinal masses
b. When there is a substantial volume of pleural fluid, but the trachea and heart show no significant shift to the opposite side or remain central or shifted to the same side as the effusion, it suggests a potential underlying lung collapse.
c. Oliver's sign, also known as the tracheal tug sign, refers to an anomalous downward displacement of the trachea during systole, indicating a possible dilation or aneurysm of the aortic arch.

Ans. 13

a. Bronchial breathing inspiration is less than or equal to expiration with a gap between the two

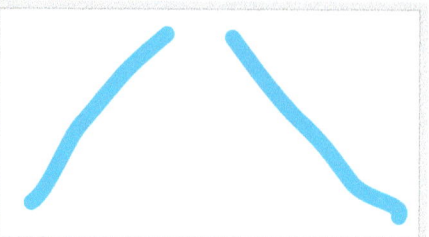

b. (1) Tubular—high-pitched—over consolidation; (2) cavernous—low pitched with hollow character—over the cavity; (3) amphoric—high-pitched with Echo or metallic quality—large cavity with small opening, pneumothorax communicating with bronchus.
c. It is normally heard anteriorly over the manubrium and posteriorly between the C7 and T3 vertebrae.

Ans. 14

a. Tension pneumothorax
b. Immediate needle decompression by inserting a large-bore (e.g., 14- or 16-gauge) needle into the second intercostal space in the midclavicular line.

Ans. 15

a. Obstructive sleep apnea (OSA)
b. Polysomnography/sleep study

Complications of OSA: These include asthma, atrial fibrillation, hypertension, cardiovascular diseases, cognitive and behavioral disorders, glucose intolerance and diabetes mellitus, and liver problems.

Ans. 16

a. Pulmonary sarcoidosis
b. Bx either from pulmonary or extrapulmonary organ revealing noncaseating granuloma and infections; malignancy should be ruled out.

Ans. 17

a. This is a skiagram of PA view of chest showing normal bony structures, with proper exposure showing a thick-walled cavity with an air–fluid level in the right upper lobe of chest.
b. Our provisional diagnosis is Lung abscess.
c. As the person is a known alcoholic so a probability is there that the lung abscess is due to aspiration of oral anaerobic flora. So the main modality of treatment is intravenous (IV) antibiotics with anaerobic coverage (i.e., inj. clindamycin)
d. *Complication of lung abscess:* Rupture into pleural space pleural fibrosis, respiratory failure, bronchopleural fistula, and pleurocutaneous fistula

Ans. 18

a. The skin lesions are red, tender nodules affecting the anterior aspect of shin which is classical for *erythema nodosum*.
b. A H/O dry cough, low-grade fever and weight loss with B/L hilar lymphadenopathy on CXR and erythema nodosum a diagnosis of sarcoidosis can be a possibility (provided TB is ruled out in Indian scenario). Investigations suggestive of sarcoidosis are peripheral lymphopenia on peripheral blood smear (PBS), cluster of differentiation 4 (CD4)/CD8 ratio in bronchoalveolar lavage (BAL) fluid >3.5. Confirmation is done by CT-guided Bx of hilar lymph node showing *noncaseating granuloma*.
c. *Scadding staging* is used for sarcoidosis: *Stage 1:* B/L hilar lymphadenopathy; *Stage 2:* B/L hilar lymphadenopathy + lung infiltrates; *Stage 3:* lung infiltrates without hilar lymphadenopathy; *Stage 4:* fibrosis.

Ans. 19

a. The above patient developed respiratory distress after the third transfusion and BP was 80/40 mm Hg and B/L crepitations were seen with whiteout lung fields. We have two possibilities: TACO/TRALI (transfusion-associated cardiac overload/transfusion-associated acute lung injury). Since the BP of the patient is not elevated so diagnosis of TACO was ruled out. So our diagnosis remains TRALI.

Management: Supportive treatment with oxygen, judicious fluid use, and ventilatory support; no role of steroids.

Ans. 20

a. This USG picture shows multiple and alternating hypoechoic and hyperechoic straight lines which are suggestive of "barcode sign" seen in pneumothorax.
b. The HRCT thorax showed multiple air filled thin lined cavities in right. Hemithorax and a collapsed lung in left hemithorax s/o emphysematous bullae in right hemithorax and pneumothorax in left hemithorax.
c. With the abovementioned clinical history of sudden-onset severe left-sided chest pain worsening on deep inspiration, with tachycardia and hypotension and hyperresonant note on percussion of left hemithorax and absent vesicular BS, a diagnosis of *tension pneumothorax with panacinar emphysema due to underlying AAT deficiency* can be made (liver Bx s/o abnormal hepatocellular cytoplasmic eosinophilic globules). The gene involved is *SERPINA1*.

Ans. 21

a. COPD
b. Prolonged expiratory phase, expiratory wheeze, tripod position, cyanosis, Hoover's sign (paradoxical inward movement of ribs cage with inspiration)
c. Beta agonists (short-acting, e.g., salbutamol; long-acting, e.g., formoterol, salmeterol, vilanterol), muscarinic antagonist (short-acting, e.g., ipratropium bromide; long-acting, e.g., glycopyrrolate, tiotropium), steroids, theophylline, phosphodiesterase 4 (PDE4) inhibitors (roflumilast).

d. To determine whether to use inhaled corticosteroid; steroid is indicated if eosinophil count is ≥300 cells/μL.

Ans. 22

a. Encysted hydropneumothorax
b. Lung abscess, hydrohemothorax, bronchopleural fistula, malignancy
c. Pigtail drain, antibiotics, physiotherapy, treatment of underlying cause, pleurodesis

Ans. 23

a. Pneumatocele
b. *Infectious:* TB and *Staphylococcus aureus*; noninfectious: trauma/positive pressure mechanical ventilation; drug abuse: IV heroin use

Ans. 24

a. Pulsus paradoxus refers to an exaggerated fall in a patient's BP during inspiration by greater than 10 mm Hg.
b. Cardiac tamponade and constrictive pericarditis
c. Acute bronchial asthma and acute exacerbation of COPD

Ans. 25

a. Thin wall cavity with the air-fluid level on the right upper lobe
b. Right upper lobe lung abscess
c. IV clindamycin 600 mg 8 hourly followed by oral 150–300 mg 6 hourly for 4–6 weeks
d. Empyema, bronchopleural fistula

Ans. 26

a. Sarcoidosis
b. Increased hydroxylation of vitamin D

Ans. 27

a. Obstructive pattern seen on PFT
b. GOLD 1—mild: FEV_1 ≥80% predicted
GOLD 2—moderate: 50% ≤FEV_1 <80% predicted
GOLD 3—severe: 30% ≤FEV_1 <50% predicted
GOLD 4—very severe: FEV_1 <30% predicted.

SECTION 14

Critical Care Medicine

QUESTIONS

Q1. A 32-year-old alcoholic male was brought to the emergency room (ER) with hyperventilation and a decreased level of consciousness, poor coordination, hypothermia, and decreased vision after drinking a countrymade liquor. Arterial blood gas (ABG) test revealed severe acidosis.

a. What is the diagnosis? *(3 marks)*
b. How would you treat? *(4 marks)*
c. What is the prognosis? *(3 marks)*

Q2. 40-year-old man presents with profuse vomiting after binge alcohol drink; heart rate (HR)—115 beats/min; blood pressure (BP) is 100/70 mm Hg.
- *Step 1:* pH normal
- *Step 2:* HCO_3 normal
- *Step 3:* Expected compensated $PaCO_2$ (partial pressure of arterial carbon dioxide) = $(1.5 \times HCO_3^-) + 8 \pm 2 = (34.5) + 8 \pm 2 = 40.5 - 44.5$
- *Step 4:* Calculate anion gap = $Na - (HCO_3 + Cl^-) = 140 - (23 + 95) = 140 - 118 = 22$ high anion gap metabolic acidosis
- *Step 5:* Delta ratio = $(\Delta AG)/(\Delta HCO_3^-) = (20 - 12)/(24 - 23) = 8$

a. What is the acid–base abnormality in the given ABG below? *(5 marks)*
b. What is etiological diagnosis as per ABG and clinical status? *(5 marks)*

pH	7.42	Na	140
pCO_2	40	K	3.0
HCO_3	23	Cl	95

(pCO_2: partial pressure of carbon dioxide)

Q3. A 23-year-old man who is a known case of type 1 diabetes mellitus (DM) with random blood sugar (RBS) reading of 480 presents with abdominal pain and breathlessness; HR—120 beats/min and BP is 96/60 mm Hg.

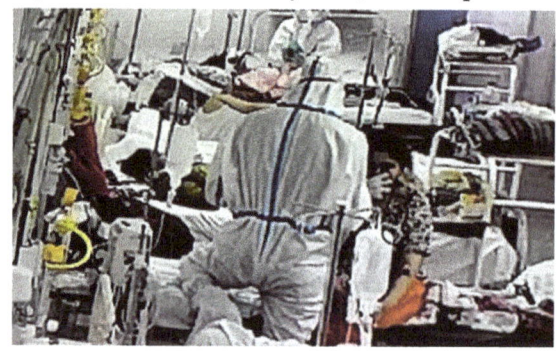

pH	7.15	Na	135
pCO₂	20	K	6.5
HCO₃	8	Cl	95

a. What is the diagnosis in terms of both etiological and acid–base abnormality? *(5 marks)*
b. What is the management of the above condition? *(5 marks)*

Q4. A 40-year-old medical health worker while working in the coronavirus disease (COVID) ward as shown in pic with inadequate ventilation for the past 6 hours has presented with severe fatigue and altered behavior. On examination, radial pulse is absent, brachial pulse rate (PR) is 110 beats/min with low pulse volume, BP—80 systolic, and temperature is 103 °F.

a. Enumerate the physical findings expected in this patient. *(3 marks)*
b. What is the diagnosis? *(2 marks)*
c. List investigations that help in diagnosis? *(2 marks)*
d. Enumerate treatment modalities in this patient. *(3 marks)*

Q5. A 30-year-old lady presented to the ER with cardiogenic shock. A screening echocardiography was done.

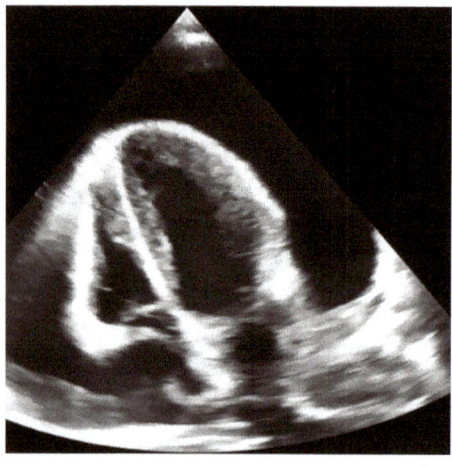
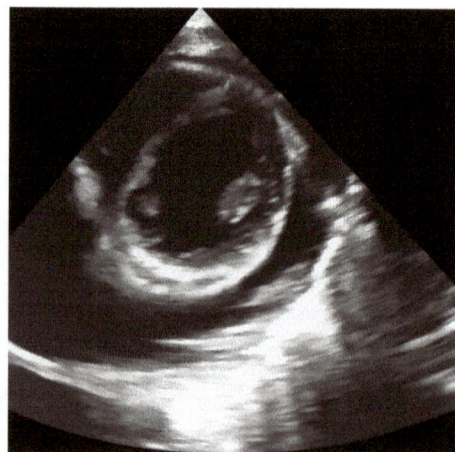

a. What is the diagnosis? *(2 marks)*
b. What are the common causes? *(2 marks)*

c. Enumerate the clinical signs. (4 marks)
d. What is immediate management? (2 marks)

Q6. The following image shows ABG of a 45-year-old woman who had poorly controlled diabetes and hypertension for the last 5 years; pH—7.421, pCO_2—30.1, HCO_3^-—19.6, blood glucose—564.
a. What acid–base disorder is present? (2 marks)
b. What is the underlying cause of these metabolic abnormalities? (2 marks)
c. Comment on anion gap in this ABG. (2 marks)
d. How will you proceed with management of this case? Mention any two steps. (4 marks)

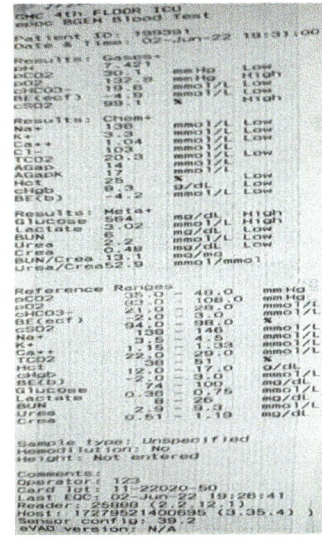

Q7. On the basis of ABG, answer the following questions.

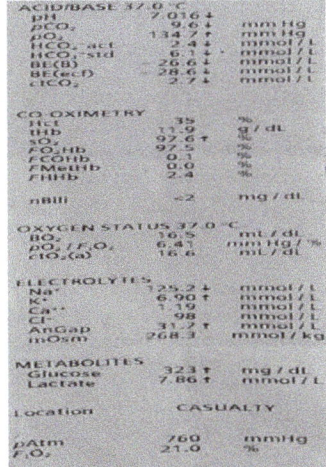

(pO_2: partial pressure of oxygen)

a. Interpretation. (5 marks)
b. Give the causes of normal anion gap metabolic acidosis. (5 marks)

Q8. A 68-year-old female, admitted with fever with chills, dysuria, flank pain, and hypotension requiring inotropic support develops the lesion shown in the image below.

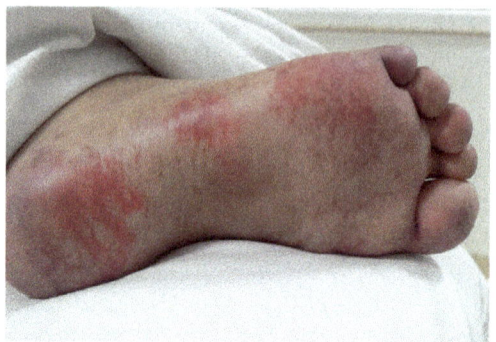

a. Identify the lesion. (5 marks)
b. Management. (5 marks)

Q9. On the basis of the ABG report, answer the following questions.

```
ACID/BASE 37.0 °C
pH            7.360
pCO₂          80.2 ↑    mm Hg
pO₂           85.6      mm Hg
HCO₃⁻act      44.3 ↑↑   mmol/L
HCO₃⁻std      39.1 ↑    mmol/L
BE(B)         15.3 ↑    mmol/L
BE(ecf)       18.8 ↑    mmol/L
ctCO₂         46.8 ↑    mmol/L

CO-OXIMETRY
Hct           36        %
tHb           12.4      g/dL
sO₂           94.7 ↓    %
FO₂Hb         93.6      %
FCOHb         0.9       %
FMetHb        0.3       %
FHHb          5.2       %

nBili         <2        mg/dL

OXYGEN STATUS 37.0 °C
BO₂           17.0      mL/dL
pO₂/F₁O₂      4.08      mmHg/%
ctO₂(a)       16.4      mL/dL

ELECTROLYTES
Na⁺           139.8     mmol/L
K⁺            3.88 ↓    mmol/L
Ca⁺⁺          1.14      mmol/L
Ca⁺⁺(7.4)     1.12      mmol/L
Cl⁻           92 ↓      mmol/L
AnGap         7.4 ↓     mmol/L
mOsm          285.5     mmol/kg

METABOLITES
Glucose       107       mg/dl
Lactate       0.95      mmol/L

pAtm          760       mm Hg
F₁O₂          21.0      %

↑, ↓ = Out of reference range
```

a. What is the possible interpretation of ABG report? (5 marks)
b. What are the contraindications of noninvasive ventilation (NIV)? (5 marks)

ANSWERS

Ans. 1

a. Methyl alcohol intoxication
b. The initial approach involves stabilizing the individual, followed by administering the antidote fomepizole. If fomepizole is unavailable, ethanol may be used instead. Hemodialysis may also be used in those where there is organ damage or a high degree of acidosis. Other treatments may include sodium bicarbonate, folate, and thiamine.
c. Long-term outcomes may include blindness and kidney failure. Death may occur even after drinking a small amount.

Ans. 2

a. High anion gap metabolic acidosis + metabolic alkalosis
b. Alcoholic ketoacidosis + vomiting

Ans. 3

a. Isolated high anion gap metabolic acidosis [diabetic ketoacidosis (DKA)]
b. *Management*:
- Confirm diagnosis (↑ serum glucose, ↑ serum β-hydroxybutyrate, metabolic acidosis).
- Admit to hospital; intensive care setting may be necessary for frequent monitoring, if pH <7.00, labored respiration, or impaired level of arousal.
- *Assess*:
    - Serum electrolytes (K^+, Na^+, Mg^{2+}, Cl^-, bicarbonate, phosphate)
    - Acid–base status—pH, HCO_3^-, pCO_2, β-hydroxybutyrate
    - Renal function (creatinine, urine output)
- *Replace fluids*: 2–3 L of 0.9% saline or lactated Ringer's over first 1–3 hours (10—20 mL/kg/h); subsequently, 0.45% saline at 250–500 mL/h; change to 5% glucose and 0.45% saline or lactated Ringer's at 150–250 mL/h when blood glucose reaches 250 mg/dL (13.9 mmol/L).
- *Administer short-acting regular insulin*: Intravenous (IV) (0.1 units/kg), then 0.1 units/kg/h by continuous IV infusion; increase two- to threefold if no response by 2–4 hours. If the initial serum potassium is <3.3 mmol/L (3.3 mEq/L), do not administer insulin until the potassium is corrected. Subcutaneous insulin may be used in uncomplicated, mild-to-moderate DKA with close monitoring.
- *Assess patient*: What precipitated the episode (noncompliance, infection, trauma, pregnancy, infarction, cocaine)? Initiate appropriate workup for precipitating event [cultures, chest X-ray (CXR), electrocardiogram (ECG), etc.].
- Measure blood glucose every 1–2 hours; measure electrolytes (especially K^+, bicarbonate, phosphate) and anion gap every 4 hours for the first 24 hours.
- Monitor blood pressure, pulse, respirations, mental status, fluid intake and output every 1–4 hours.
- *Replace K^+*: 10 mEq/h when plasma K^+ <5.0–52 mEq/L (or 20–30 mEq/L of infusion fluid), ECG normal, urine flow, and normal creatinine documented; administer

40–80 mEq/h when plasma K⁺ <3.5 mEq/L or if bicarbonate is given. If initial serum potassium is >5.2 mmol/L (5.2 mEq/L), do not supplement K⁺ until the potassium is corrected.

Ans. 4

a. Tachycardia, hypotension, cold and clammy extremities, low jugular venous pressure (JVP)
b. Hyperthermia, severe dehydration, and hypovolemic shock
c. Complete blood count (CBC), renal function test (RFT), ABG, and serum electrolyte
d. Secure airway and breathing, take off personal protective equipment (PPE), cooling of body temperature by cold sponging, and intravenous fluid (IVF) 2–3 L stat

Ans. 5

a. Massive pericardial effusion causing tamponade
b. Common causes are:
   - Malignancy
   - Uremia
   - Idiopathic pericarditis
   - Cardiac rupture
   - Proximal aortic dissection with rupture
c. Common clinical signs are:
   - Tachycardia
   - Tachypnea with clear lung
   - Beck's triad (distended JVP, distant cardiac sound, hypotension)
   - Pulsus paradoxus
d. Urgent pericardiocentesis

Ans. 6

a. Uncompensated metabolic acidosis with respiratory alkalosis
b. Type 2 DM presenting with uncontrolled hyperglycemia (? Diabetic ketoacidosis)
c. High anion gap
d. *Management:*
   - Replacement of fluids 2–3 L of 0.9% normal saline (NS) or Ringer's lactate over 1–3 hours subsequently 250–500 mL/h
   - Insulin infusion 0.1 units/kg/h continued until acidosis resolves and patient is metabolically stable. Patient overlapped and switched to subcutaneous insulin as soon as eating resumed.
   - Treatment of precipitating causes
   - Monitoring—BP, PR, respiratory rate (RR), mental status, fluid intake and output, blood glucose, serum electrolytes
   - Potassium correction

Ans. 7

a. High anion gap
b. Metabolic acidosis

Ans. 8

a. Purpura fulminans
b. Treatment of underlying sepsis

Ans. 9

a. Compensated respiratory acidosis
b. *Contraindications for NIV:*
    - Facial trauma/burns/recent facial, upper airway, or upper gastrointestinal tract surgery
    - Upper airway obstruction
    - Inability to protect airway and clear respiratory secretions
    - Impaired consciousness [Glasgow Coma Scale (GCS) <10]
    - Severe confusion/agitation
    - Vomiting and risk of aspiration
    - Allergy or sensitivity to mask materials

SECTION 15

Poisoning and Toxicology

QUESTIONS

Q1. A 17-year-old girl presents to the emergency department after an argument with her boyfriend. He says that she took lots of tablets. She denies this. You persuade her to let you do an arterial blood gas (ABG) test:
- pH: 7.46 (7.35–7.45)
- Partial pressure of oxygen (pO_2): 12.5 (10–14)
- Partial pressure of carbon dioxide (pCO_2): 3.5 (4.5–6.0)
- Bicarbonate (HCO_3): 22 (22–26)
- Base excess (BE): +1 (−2 to +2)
- Other values within normal range

A few hours later she says she feels increasingly unwell and is complaining of ringing in her ears. A repeat ABG shows:
- pH: 7.15 (7.35–7.45)
- pO_2: 11.0 (10–14)
- pCO_2: 3.2 (4.5–6.0)
- HCO_3: 9 (22–26)
- BE: −18 (−2 to +2)
- Other values within normal range

a. What is the abnormality? (2 marks)
b. What is the diagnosis? (4 marks)
c. How will you manage? (4 marks)

Q2. A 64-year-old gentlemen who is known diabetic for last 16 years presented to medical outpatient department (MOPD) with mild bipedal edema and decreased urine output. His past history revealed that he had lower respiratory tract infection (LRTI) 2 weeks ago for which he took some over the counter medication. His urine microscopy showed following finding:

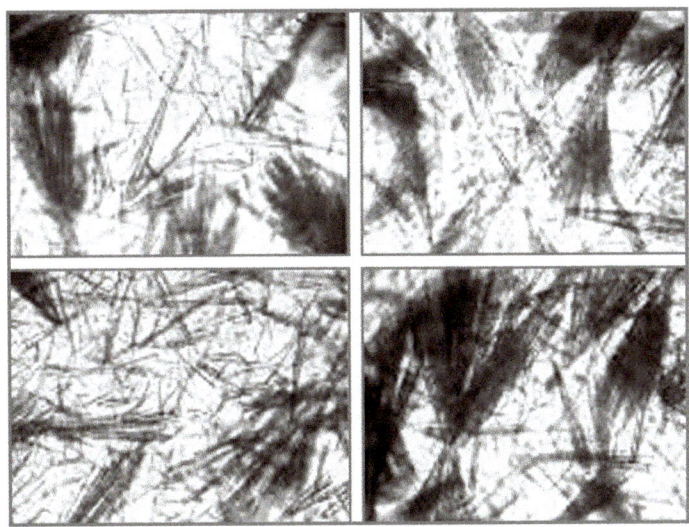

a. What is the diagnosis? (1 mark)
b. What are the other extra renal adverse effects of the causative factor? (4 marks)
c. What are the drugs that can give rise to such situation? (5 marks)

Q3. A 26-year-old male presented in the nephrology clinic with a history of (H/O) swelling feet, low-grade fever, and myalgia for 3 weeks. The swelling worsened during the evening and improved on resting.

Symmetrical pitting edema affects both lower limbs from ankles to scrotum and abdominal wall. Notable cutaneous flush, tenderness, and blanching of edematous areas with sensations of burning, itching, and paresthesia were noted. Laboratory investigations yielded no significant findings. Similar complaints were reported in her local area.

a. What is the diagnosis? (2 marks)
b. What is the etiology and pathogenesis? (3 marks)
c. Enumerate two differential diagnosis (D/D). (2 marks)
d. Enumerate the management strategy. (3 marks)

Q4. A 25-year-old was brought in the emergency room (ER) with frothing and pinpoint pupils after an alleged insecticide intake. The senior resident tested the knowledge of the second year student with the following questions.

a. Name two symptoms/signs depicting the action on different receptors. (4 marks)
b. Enumerate three late manifestations/sequelae of this condition. (3 marks)
c. Enlist two therapies and their action sites. (2 marks)
d. What is the most common cause of death? (1 mark)

Q5. A 28-year-old unemployed youth was brought to ER at 4 PM with nausea, vomiting, stomach burning feeling, dizziness, weakness, abdominal pain, and diarrhea. An urgent electrocardiogram (ECG) done is shown below.

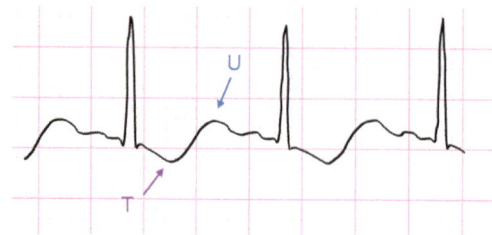

a. Describe the ECG findings and the diagnosis. *(3 marks)*
b. Which poisoning could have resulted in this ECG change? *(2 marks)*
c. How would you manage? *(5 marks)*

Q6. A village sarpanch organized a party after his election win. Following the party next morning 17 were reported to have died of "Hooch tragedy".
a. What is the mechanism of action and routes of toxicity of this chemical? *(4 marks)*
b. Name three clinical signs elicited in this poisoning. *(3 marks)*
c. How would you manage? *(3 marks)*

Q7. A 43-year-old recently diagnosed as type 2 diabetes mellitus (DM) started alternative therapy from a "hakim". He was admitted in gastrointestinal (GI) ER with severe constipation and intestinal pseudo-obstruction. On examination (O/E) he had diminished ankle reflexes. His hemoglobin (Hb) was estimated to be 10 g%. A smart resident made the diagnosis after a thorough general physical examination (GPE).

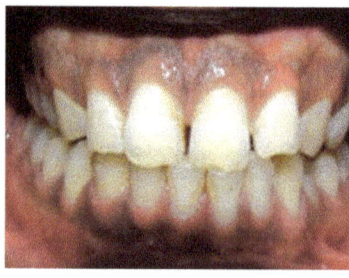

a. Name the abnormality on GPE and the diagnosis. *(4 marks)*
b. Name three other symptoms of this disorder. *(3 marks)*
c. How would you manage? *(3 marks)*

Q8. Aman is brought to the emergency department by his coworkers who found him collapsed in a field where he was spraying pesticides. On arrival, he is agitated, confused, and experiencing difficulty in breathing. According to witnesses, he was not wearing appropriate protective gear during pesticide application. His symptoms started approximately 2 hours ago with weakness, sweating, and excessive salivation.
a. What is the provisional diagnosis? *(3 marks)*

b. What is the antidote? (4 marks)
c. What is the expected pupil change? (3 marks)

Q9. A 34-year-old housewife was brought to the hospital with an alleged H/O consumption of about 100 mL of insecticide solution containing malathion. Prior to coming here, she was immediately taken to a primary health center (PHC) where a stomach wash was given, followed by intravenous (IV) fluids and 1.2-mg inj. atropine. She has a pulse of 66 beats/min, blood pressure 100/60 mm Hg, bilateral dilated pupils, with bilateral chest wheeze.

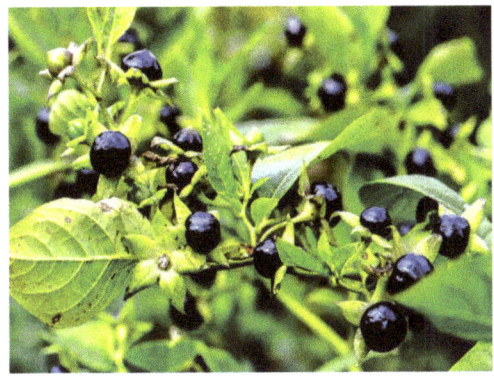

a. Identify the above plant from which atropine is derived? (1 mark)
b. What is the end point of giving atropine to this patient? (3 marks)
c. Enumerate the likely side effects of atropinization? (2 marks)
d. What are the other alternatives which can be used in place of atropine? (2 marks)
e. What is the mechanism of action of atropine in organophosphorous (OP) poisoning? (2 marks)

Q10. A 22-year-old lady staying in a rural area had a quarrel with her parents and thereafter consumed some pesticides. She developed recurrent vomiting, profuse sweating, and frequent urination after which she became drowsy. She was urgently taken to a local hospital where she was found to be comatose with response to only painful stimuli, with bradycardia and hypotension. Clinical examination also revealed the following finding in the pupillary size.

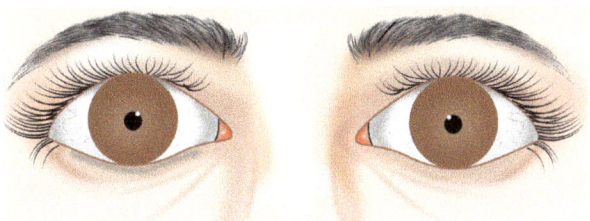

a. Identify the pupillary abnormality. (1 mark)
b. Enumerate some neurological conditions which can cause this finding? (2 marks)
c. Enumerate some poisons which can cause this finding? (2 marks)
d. What is the likely agent causing the poisoning? (1 mark)
e. Enumerate other common features of this poising? (4 marks)

Q11 A 42-year-old chronic alcohol consumer visited a country liquor shop and consumed large quantity of illicit country liquor. He complained of blurring of vision followed by drowsiness, altered sensorium, and became comatose. He was rushed to a nearby hospital where an urgent ABG was done as given below.

ABG
pH—7.06
O_2—82
CO_2—48
HCO_3—4
Na—134
Cl—104
K—3.5
Ca—1.11
Lactate—2.2
Glucose—92

a. Identify the common poisonous agent in illicit liquor (1 mark)
b. Identify the most prominent acid base disorder in the ABG? (1 mark)
c. Enumerate the other clinical features in this poisoning? (3 marks)
d. Mention the antidote, mode of action and its dose in methanol poisoning? (3 marks)
e. What is the likely cause of blindness in methanol poisoning? (2 marks)

Q12. A 27-year-old housewife was brought to the hospital with an alleged H/O consumption of about 50 mL of insecticide solution containing malathion. She was immediately taken to a PHC where a stomach wash was given followed by IV fluids and was then referred to higher center. The image below shows the normal functioning of a synapse at a myoneural junction.

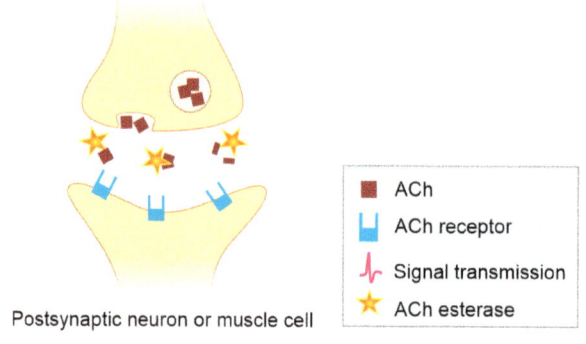

(ACh: acetylcholine)

a. Identify the likely type/class of poison? (1 mark)
b. Which component of the myoneural junction affected by this poison and how? (3 marks)
c. Enumerate the other poisonings which can occur with insecticide consumption? (3 marks)
d. What is the line of management in this type of poisoning? (3 marks)

Q13. A 22-year-old boy consumed a rodenticide poison with a suicidal intent as given in the photograph. He was initially scared and did not tell anyone. But after few hours, he developed fatigue, tiredness, dyspnea, nausea, vomiting, with a garlic odor in the breath; followed by loss of consciousness. He was rushed to a nearby hospital.

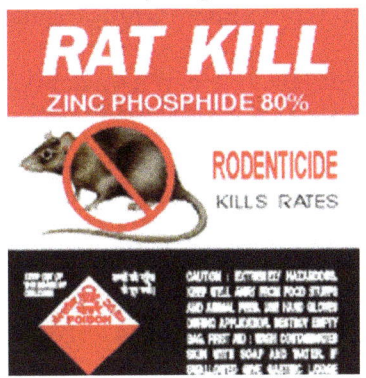

a. Identify the common poisonous substances in rodenticides. *(2 marks)*
b. Enumerate the clinical features of zinc phosphide poisoning? *(3 marks)*
c. What is the mechanism of action of zinc phosphide poisoning? *(2 marks)*
d. How is zinc phosphide poisoning managed? *(3 marks)*

Q14.

a. What is your interpretation? *(5 marks)*
b. What is the cause of this situation? *(5 marks)*

ANSWERS

Ans. 1

a. This is the classic picture of aspirin overdose.
b. There is an initial respiratory alkalosis due to central respiratory center stimulation causing increased respiratory drive.
c. In the later stages a metabolic acidosis develops alongside the respiratory alkalosis as a result of direct effect of the metabolite salicylic acid and more complex disruption of normal cellular metabolism.

Ans. 2

a. Amoxicillin-induced drug crystal
b. Skin rash, diarrhea, nausea, vomiting, Stevens–Johnson syndrome (SJS)
c. Ciprofloxacin, acyclovir, indinavir, sulfadiazine

Ans. 3

a. Epidemic dropsy
b. Epidemic dropsy is attributed to argemone oil, often stemming from the use of adulterated mustard oil, with which argemone oil is fully miscible. The primary toxic component in argemone oil is the alkaloid sanguinarine. Sanguinarine has demonstrated the ability to induce widespread capillary dilation along with increased capillary permeability.
c. It is essential to differentiate epidemic dropsy from conditions such as hypoproteinemia, filariasis, venous insufficiency, beriberi, hypothyroidism, and nephrotic syndrome.
d. The initial crucial step in managing epidemic dropsy involves discontinuing the use of contaminated cooking oil. Supportive measures like bed rest with leg elevation and a protein-rich diet prove beneficial. Additionally, supplements such as calcium, antioxidants (vitamins C and E), and thiamine, along with other B vitamins, are commonly employed.

Ans. 4

a. Muscarinic—D = Defecation/diaphoresis, U = Urination, M = Miosis, B = Bronchospasm/bronchorrhea, E = Emesis, L = Lacrimation, S = Salivation
   Nicotinic signs and symptoms include muscle fasciculations, cramping, weakness, and diaphragmatic failure.
b. Confusion, impairment in memory, lethargy, psychosis, peripheral neuropathy
c. Atropine—muscarinic, pralidoxime (2-PAM) also should be given to affect the nicotinic receptors since atropine only works on muscarinic.
d. Respiratory failure

Ans. 5

a. Hypokalemia is evident with a serum potassium level of 1.8/L, and the ECG displays characteristic alterations, including PR interval prolongation, ST segment depression (0.05–0.6 mV) with U waves (up to 1.0 mv), and t wave inversion.
b. Barium chloride poisoning

c. To counter the presence of barium ions in the intestines, precipitation can be induced through oral administration of sodium sulfate, sodium thiosulfate, or magnesium sulfate.
   - Magnesium ions play a role in maintaining normal intracellular potassium levels and enhancing potassium retention in potassium-deficient conditions. Thus, oral magnesium supplementation is recommended for patients with hypokalemia.
   - Clinically, potassium infusion is employed to reverse the toxic effects of barium.

Ans. 6

a. Methanol gets converted to formaldehyde and formic acid causing severe metabolic acidosis, circulatory, and tissue hypoxia, resulting in death.
b. Physical examination findings may reveal tachypnea, while eye examination may indicate dilated pupils with hyperemia of the optic disc and retinal edema. Tachycardia and hypotension may also be observed.
c. Management of methanol poisoning involves the use of fomepizole. In cases where fomepizole is unavailable, ethanol can serve as an alternative.
   - Additional therapeutic measures include the administration of sodium bicarbonate to address metabolic acidosis.
   - Hemodialysis or hemodiafiltration is employed to eliminate methanol and formate from the bloodstream.
   - Folinic acid or folic acid may be administered to enhance the metabolism of formate.

Ans. 7

a. High BP and lead line in the gingiva lead to the diagnosis of lead toxicity.
b. Irritability, lethargy, myalgia or paresthesia, difficulty concentrating/muscular exhaustibility
c. Withdrawing the offending agent, chelation therapy if lead levels are >45 ug/dL.
   The drugs used as chelating agents for lead include dimercaptosuccinic acid (DMSA), dimercaptopropane sulfonate (DMPS), dimercaprol [British anti-Lewisite (BAL)], penicillamine, and CaNa2EDTA (edetate calcium disodium)

Ans. 8

a. Organophosphorous poisoning
b. Atropine
c. Pinpoint pupil

Ans. 9

a. *Atropa belladonna*
b. *The end points of atropinization:* Clear chest on auscultation with no wheeze, heart rate >80 beats/min, pupils no longer pinpoint, dry axilla, systolic blood pressure >80 mm Hg
c. The presence of these indicates atropine excess: confusion, pyrexia, and absent bowel sounds.
   Apart from these, patient is also likely to have other anticholinergic effects.
d. Glycopyrrolate, Scopolamine
e. Atropine is a cholinergic muscarinic antagonist. It works by blocking the chemical acetylcholine, including excess acetylcholine caused by OP poisoning.

Ans. 10

a. Pinpoint pupils (miosis)
b. Pontine hemorrhage, Horner syndrome, Use of miotic eye drops, Iritis, Elevated body temperature, Narcotic substance abuse
c. OP compounds, carbamates, barbiturates, morphine, opiates, fentanyl, heroin
d. OP poisons or carbamates
e. SLUDGED: Salivation, Lacrimation, Urination, Defecation, GI symptoms, Emesis, Bronchorrhea, Bronchospasm, Bradycardia
  Others include fasciculations, cramps, weakness, miosis, blurred vision, bradycardia, hypotension, arrhythmias

Ans. 11

a. Methanol poisoning
b. High anion gap metabolic acidosis (HAGMA)
c. Neurological—inebriation progressing to coma, convulsions; visual—blurred vision, photophobia, visual acuity loss, optic nerve edema, gastrointestinal tract (GIT)—nausea, vomiting; cardiac—tachycardia, hypertension progressing to hypotension and cardiogenic shock; respiratory—tachypnea
d. Fomepizole
  Action: Fomepizole is a competitive inhibitor of alcohol dehydrogenase, and prevents the conversion of methanol to their toxic metabolites.
  Dosing: A loading dose of 15 mg/kg should be administered, followed by doses of 10 mg/kg every 12 hours for 4 doses, then 15 mg/kg every 12 hours
e. Methanol is converted to active metabolites like formic acid which are toxic to the optic nerve and may cause direct damage to the optic nerve and to both the outer and inner retinal layers, causing blindness.

Ans. 12

a. OP poisoning (OP poison)
b. *OP affect the anticholinesterases:* OP attaches to serine hydroxyl group of esteratic site of AChE, cause phosphorylation of enzyme, $t_{½}$ of reactivation of enzyme increases more than the regeneration time of enzyme, the phosphorylated enzyme undergoes "aging", and there is accumulation of ACh at nerve endings leading to excessive muscarinic and nicotinic effects.
c. OP compounds, carbamates, organochlorous componds, pyrethroids, nicotinoids, biological poisons
d. *Source control:* Washing body, removing clothes, gastric lavage; hemodynamic stabilization, inj. atropine 0.02–0.04 mg/kg bolus followed by 0.02–0.08 mg/kg/h titrated to effect, inj. pralidoxime 30 mg/kg loading dose over 10–20 minutes followed by 8–10 mg/kg/h.

Ans. 13

a. Phosphorous, struchnine, metal phosphides, sodium monofluoroacetate, arsenic, cholecalciferol, warfarin, superwarfarins, bromethalin

b. Early symptoms involve gastrointestinal distress and garlic breath, progressing to severe complications such as circulatory collapse, myocarditis, acute pulmonary edema, and organ failures.
c. Phosphides, reacting in the stomach, release phosphine gas that disrupts oxidative respiration, decreases mitochondrial membrane potential, and induces cell death through hydroxyl radical-mediated lipid peroxidation.
d. Gastric lavage is debated for oral phosphide poisoning; alternatives like vegetable oils are tried. Intensive care unit (ICU) care involves ventilation, organ support, vasoactive drugs, and correcting electrolyte imbalances. N-acetyl cysteine is used in acute liver failure (ALF) from phosphide poisoning. Pralidoxime shows limited benefit.

Ans. 14

a. HAGMA with inadequate respiratory compensation
b. Most likely suspected poisoning, rule out other causes of HAGMA

SECTION 16

Diagnostic Imaging

QUESTIONS

Q1.

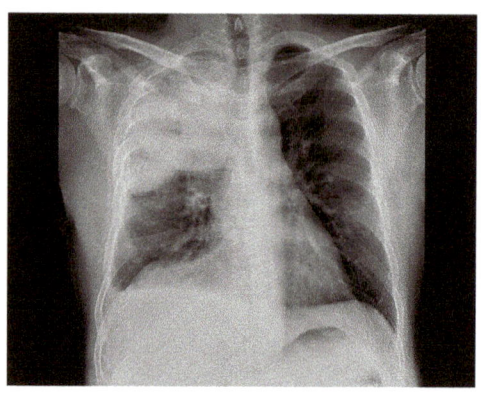

a. Sign depicted in given chest X-ray? (5 marks)
b. Name the organism associated with given condition. (5 marks)

Q2. A 5-year-old male presenting with pain in the legs, some bowing, with irritable behavior.
a. Name the first radiological investigation to be asked for. (4 marks)
b. What are the findings in the X-ray? (3 marks)
c. What is the diagnosis? (3 marks)

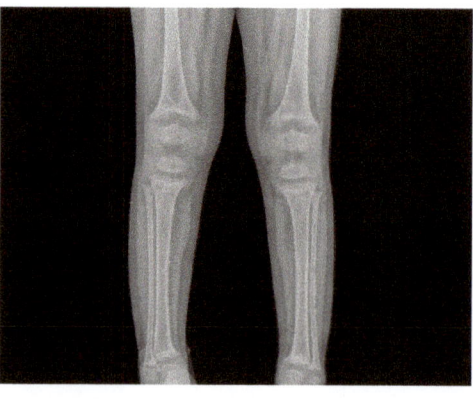

Q3. A 62-year-old male, a diabetic, presenting with acute onset of right-sided weakness.

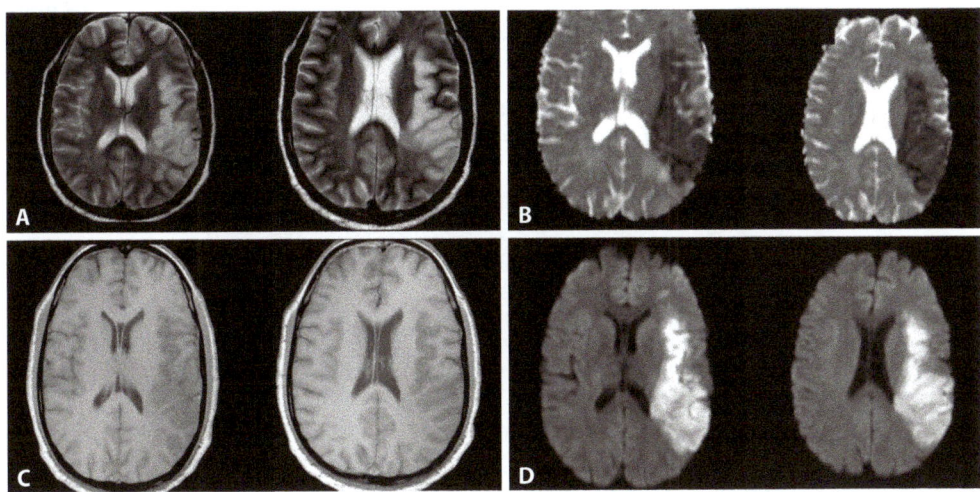

a. Name the investigation enclosed and identify different types of images. *(4 marks)*
b. What are the findings? *(3 marks)*
c. What is the diagnosis? *(3 marks)*

Q4. A 25-year-old male presenting with seizures.

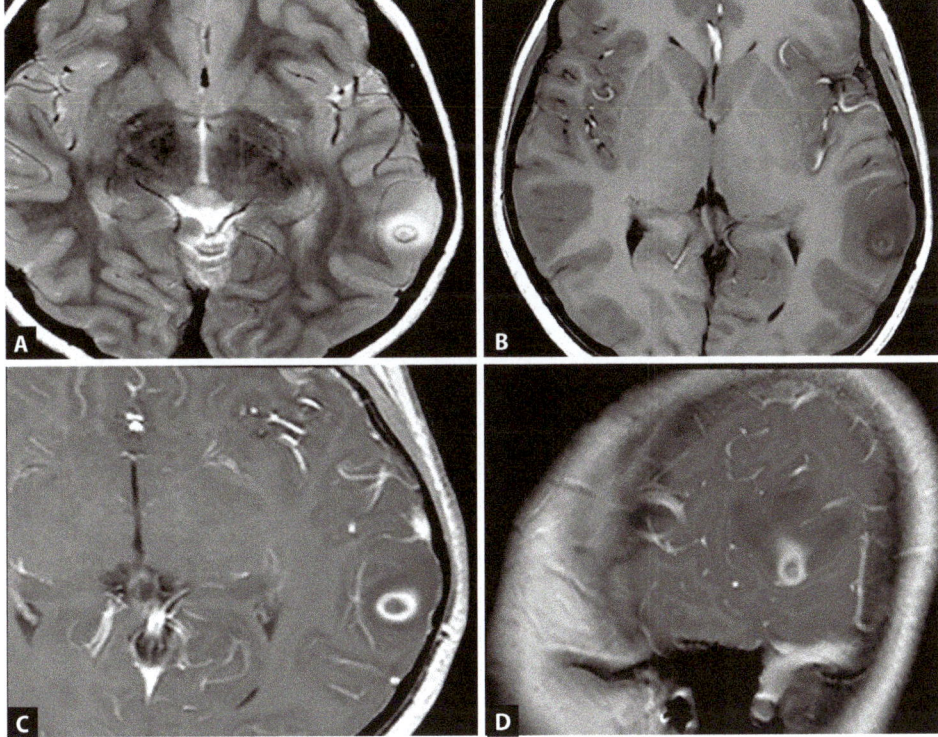

a. What should be the investigation of choice? (4 marks)
b. What are the findings? (3 marks)
c. What is the diagnosis and differential diagnosis (D/D)? (3 marks)

Q5. A 55-year-old hypertensive known case of coronary artery disease presented to emergency with chest pain and difficulty in breathing.

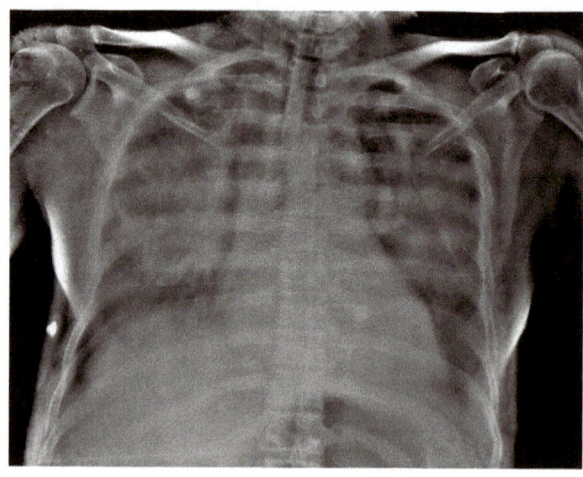

a. First radiological investigation. (2 marks)
b. What are the findings? (4 marks)
c. What is the diagnosis and D/D? (4 marks)

Q6. A 45-year-old male presenting with acute onset of breathlessness in emergency.

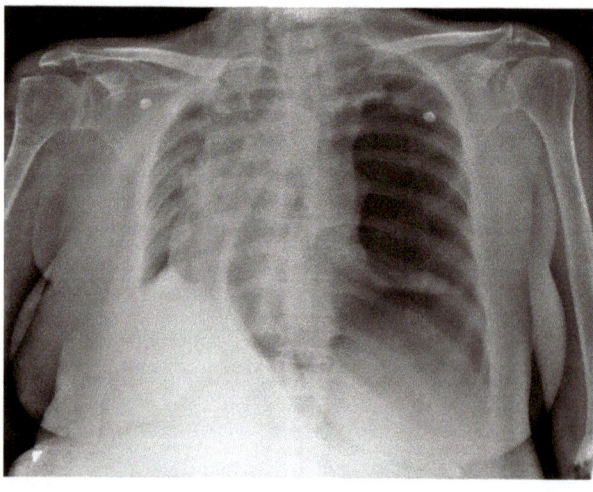

a. First radiological investigation. (2 marks)
b. What are the findings? (4 marks)
c. What is the diagnosis? (4 marks)

Q7. A 45-year-old male, an alcoholic, presents with acute pain abdomen in emergency.

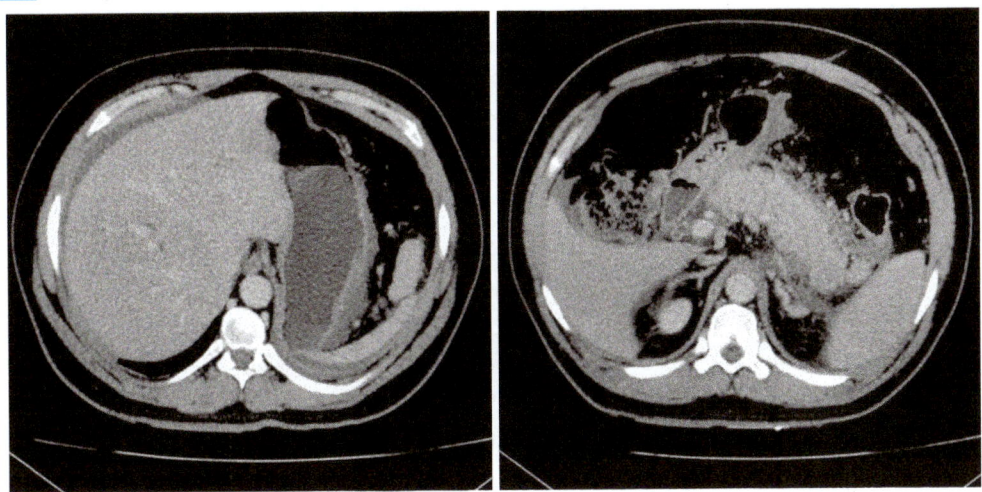

a. What is the first investigation to be asked for? *(2 marks)*
b. The first investigation was nonconclusive, what should be the next investigation? *(3 marks)*
c. What are the findings? *(3 marks)*
d. What is the diagnosis? *(2 marks)*

Q8. A 35-year-old female presenting with acute pain abdomen with mild derangement of liver function.

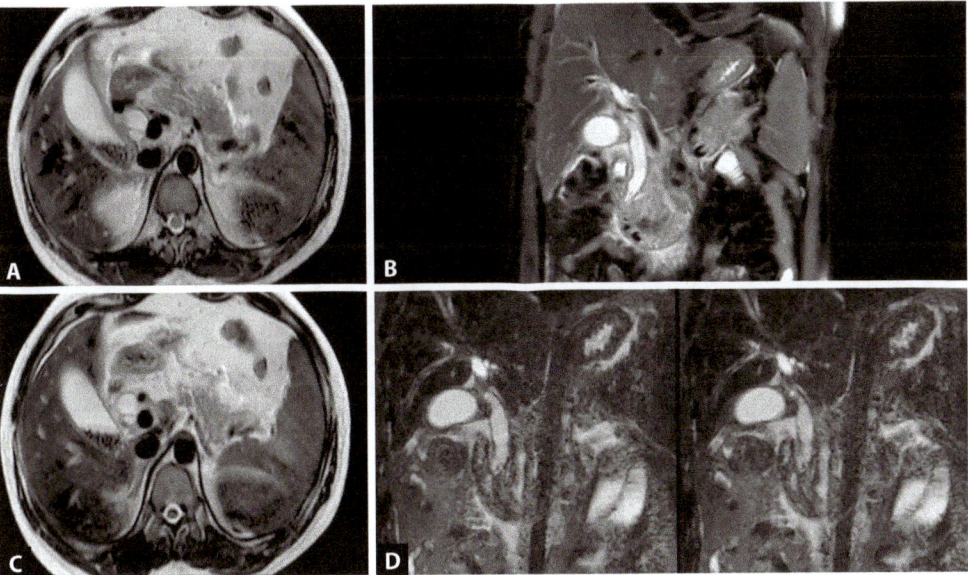

a. Name the investigation and the types of images. *(3 marks)*
b. What are the findings? *(3 marks)*
c. What is the diagnosis? *(4 marks)*

Q9. A 62-year-old male presenting with persistent cough and an episode of hemoptysis. There is history of pulmonary tuberculosis in the past for which he was treated.

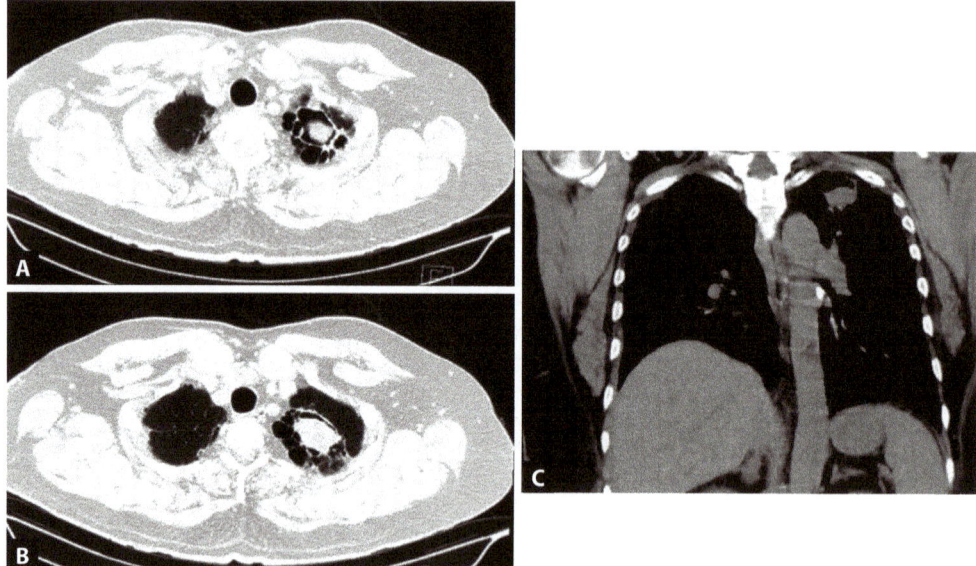

a. Name the investigation. (4 marks)
b. What are the findings? (3 marks)
c. What is the diagnosis? (3 marks)

Q10. A 60-year-old female presenting with acute abdominal pain in right hypochondrium.

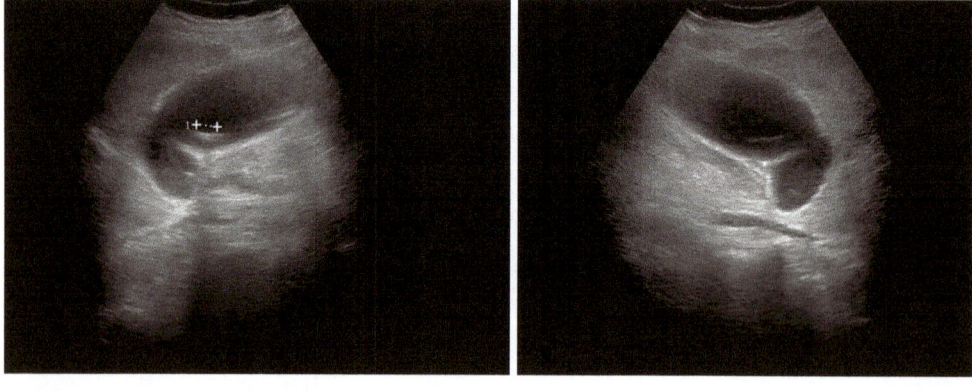

a. First radiological investigation. (2 marks)
b. Describe the findings. (3 marks)
c. What is the diagnosis? (3 marks)
d. What is the next preferable radiological investigation before surgery? (2 marks)

Q11. A 40-year-old male presenting with abdominal pain in right lower quadrant with nausea. Complete blood count (CBC) showed mild leukocytosis.

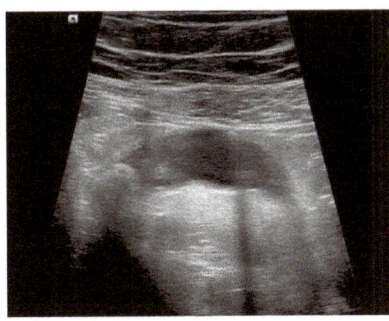

a. What is the initial radiological investigation? (3 marks)
b. What are the findings? (3 marks)
c. What is the diagnosis? (4 marks)

Q12. A 32-year-old male recently recovered from COVID presents with complaints of breathlessness with raised D dimer.

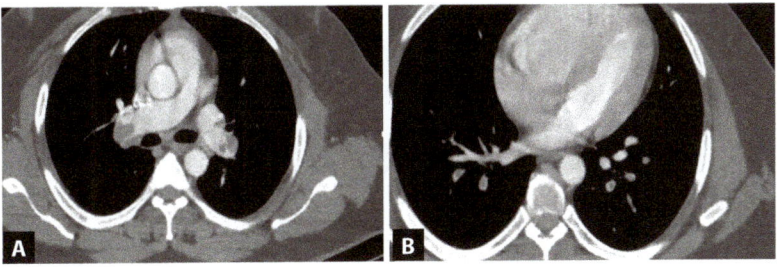

a. Name the investigation. (2 marks)
b. Explain the findings. (4 marks)
c. What is the diagnosis? (4 marks)

Q13. A 4-year-old male presenting with choreoathetosis.

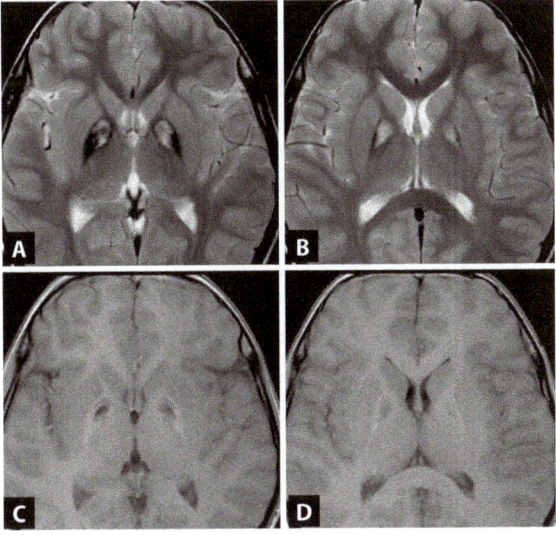

a. Name the radiological investigation of choice. (2 marks)
b. What are the findings? (4 marks)
c. What is the diagnosis? (4 marks)

Q14. An elderly male presented with cough and fever. Clinical examination revealed the presence of decreased breath sounds in the right infrascapular area and lower part of both the right axillary and mammary areas. Examination of the abdomen revealed the presence of resonance in the right hypochondrium. Chest X-ray (posteroanterior view) was taken.

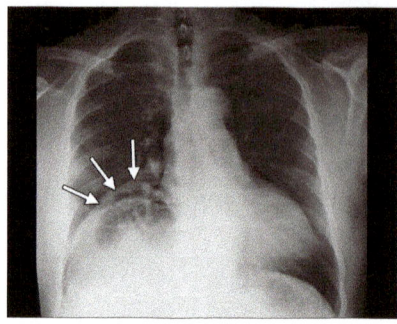

a. What does the X-ray show (see arrows)? (2 marks)
b. What is this sign called? (2 marks)
c. Suggest another investigation to confirm the diagnosis. (2 marks)
d. What is the treatment of this condition? (4 marks)

Q15. A 12-year-old male presenting with two episodes of focal seizures. EEG showed localization in the right parietal lobe.
a. Name the sequences shown. (3 marks)
b. What are the findings? (3 marks)
c. What is the diagnosis and D/D? (4 marks)

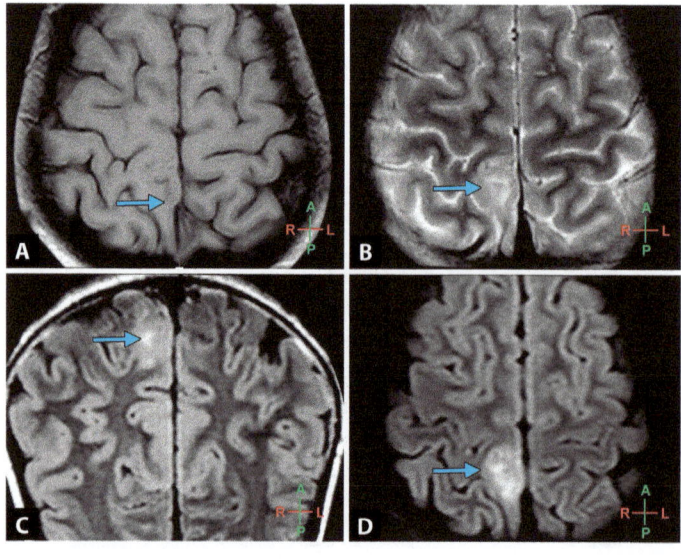

ANSWERS

Ans. 1
a. Bulging fissure sign
b. *Klebsiella pneumonia*

Ans. 2
a. X-ray leg—anteroposterior (AP) view
b. Metaphyseal splaying—widening of the metaphyseal ends, cupping—concavity of metaphysis, and fraying—indistinct margins metaphysis. Changes best seen in the distal end of femur but also seen in proximal and distal tibia.
c. Rickets
   Rickets is a result of deficient mineralization of the growth plate in the growing pediatric group. Although can be due to a number of causes, the most common cause in our country is vitamin D deficiency, which may be due to diet deficiency, poor sun exposure, or malabsorption. The disease can be treated easily if detected early by diet changes, supplementing the diet with vitamin D, improving sun exposure, and treating malabsorption if there.

Ans. 3
a. Investigation enclosed is magnetic resonance imaging (MRI). Four different types of images due to different sequences: (A) T2 weighted (T2W), (B) ADC images, (C) T1-weighted images, and (D) diffusion weighted images.
b. Focal area of hyperintense signal on T2W images (A) in the left parietal lobe involving sylvian, perisylvian region, which is low intense on T1 images (C), ADC images, and hyperintense on diffusion weighted images (D).
c. Ischemic stroke
   Ischemic stroke refers to neurological dysfunction due to focal ischemia in the part of brain due to arterial occlusion due to thrombosis or embolization. It is essential to differentiate between ischemic from hemorrhagic stroke.

Ans. 4
a. MRI with epilepsy protocol
b. A well-defined lesion in the left temporal lobe showing central hyperintense signal with peripheral low-intense signal on T2W (A) images. Small low-intense eccentric nodule is seen. Postcontrast T1 W images (C and D) showing peripheral rim enhancement. There is mild perilesional edema seen as hyperintense signal around this lesion on T2W images.
c. Degenerating cysticercosis. D/D is tuberculoma.

Ans. 5
a. X-ray of chest
b. Mild cardiomegaly with bilateral perihilar consolidation in a Bat-wing pattern with blunting of left cerebellopontine (CP) angle.

c. Pulmonary edema likely cardiogenic. D/D of Bat-wing opacities include pneumonia, inhalational injury, pulmonary alveolar proteinosis, lymphoma, leukaemia, and bronchoalveolar carcinoma.

Ans. 6

a. X-ray of chest
b. X-ray of chest reveals large left pneumothorax evidenced by lucency of left hemithorax associated with gross mediastinal shift contralaterally. There is no obvious lesion seen in the right lung.
c. *Tension pneumothorax:* It is a medical emergency, which results from progressive intrapleural accumulation with hemodynamic compromise. It needs rapid recognition and prompt treatment.

Ans. 7

a. *Ultrasonography (USG):* USG in this patient revealed normally distended gallbladder. Liver was fatty. There was minimal fluid in the peritoneal cavity. Pancreas and retroperitoneum could not be commented due to gaseous abdomen.
b. Computed tomography
c. The liver is fatty; pancreas appears bulky with peripancreatic edema and inflammatory changes. However, no defined collection is seen. There is small amount of fluid in the peritoneal cavity.
d. Acute pancreatitis

Ans. 8

a. MRI with magnetic resonance cholangiopancreaticography (MRCP). Images shown are: (A and C) Axial T2W, (B) Coronal T2W, and (D) Raw data of MRCP.
b. Gallbladder is normally distended and shows multiple small low-intense intraluminal foci. Pancreas is mildly bulky with subtle hyperintense signal and peripancreatic edema. The common bile duct is mildly dilated with low-intense filling defects in the distal end.
c. Cholelithiasis with choledocholithiasis with mild acute pancreatitis

   Magnetic resonance cholangiopancreaticography is a noninvasive technique to evaluate the biliary ductal system as well as pancreatic duct. There is no radiation and no contrast requirement.

Ans. 9

a. Axial (A and B) scan through upper zone and multiplanar reformation (MPR) coronal (C) CT image
b. There is a thin smooth thin-walled cavity in the left upper zone with a well-defined soft tissue density intracavitary mass. There are associated fibro cavitatory changes around. There is pleural thickening in the right upper zone.
c. Aspergilloma

   Aspergilloma is a mass-like fungal ball usually composed of *Aspergillus fumigatus*. They occur in patients with normal immunity but structurally abnormal lung with preexisting cavitary lesion. Tuberculosis is the most common underlying condition, other uncommon underlying pathology may be sarcoidosis, bronchiectasis due to any cause, or any other pulmonary cavity.

Ans. 10

a. Ultrasound abdomen
b. Gallbladder is distended with smooth thickened echogenic walls. There is thin streak of pericholecystic fluid. There is a small calculus showing distal acoustic shadowing.
c. Acute cholecystitis with cholelithiasis
d. MRCP to assess the status of cystic duct and common bile duct

Ans. 11

a. Ultrasound abdomen
b. Dilated thick-walled, blind-ending, tubular structure arising from the base of cecum. There is focal lesion within showing distal shadowing, suggestive of appendicolith. On the dynamic study, this will be noncompressible aperistaltic.
c. Acute appendicitis
   Acute appendicitis is the acute inflammation of vermiform appendix, usually presenting with pain in right lower quadrant/periumbilical region. USG should be the initial modality of choice. In nonconclusive cases, noncontrast computed tomography (NCCT) shall be performed. The common USG findings include: (1) Dilated >6 mm, aperistaltic, noncompressible appendix, (2) appendicolith seen as hyperechoic lesion with distal acoustic shadowing, (3) pericecal periappendiceal fat echogenicity, (4) fluid collection around appendix, (5) target appearance in axial view, (6) node prominence/enlargement around appendix, (7) wall thickening of >3 mm, etc.

Ans. 12

a. CT pulmonary angiography
b. Filling defects seen in the right as well as left pulmonary artery (A) as well as in segmental branches (B).
c. *Pulmonary thromboembolism:* Pulmonary embolism is embolic occlusion of the pulmonary arterial system. The most common source of embolus is deep venous thrombosis of the legs. The incidence was found to be increased in post COVID recovered patients.

Ans. 13

a. MRI
b. T2W images (upper two) showing low-intense globus pallidus with hyperintense signal in the center and relatively mildly hyperintense signal on T1 with low-intense signal in the center.
c. *Hallervorden–Spatz syndrome:* This syndrome is a neurodegenerative disorder with brain iron accumulation. This is an autosomal disorder due to pantothenate kinase-associated neurodegeneration, resulting in involuntary spasticity and progressive dementia.

Ans. 14

a. Hepatic flexure of the colon interposed between the elevated right hemidiaphragm and the liver
b. Chilaiditi's sign
c. CT scan
d. It requires no treatment.

Ans. 15

a. Axial T1W (A), T2W (B), coronal (C), and axial (D) FLAIR MR images
b. Focal area of cortical thickening with signal alteration in the right parietal lobe in parafalcine location showing mildly low-intense signal on T1 (A) and mildly hyperintense on T2W (B), and FLAIR (C and D) images. There is no perilesional edema.
c. Focal cortical dysplasia. D/D include cortex-based tumor or granulomatous lesion.

SECTION 17

Dermatology

QUESTIONS

Q1. A 55-year-old lady presented with abrupt onset fever, arthralgia, erythematous, tender, nonpruritic, papules, nodules, and plaques with predominantly head, neck, and upper trunk distribution (see image below). Laboratory test revealed neutrophilic leukocytosis.

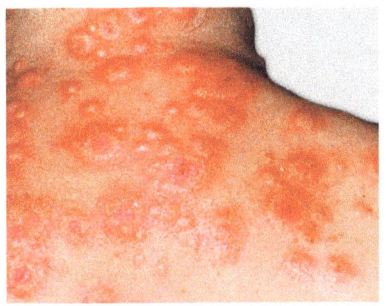

a. What is the diagnosis? (4 marks)
b. Name three risk factors. (3 marks)
c. How do you confirm the diagnosis? (2 marks)
d. Write two treatment strategies. (2 marks)

Q2. A 60-year-old woman with a 5-year history of uncontrolled diabetes mellitus presented with an ulcerating rash (see images), primarily on the shins, groin, and face; cheilitis; and glossitis. Her symptoms had been worsening for 4 years despite specialized wound care. In addition, she noted concurrent, severe weight loss, depression, abdominal pain, and intractable nausea. Computed tomography (CT) scan of abdomen reveals a pancreatic mass.

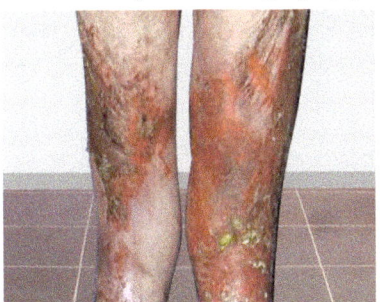 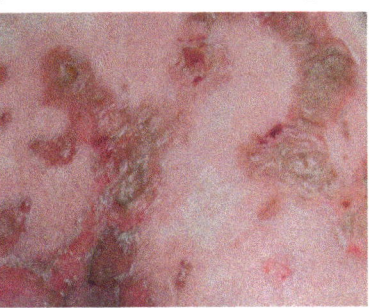

a. Write the diagnosis and finding. (2 marks)
b. Write the triad. (2 marks)
c. Name the syndrome related to it. (2 marks)
d. Name the functional imaging modality of choice for staging and localization of tumor. (4 marks)

Q3. A 52-year-old male tobacco chewer was prescribed minocycline for his chronic obstructive pulmonary disease (COPD) 10 days following that he presented to the general physician (GP) with complaint of (c/o) black tongue (see image below).

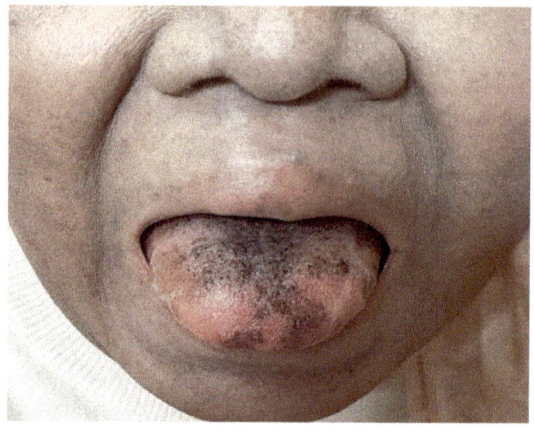

a. What is the diagnosis? (3 marks)
b. What are the risk factors? (3 marks)
c. How would you manage? (4 marks)

Q4.

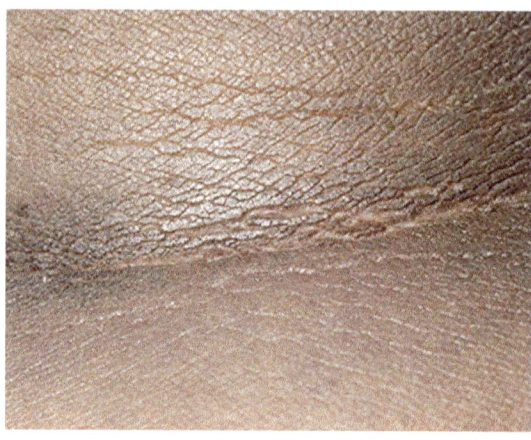

a. Describe skin lesion and diagnosis. (2 marks)
b. Write four causes. (4 marks)
c. Write four features suggestive of underling malignancy. (4 marks)

Q5.

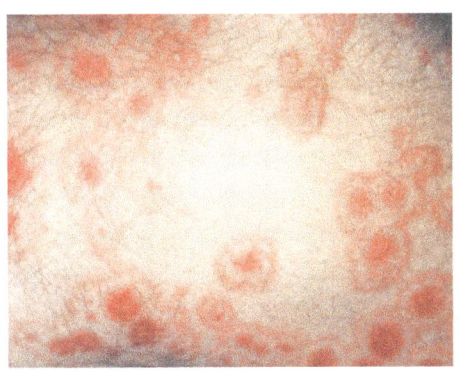

a. Describe the lesion. (3 marks)
b. List two infectious and noninfectious causes. (4 marks)
c. What is the typical course? (3 marks)

Q6.

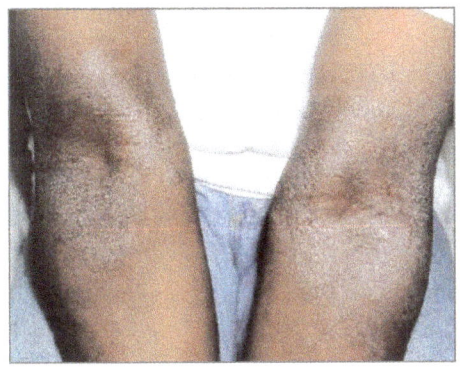

a. Describe the lesion. (3 marks)
b. What is the diagnosis? (4 marks)
c. How would you treat? (3 marks)

Q7.

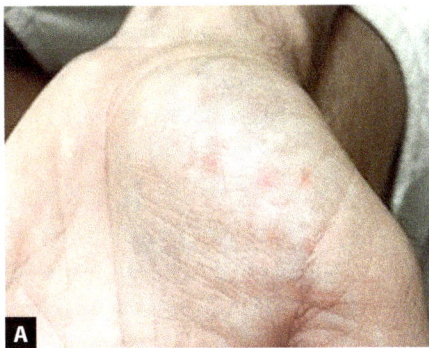
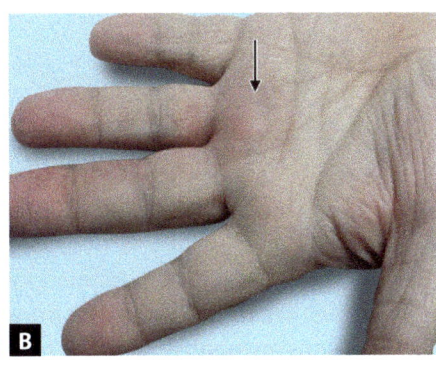

a. Identify the Images A and B. (5 marks)
b. Discuss the criteria used for the disease. (5 marks)

Q8. A 39-year-old lady presents with rashes over face and neck for 6 months. Clinical examination rules out any articular or neuromuscular pathology.

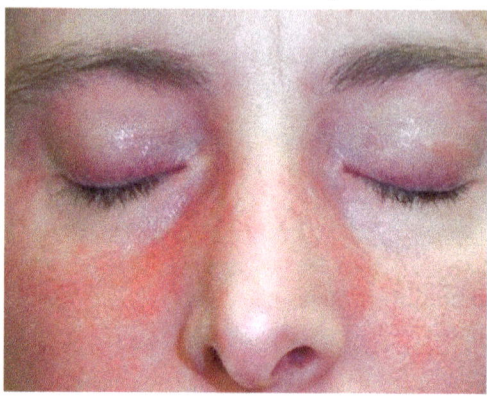

a. Describe the skin finding. (3 marks)
b. What is the diagnosis? (3 marks)
c. Discuss the treatment of patients with severe cutaneous manifestations with this disorder. (4 marks)

Q9. A 54-year-old alcoholic male presented with pain in abdomen. Ascitic fluid study (atraumatic tap) showed plenty of red blood cell (RBC) with high serum-ascites albumin gradient (SAAG) ascites.

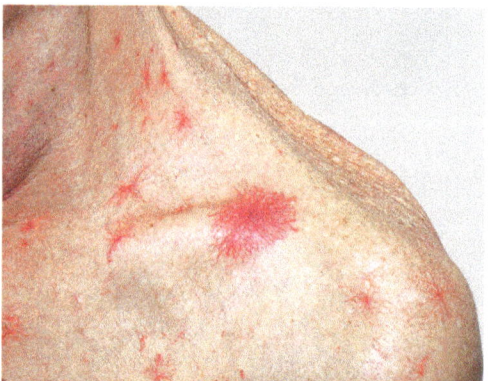

a. Write the diagnosis of the skin finding. (3 marks)
b. What is the possible cause of RBC in ascitic fluid in this patient? (4 marks)
c. How spontaneous bacterial peritonitis (SBP) is diagnosed? (3 marks)

Q10. A 68-year-old gentleman presented to his physician with skin eruptions in both legs and a mild burning sensation. He took some ayurvedic medications very recently. On clinical examination, lesions are nonblanching in nature.

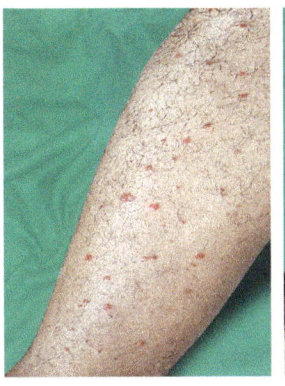
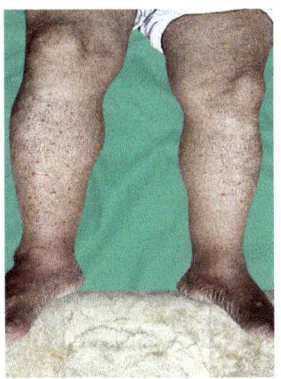

a. Describe the lesion. *(3 marks)*
b. What is the diagnosis? *(2 marks)*
c. Enumerate the causes. *(5 marks)*

Q11.

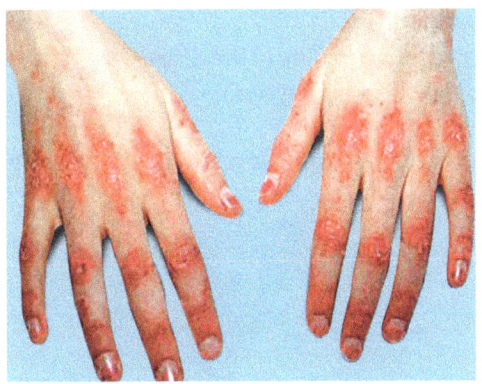

a. Identify the sign. *(2 marks)*
b. IOC of condition in which these papules are seen. *(4 marks)*
c. Distal muscle is predominantly involved. (True or False) *(4 marks)*

Q12.

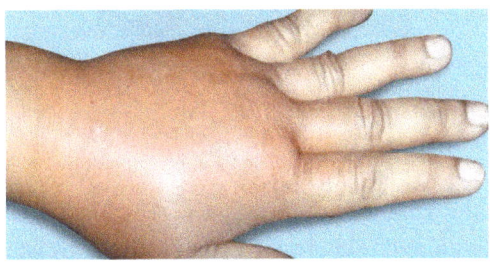

An alcoholic patient took nonvegetarian diet and got the manifestations shown in image.
a. Describe the findings in the image. *(5 marks)*
b. Write differential diagnoses (D/D). *(5 marks)*

Q13. A 35-year-old male presented to the medicine OPD with c/o greasy stools for last 2 years, which is exacerbated on taking chapatis. Now he felt of consulting a doctor after getting severe itchy rashes over back and dorsum of elbow. Biopsy was taken for histopathological examination (HPE), which shows as follows.

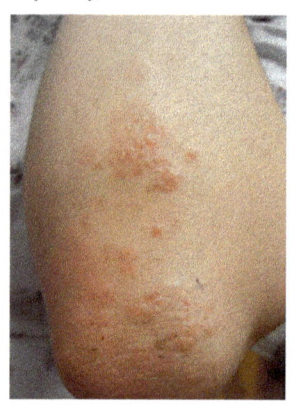
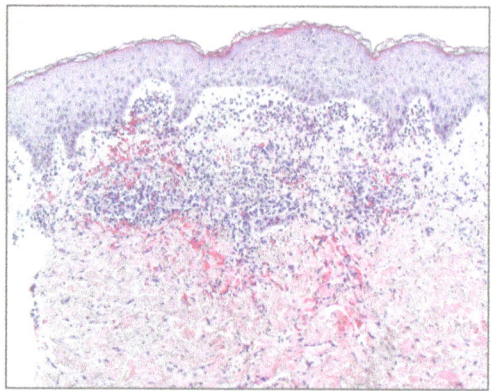

a. What is the clinical condition? (4 marks)
b. What is the antibody used for screening of the disease process? (3 marks)
c. What is the histopathological grading system? (3 marks)

Q14. An 18-year-old female referred from dermatologist, with a lipid profile report.

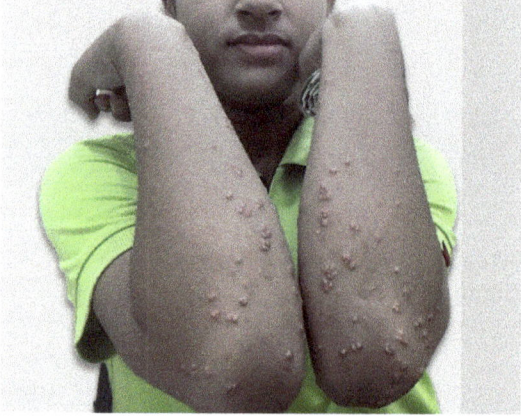

a. What is your diagnosis? (3 marks)
b. What are the D/D? (3 marks)
c. What is the management? (3 marks)

Q15. A 48-year-old male from remote village of South 24 PGS of West Bengal (WB) complaining of asymptomatic such skin lesions all over the body except head, neck, and face. Similar skin lesions are present in his all other three family members and few persons of same village.

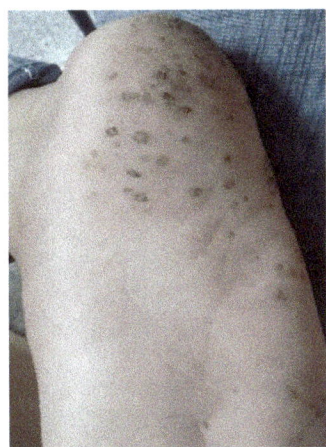

a. What will be the D/D? (3 marks)
b. Suggest three investigations to confirm the diagnosis. (3 marks)
c. List four complications of this condition. (4 marks)

Q16. A 34-year-old human immunodeficiency virus (HIV)-positive female from the remote village of Malda district of WB, complaining of asymptomatic skin lesions all over the body with fever for 2 months. On examination, she had pallor and hepatosplenomegaly.

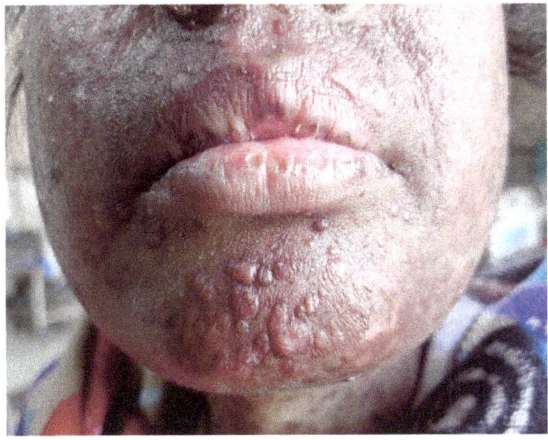

a. What will be the D/D? (3 marks)
b. How will you confirm the diagnosis? (2 marks)
c. How will you treat the patient? (4 marks)
d. Write one life-threatening complication of this condition. (1 mark)

Q17. A 55-year-old female presented with a rash, 1 week after being started on a medication for a seronegative inflammatory arthritis. Please find below images of her rash and full blood count report.

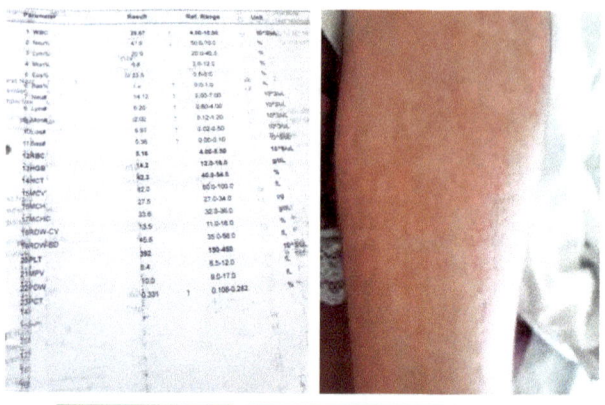

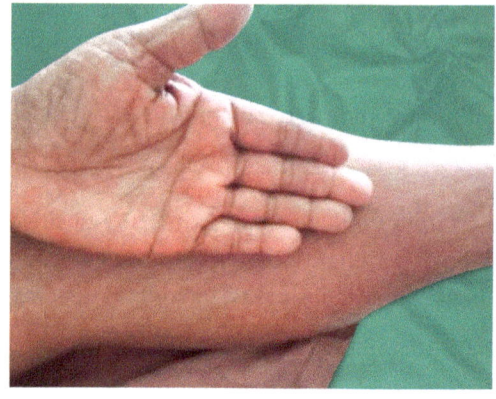

a. What is the diagnosis? (2 marks)
b. What other physical signs may be present? (3 marks)
c. What are the probable causative agent/s? (2 marks)
d. List three complications of this condition. (3 marks)

Q18.

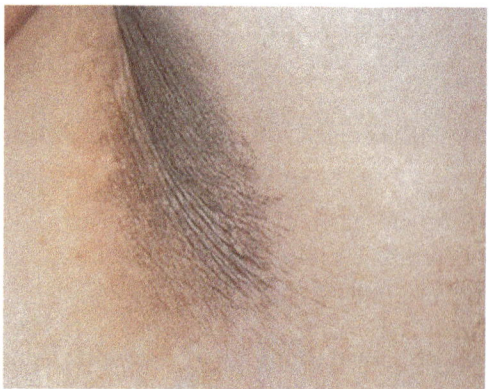

a. What is the name of the condition? (2 marks)
b. Name six causes for this condition. (6 marks)
c. Mention the principle of management of the conditions. (2 marks)

Q19. A 22-year-old female presented with the above skin lesions on her forehead (Image A) scalp, upper arms, chest, back, knees, elbows, and behind the ear, which had a strong odor, and had flares. Her nails showed the findings as in Image B. She had mild intellectual disability and seizure disorder.

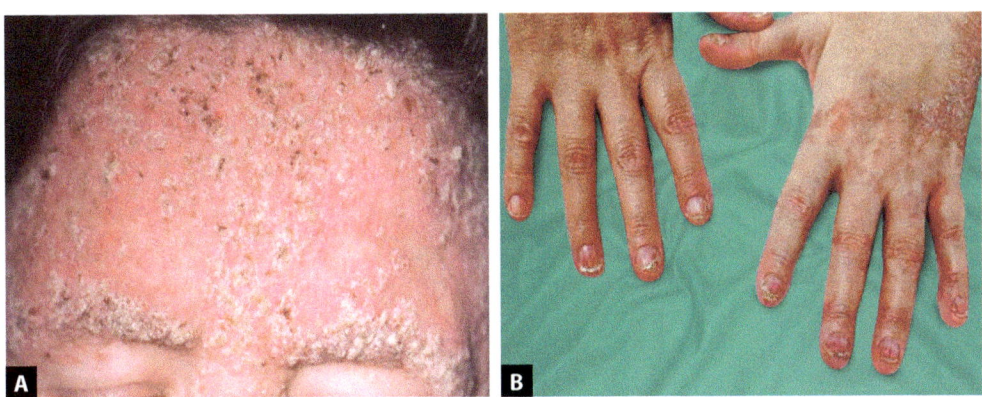

a. Identify the disease. *(2 mark)*
b. What is its inheritance? *(3 mark)*
c. What is the defective gene, where is that gene located, and which enzyme does it code for? *(2 + 2 + 1 marks)*

ANSWERS

Ans. 1
a. Sweet syndrome
b. Leukemia or lymphoma, ulcerative colitis or Crohn's disease, chest infection, and colon or breast cancer
c. Skin biopsy demonstrating neutrophilic infiltration
d. Heals spontaneously, corticosteroids may help and treat the underlying condition

Ans. 2
a. Glucagonoma; necrotic migratory erythema
b. Necrolytic migratory erythema as seen on examination + weight loss + diabetes mellitus (DM)
c. Multiple endocrine neoplasm syndrome type 1 (MEN1)
d. Ga-68 DOTATOC

Ans. 3
a. Black hairy tongue. Hairy tongue is a benign condition that involves elongation and discoloration of the filiform papillae on the dorsal aspect of the tongue.
b. Risk factors include smoking, dehydration, poor oral hygiene, and antimicrobial use.
c. Advise the patient to maintain oral dental hygiene, gently scrub the surface of his tongue with a toothbrush 3–4 times daily, stay hydrated, and smoking cessation.

Ans. 4
a. *Acanthosis nigricans*—hyperpigmented velvety plaques
b. Obesity, DM, polycystic ovarian disease (PCOD), malignancy, and glucocorticoids
c. Rapid onset of skin lesions, additional paraneoplastic findings [e.g., rapid growth or inflammation of seborrheic keratoses (the sign of Leser-Trélat) or the presence of tripe palms], extensive involvement, lesions in atypical sites (e.g., mucous membranes, palms, or soles), unexplained weight loss, and older adult.

Ans. 5
a. Erythema multiforme—multiple erythematous plaques with a target or iris morphology
b. *Infectious—herpes simplex virus (HSV) and mycoplasma; noninfectious—nonsteroidal anti-inflammatory drugs (NSAIDs) and sulfonamides*
c. Usually appear over the course of 3–5 days and resolve within approximately 1 week. Although the skin lesions do not scar, postinflammatory hyperpigmentation may remain for months after resolution, particularly in patients with dark skin.

Ans. 6
a. Hyperpigmentation, lichenification, and scaling in the antecubital fossae
b. Atopic dermatitis
c. Avoidance of allergens, topical glucocorticoids, topical tacrolimus, treat secondary infections

Ans. 7

a. Janeway lesion and Osler nodes
b. Duke's criteria

Ans. 8

a. Heliotrope rash
b. Dermatomyositis sine myositis
c. *Treatment:* Methotrexate and hydroxychloroquin

Ans. 9

a. Spider angioma
b. *Causes:* Malignancy, rupture of peritoneal varix, and infection (rare)
c. *Diagnosis of SBP:* A positive ascitic fluid bacterial culture and an ascitic fluid absolute polymorphonuclear neutrophil (PMN) count ≥250 cells/mm^3

Ans. 10

a. Multiple, red-colored nonblanching slightly elevated round-shaped lesions of varying sizes with regular margins involving both the lower limbs
b. Palpable purpura
c. Causes of palpable purpura are:
   - Vasculitis—leukocytoclastic vasculitis or small vessel vasculitis [drugs, connective tissue disease (CTD), Henoch-Schönlein purpura (HSP), hepatitis C virus (HCV)], and polyarteritis nodosa
   - Embolic—acute meningococcemia and disseminated gonococcal infection.

Ans. 11

a. Gottron papules
b. Muscle biopsy
c. False

Ans. 12

a. Red hand with edema showing sign of inflammation—rubor, calor, tumor, and dolor
b. *D/D:* Acute gout, trauma, and cellulitis

Ans. 13

a. The clinical condition is known as *Dermatitis Herpetiformis (DH)*. It is an extremely itchy maculopapular rash involving the extensor surface of arms and back and mainly occurs due to underlying malabsorption syndrome like celiac disease, which is evident in the above case as there is a history of semisolid stool after eating chapatis.
b. The antibody used to screen the disease process is *antitissue transglutaminase IgA (anti-tTG IgA)*.
c. Histopathological grading system: *Marsh grading*

Type	Intraepithelial lymphocytes per 100 enterocytes	Crypts	Villi
0	<40	Normal	Normal
1	>40	Normal	Normal
2	>40	Increased	Normal
3a	>40	Increased	Mild atrophy
3b	>40	Increased	Marked atrophy
3c	>40	Increased	Absent

Ans. 14

a. Her lipid profile was:
   - Cholesterol: 670 mg/dL
   - Low-density lipoprotein (LDL): 235 mg/dL
   - High-density lipoprotein (HDL): 17 mg/dL
   - Very LDL: 418 mg/dL
   - Triglyceride (TG): 6,539 mg/dL
b. *Diagnosis:* Eruptive xanthoma
   Differential diagnoses:
   - Molluscum contagiosum
   - Syringoma
   - Sebaceous hyperplasia
c. *Management:* Fenofibrate

Ans. 15

a. Chronic arsenicosis, melanin deposition, and secondary syphilis
b. Arsenic estimation from patient's hair, nail, and consumed water, serum venereal disease research laboratory test (VDRL), and skin biopsy.
c. Basal cell carcinoma (BCC), squamous cell carcinoma (SCC), hepatic involvement, and cardiac and pulmonary involvement.

Ans. 16

a. Histoplasmosis, talaromyces marneffei, and cryptococcosis
b. Slit skin smear and skin biopsy for histopathological examination with fungal stain
c. Injection liposomal amphotericin B for 2 weeks followed by tablet itraconazole till the CD4 count rises above 250 for consecutive two occasions.
d. Adrenal insufficiency

Ans. 17

a. Drug reaction with eosinophilia and systemic symptoms (DRESS) syndrome
b. Hepatomegaly, lymphadenopathy, fever, and facial edema

c. Sulfasalazine and allopurinol
d. Acute liver failure, acute interstitial nephritis, acute interstitial pneumonia, and eosinophilic myocarditis

Ans. 18

a. *Acanthosis nigricans*
b. Polycystic ovarian syndrome (PCOS), type 2 DM, metabolic syndrome, gastric adenocarcinoma, Cushing syndrome, acromegaly, lymphoma, obesity, and idiopathic
c. Management of the underlying cause

Ans. 19

a. Darier disease
b. Autosomal dominant
c. The abnormal gene in Darier disease has been identified as ATP2A2, found on chromosome 12Q23-24.1. This gene codes for the SERCA enzyme or pump (SarcoEndoplasmic Reticulum Calcium ATPase) that is required to transport calcium within the cell.

SECTION 18

Medical Genetics

QUESTIONS

Q1. A 46-year-old male, a case of rheumatic heart disease (RHD) with mitral stenosis (MS) and atrial fibrillation, is being prescribes warfarin. An enthusiastic resident explains the precautions while taking the drug. He also suggested a genetic testing.
a. Enumerate four instructions to be taken before prescribing warfarin. *(4 marks)*
b. Why did the resident order a genetic testing and explain the actual test? *(3 marks)*
c. Explain the mechanism of warfarin-induced skin necrosis. *(3 marks)*

Q2. A 14-year-old boy was brought to the outpatient department by his mother with history of (h/o) progressive difficulty in getting up from squatting position. His initial evaluation revealed a threefold rise in creatine phosphokinase (CPK) levels.
a. What is the diagnosis? *(2 marks)*
b. What is peculiar about the calf muscles in them? *(2 marks)*
c. What is the molecular cause of the disease? *(2 marks)*
d. Why was 2D Echo ordered in this case? *(2 marks)*
e. What is the life span of such patients? *(2 marks)*

Q3. A 38-year-old male presented to the neurologist with h/o progressive dystonia. He reported early death of his father due to some neurological disease. The neurologist ordered an imaging and some genetics test.
a. What diagnosis is being considered by a neurologist? What changes is he expecting on imaging? *(4 marks)*
b. How is it transmitted and what is the molecular basis? *(3 marks)*
c. What is the triad of symptoms with which they can present? *(3 marks)*

Q4. A 67-year-old male was brought to the emergency room (ER) by the family members with a H/O sudden onset of a severe headache, accompanied with nausea, vomiting, and a loss of consciousness. He was a known hypertensive and a dedicated ER resident while doing the examination of the patient observed bilateral abdominal lumps. He made the diagnosis and advised neuroimaging.
a. What has the patient presented with? What is the underlying diagnosis? *(4 marks)*
b. What is the cause of this disease? *(3 marks)*
c. Name a medication that has been shown to decrease the progress of this disease. *(3 marks)*

Q5. A 27-year-old asymptomatic female while being evaluated for her pregnancy was found to have an Hb of 9.7 g%. Her peripheral smear demonstrated microscopic hypochromic anemia. Her transferrin saturation was found to be 28.

a. What is the like cause for her anemia? How will you confirm the diagnosis? *(5 marks)*
b. Name three differential diagnoses (D/D) of this peripheral smear. *(3 marks)*
c. How do you manage this condition? *(2 marks)*

Q6. A 42-year-old presented to emergency with h/o sudden-onset palpitations at night. He had tachycardia and a BP of 100/60 mg Hg. He reported sudden death in a family. His ECG is shown in image below.

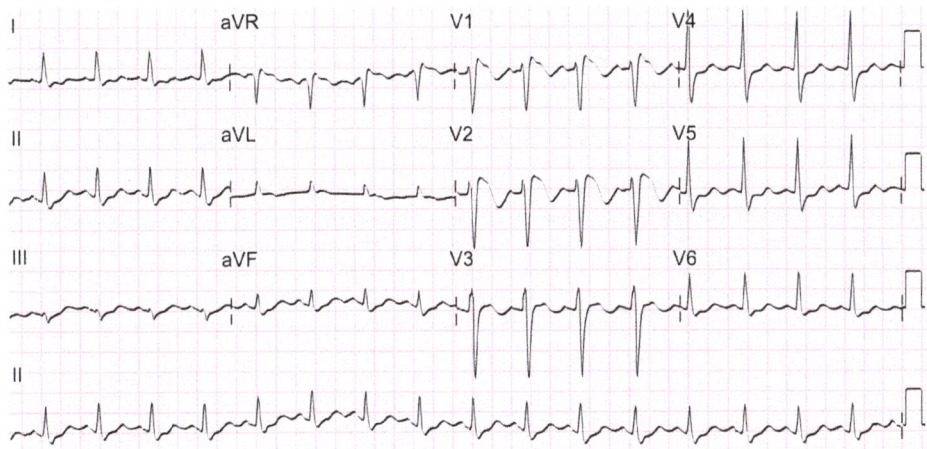

a. Describe the ECG findings. *(2 marks)*
b. What is the diagnosis? How is the mechanism of the disorder? *(3 marks)*
c. What is the etiology and risk factors for more malignant occurrence? *(3 marks)*
d. What is the definitive treatment? *(2 marks)*

Q7.

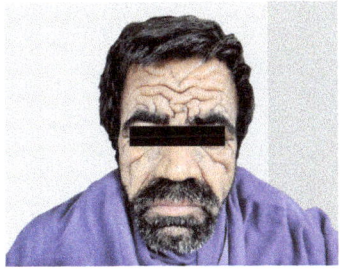
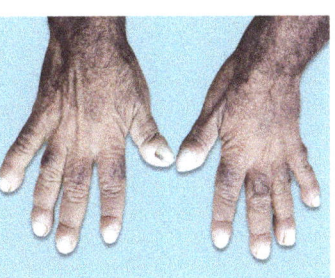

a. What is the possible diagnosis? *(2 marks)*
b. State the clinical changes. *(2 marks)*
c. How will you confirm the diagnosis? *(2 marks)*
d. Mention four differential diagnoses. *(2 marks)*
e. State most important clinical impacts. *(2 marks)*

Q8.

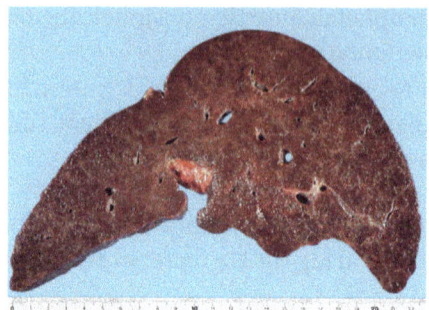

a. Describe the disorder. (2 marks)
b. How is it transmitted? (4 marks)
c. What is the finding? (4 marks)

Q9.
A 30-year-old male was seen in the fertility clinic for evaluation. His history was suggested of repeated bouts of chest infection and H/O ear discharge. He had grade 3 digital clubbing. The resident could not locate the apical impulse.

a. What is the diagnosis? (2 marks)
b. How is the disease transmitted? (2 marks)
c. Enumerate three important tests and expected findings. (6 marks)

Q10.
A 27-year-old female presented with a H/O intermittent episode of acute colicky pain in the epigastrium for several weeks. Her past history was significant of surgical H/O appendicectomy. On examination (O/E), she was anxious and looking depressed and had absent lower limb reflexes.

a. What is the diagnosis? (2 marks)
b. How is it transmitted? What is the underlying pathogenetic pathway? (2 marks)
c. What are the triggering factors? (2 marks)
d. List two management strategies. (4 marks)

Q11.

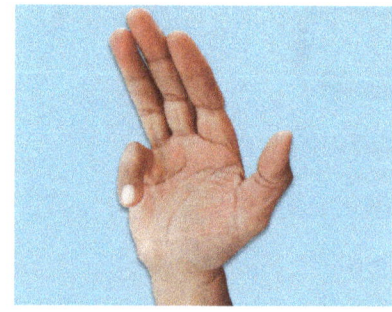

a. Identify the finding. (5 marks)
b. Other peripheral findings seen in the condition. (5 marks)

Q12. A 25-year-old male patient who presents with a combination of neurological symptoms, such as tremors, dysarthria, and dystonia. On further evaluation, laboratory tests reveal elevated liver enzymes along with low serum ceruloplasmin levels and increased urinary copper excretion. Additionally, abdominal ultrasound shows hepatomegaly.

a. What is the diagnosis? *(2 marks)*
b. Name the gene responsible for this condition and its inheritance pattern? *(3 marks)*
c. Name the tremor and pathognomonic ocular manifestation that is characteristic in this condition? *(2 marks)*
d. What medications are available for management of this condition? *(3 marks)*

Q13. Phenotypically female of 13 years age, presented with c/o nondevelopment of secondary sex characters.

a. Describe the apparent clinical features present over facies. *(3 marks)*
b. What is provisional diagnosis? *(3 marks)*
c. Discuss plan of management. *(4 marks)*

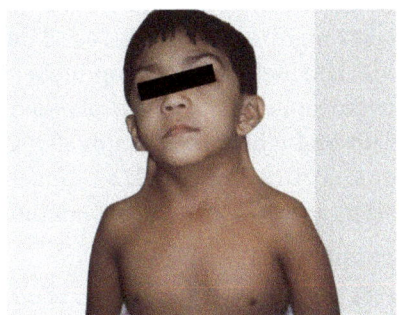

Q14. A 13-year-old boy presented in a city hospital with generalized tonic–clonic seizure (GTCS) for 2 days. As he had persistent features of hypocalcemia, laboratory reports were repeated after 2 days duration.

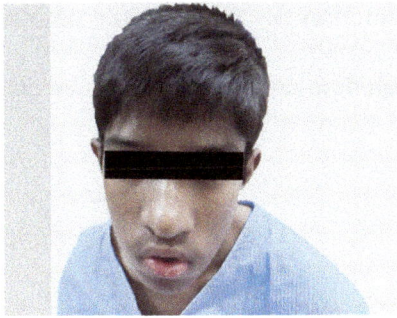

The following are the biochemistry:
- Ca—6.9 mg/dL (8.4-10.4), phosphate-5.2 mg/dL (2.6-4.5), Mg—1.6 mEq/L
- Na—144 mEq/L/, K—4.0 mEq/L
- 25(OH)D—12 ng/mL (30-100)

- Morning cortisol (9 am)—28 µg/dL
- Parathyroid hormone (PTH)—10.20 pg/mL (refer range: 15–68.3)
- HRCT thorax—no appreciable thymus tissue

a. What is the facial abnormality? (3 marks)
b. What is the provisional diagnosis? (3 marks)
c. How you manage his biochemical abnormalities? (4 marks)

Q15. A 23-year-old tall stature male with gynecomastia and small firm testes attends your clinic.

a. What is the probable disease that he is suffering from? (1 mark)
b. What is the common karyotype in this disease? (1 mark)
c. He is at an increased risk of cancer of which organ? (1 mark)
d. Which endocrinal disease occurs in them, especially in later life? (1 mark)
e. What is the treatment of such case? (1 mark)

Q16. A 58-year-old obese woman diagnosed with coronary artery disease. Her lipids were found to be total cholesterol—327 mg/dL, triglycerides—257 mg/dL, low-density lipoprotein (LDL) cholesterol—180.2 mg/dL, and high-density lipoprotein (HDL) cholesterol—31 mg/dL. She was advised for further investigations. Patient was planned to start on tablet clopidogrel 150 mg/aspirin 75 mg once daily and tablet atorvastatin 80 mg once daily. She was advised to undergo genetic testing for *CYP2C19* and *SLCO1B1*. Genetic testing reports revealed—CYPC2C19*2*2 (poor metabolizer) and SLCO1B1*5/*5 (poor function).

Based on this, answer the below questions:

a. What is the significance of genetic testing with CYPC2C19 and what is the effect of CYPC2C19*2*2—poor metabolizer on clopidogrel pharmacokinetics and pharmacodynamics? (3 marks)
b. What alternative drugs for clopidogrel can be prescribed for this patient? Which proton pump inhibitors to be avoided in this patient? (2 marks)
c. What is the significance of genetic testing with *SLCO1B1* and what is the effect of SLCO1B1*5/*5—poor function on atorvastatin pharmacokinetics and pharmacodynamics? (3 marks)
d. What alternative drug to high-dose atorvastatin can be prescribed in this patient? (2 marks)

ANSWERS

Ans. 1
a. Bleeding precautions, regular monitoring, drug interactions, and dietary considerations
b. Genetics can play a significant role in determining an individual's response to warfarin and their susceptibility to side effects. Specifically, individuals with specific CYP2C9 variants may metabolize warfarin more slowly, resulting in a longer-lasting effect and a higher risk of bleeding.
c. Although the exact mechanism of warfarin-induced skin necrosis is not thoroughly elucidated. It is hypothesized that this complication stems from the procoagulant effect initiated by warfarin. This effect leads to the formation of fibrin clots within the microvasculature. Consequently, these blood clots disrupt the blood supply to the skin, ultimately resulting in necrosis.

Ans. 2
a. Becker muscular dystrophy (BMD) is one of the nine forms of muscular dystrophies, which constitute a collection of genetic and degenerative conditions primarily impacting voluntary muscles.
b. The enlargement of calf muscles observed in BMD is explained by the accumulation of fat and connective tissue, leading to the coined term pseudohypertrophic muscular paralysis.
c. Mutations in the human dystrophin gene
d. To rule out (r/o) dilated cardiomyopathy
e. Individuals affected by BMD typically survive beyond 30 years of age, with a mean age of death in their mid-40s. The primary reason for mortality in BMD patients is heart failure resulting from dilated cardiomyopathy.

Ans. 3
a. Huntington's disease. Magnetic resonance imaging (MRI) proves valuable in diagnosing Huntington's disease. MRI abnormalities are detectable prior to the onset of noticeable clinical symptoms. In cases of adult-onset Huntington's disease, early striatal atrophy in the caudate nucleus is a distinctive feature, with cerebellar and cortical atrophy becoming evident in the later stages of the disease.
b. It is transmitted through autosomal dominant inheritance. It arises due to repetitions of cytosine, adenine, and guanine (CAG) trinucleotides on the short arm of chromosome 4p16.3 within the Huntingtin (*HTT*) gene. This genetic mutation results in an unusually prolonged expansion of the polyglutamine in the HTT protein, initiating the process of neurodegeneration.
c. Motor disturbances, behavior and psychiatric symptoms, and cognitive disturbances.

Ans. 4
a. Patient has presented with subarachnoid hemorrhage (SAH). He is suffering from autosomal dominant polycystic kidney disease (ADPKD).
b. ADPKD stands as the most prevalent inherited kidney ailment, impacting approximately 1 in 400 to 1 in 1,000 individuals. The majority of cases result from mutations occurring in either PKD1 (located on chromosome 16p13.3) or PKD2 (located on chromosome 4q22.1).

c. Tolvaptan, a specific antagonist of the vasopressin V2 receptor, effectively postpones the escalation of kidney volume (a surrogate indicator of disease progression), decelerates the deterioration in renal function, and alleviates pain in individuals with ADPKD who have relatively preserved renal function.

Ans. 5

a. *Thalassemia minor:* The diagnosis and categorization of thalassemia are best achieved through hemoglobin electrophoresis, considered the standard method. Quantitative assessment of HbA2 can be conducted using either electrophoresis or high-pressure liquid chromatography.
b. Iron deficiency anemia, thalassemia, and sideroblastic anemia
c. Individuals with thalassemia minor typically do not necessitate specific treatment. It is important to communicate to patients that this condition is hereditary and may sometimes be misidentified as iron deficiency by healthcare providers.

Ans. 6

a. J elevation ≥2 mm (0.2 mV), a coved-type ST-segment followed by a negative T-wave in V1, V2, and V3.
b. *Brugada syndrome* is an inherited condition inherited in an autosomal dominant manner and is linked to a heightened risk of sudden cardiac death (SCD). It is identified by distinctive ECG abnormalities, specifically ST-segment elevation in the precordial leads.
c. Genetic anomalies in the (*SCN5A*) gene, responsible for encoding the cardiac sodium channel with a loss-of-function mutation, are detectable in only around 30% of patients. Mutations may also be present in the *GPD1L* gene, likely impacting cardiac sodium channel function, or in genes encoding cardiac calcium channels (*CACNxxx*)
d. Implantable cardioverter-defibrillators (ICDs) can effectively prevent SCD in patients with Brugada syndrome.

Ans. 7

a. Pachydermoperiostosis/acromegaloid features/Touraine–Solente–Gole syndrome.
b. Thickening of the skin (pachyderma), thick lip, prominent rugae, excessive sweating, pseudoclubbing, increase hand and foot size, and prognathism
c. Serum insulin-like growth factor-1 (IGF-1) and growth hormone (GH) hormone suppression test with 75 g oral glucose load
d. Secondary hypertrophic osteoarthropathy, psoriatic arthritis, rheumatoid arthritis, thyroid arthropathy, and acromegaly
e. Cardiomyopathy, arrhythmias, left ventricular hypertrophy (LVH), decreased diastolic dysfunctions, and systemic hypertension.

Ans. 8

a. Primary disorders leading to iron overload are typically associated with genetic mutations that disrupt iron homeostasis in the gastrointestinal tract and liver. Examples include classic HFE-related hereditary hemochromatosis (HH), non-HFE HH, aceruloplasminemia, and others.

b. Classic HFE-related HH follows an autosomal recessive pattern and stands as the most prevalent genetic disorder. The initial histological abnormality involves detectable iron in the periportal hepatocytes. With increasing iron accumulation, parenchymal siderosis emerges and, if untreated, can advance to cirrhosis as fibrosis and hepatocellular hyperplasia develop.
c. The provided image illustrates micronodular cirrhosis in a case of HH.

Ans. 9

a. Primary ciliary dyskinesia—Kartagener's syndrome
b. Primary ciliary dyskinesia is genetically determined, following an autosomal recessive inheritance pattern.
c. In postpubescent males, semen analysis may indicate irregular sperm motility and ultrastructure. Chest radiographs might show early signs of chronic infection, such as bronchial wall thickening along with manifestations like hyperinflation, atelectasis, and bronchiectasis. ECG results may reveal dextrocardia.

Ans. 10

a. Acute intermittent porphyria (AIP)
b. It is a rare autosomal dominant disease characterized by a deficiency of hydroxymethyl-bilane synthase (HMBS), the third enzyme in heme synthesis. The acute attacks of AIP are a result of the uncontrolled upregulation of the aminolevulinic acid (ALA) synthase enzyme
c. The acute attacks of AIP are typically triggered by certain factors, which include several drugs, infection, fasting, alcohol, and use of steroidal hormone
d. First approach is to load the patient with a high carbohydrate diet or intravenously administered dextrose to inhibit hepatic ALAS1 transcription. Intravenous administration of heme is the specific therapy.

Ans. 11

a. Dupuytren's contracture
b. Other peripheral findings seen:
   - Palmar erythema
   - Dupuytren's contracture
   - Gynecomastia
   - Dilated veins/caput medusae

Ans. 12

a. Wilson's disease
b. Mutation of *ATP7B* gene. Autosomal recessive condition
c. Wing-beating tremor. Kayser–Fleischer ring
d. D-penicillamine, trientine hydrochloride, tetraethyl molybdate (TM), and zinc acetate

Ans. 13

a. Webbing of neck, shield chest, low set ears, hypertelorism, and micrognathia
b. Turner syndrome

c. Estrogen priming of uterus followed by EP pills to prevent osteoporosis, pubertal GH therapy in selected subjects.

Ans. 14

a. Midfacial hypoplasia with underdeveloped chin, low set ears, and wide set eyes
b. DiGeorge's syndrome (absent thymus, low calcium due to hypoparathyroidism, this boy has no cardiac abnormality)
c. For hypocalcemia, active form of vitamin D, 1,25-dihydroxycholecalciferol (1,25-DHCC) is to administered in a dose of 0.25 µg is to be given, either once or twice daily

Ans. 15

a. Klinefelter's syndrome
b. 47XXY
c. Breast
d. Type 2 diabetes mellitus (T2DM)
e. Androgen replacement therapy

Ans. 16

a. Clopidogrel must be metabolized by *CYP2C19* to generate the active metabolite which inhibits platelet aggregation.
   - The metabolism of clopidogrel to its active metabolite can be impaired by genetic variations leading to loss of function of *CYP2C19*.
   - In our patient, as her genetic testing reveals a poor metabolizer, if clopidogrel is continued patient may be at increased risk of myocardial infarction (MI) or acute coronary syndrome (ACS) because of therapeutic failure of clopidogrel.
   - If genetic testing of *CYP2C19* reports—poor or intermediate metabolizer. Clinical Pharmacogenetics Implementation Consortium (CPIC) 2022 guideline recommends use of alternate platelet inhibitors.

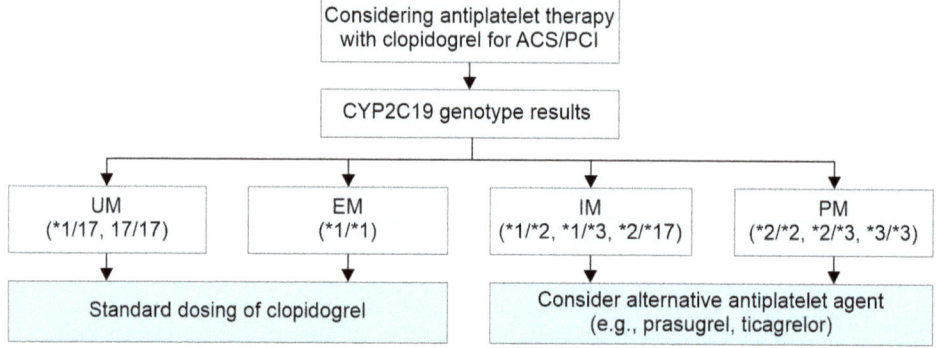

(ACS: acute coronary syndrome; PCI: percutaneous coronary intervention)
Source: Adapted from Clinical Pharmacogenetics Implementation Consortium guidelines for *CYP2C19* Genotype and Clopidogrel Therapy: 2013 Update.

b. Ticagrelor or prasugrel may be prescribed as an alternative to this patient. Ticagrelor is an active drug and *CYP2C19* genetic variations have no effect on its therapeutic effect and pharmacokinetics.

The metabolism of clopidogrel can also be impaired by drugs that inhibit *CYP2C19*, such as omeprazole and esomeprazole. Hence, concomitant prescription of these drugs is to be avoided.

c. *SLCO1B1* is a membrane transporter which facilitates the hepatic uptake of statins. Decreased function of this transporter can markedly increase the systemic exposure to atorvastatin, which can increase the risk of statin-associated musculoskeletal symptom (SAMS).

Notes: As this patient is found to have poor function of *SLCO1B1*, which means that very little atorvastatin will be taken by hepatocytes (the site of action—inhibition of HMG-CoA), majority of the drug might get systemically absorbed resulting in increased concentration of drug in muscle—leading to increased risk of SAMS.

d. Rosuvastatin 10–20 mg may be prescribed in this patient, as it has less risk of SAMS.

SECTION 19

Psychiatry

QUESTIONS

Q1. You are a resident on the inpatient psychiatric unit. A 32-year-old male patient with a history of (H/O) schizophrenia has recently been started on a new antipsychotic medication. He is brought back by the care giver with additional symptoms of very high fever (102–104 °F), fluctuating blood pressure, irregular pulse, accelerated heartbeat, increased rate of respiration (tachypnea), muscle rigidity, and altered mental status.
a. What additional complication has developed? *(3 marks)*
b. What additional tests would help? *(3 marks)*
c. Name four drugs that can cause this complication. *(2 marks)*
d. Name additional risk factors. *(2 marks)*

Q2. A resident saw a case of bipolar disorder in the OPD. The consultant asked him the following questions.
a. Describe two symptoms, each depicting the opposite moods. *(4 marks)*
b. Name three risk factors. *(3 marks)*
c. What is the overall prognosis? Name two reasons for poor outcome. *(3 marks)*

Q3. You are a resident assessing a 35-year-old patient who has a long H/O excessive health-related concerns. She frequently interprets minor physical symptoms as evidence of serious diseases and has sought medical attention repeatedly, despite multiple negative test results. The patient is convinced that her symptoms are being overlooked by healthcare providers.
a. What is your diagnosis? What was it earlier known as? *(3 marks)*
b. Name three criteria. *(3 marks)*
c. Name steps to manage this patient's condition? *(4 marks)*

Q4. You are a healthcare administrator in a mental health facility. As part of your role, you need to ensure compliance with the Mental Healthcare Act.
a. Which year was it enacted? *(2 marks)*
b. Describe the Act. *(4 marks)*
c. Enumerate three key changes from the previous Act. *(4 marks)*

Q5. A 23-year-old lady from a hilly area was brought to the OPD with complaint of (c/o) being easily startled, feeling tense, on guard, or on edge, having difficulty concentrating, and

loss of interest in previous activities for 6 weeks. The family members shared a cloud burst in their area, which was followed by disruption for 10 day around 3 months back.
a. What is the lady suffering from? (2 marks)
b. What are the components and criteria for this diagnosis? (5 marks)
c. Name two management strategies. (3 marks)

Q6. A young male presented to the medical OPD with H/O experiencing uncontrollable and recurring thoughts, engaging in repetitive behaviors. These were time-consuming symptoms and caused significant distress or interfere with daily life.
a. What is the diagnosis? (3 marks)
b. What are the risk factors for this illness? (3 marks)
c. Enumerate the management strategies. (4 marks)

Q7. A 30-year-old female presented with chronic or frequently recurring abdominal pain that initially improved with opioids. She was investigated for the cause of pain but no cause could be elucidated.
a. What is the diagnosis? (3 marks)
b. Enumerate the diagnostic criteria. (4 marks)
c. How would you manage? (3 marks)

Q8. A 13-year-old girl presented with abdominal pain, nausea, vomiting, early satiety, and loss of appetite for 3 months. On examination (O/E), she was found to have distended abdomen and a large abdominal lump reaching up to the umbilicus. She underwent a surgical procedure where a large mass was found.
a. What is the likely diagnosis? (3 marks)
b. What are the predisposing conditions? (4 marks)
c. Name the condition when it extends to small intestine. (3 marks)

Q9. A 26-year-old woman residing in a rural village, who recently delivered her first child at a primary healthcare center, presented to the medical outpatient department. She reported experiencing symptoms such as low energy, fatigue, difficulties in concentration and awareness, a bleak and pessimistic outlook on the future, disrupted sleep, and loss of appetite. The EDPS score recorded was 17.
a. What is the diagnosis? (3 marks)
b. Explain the full form of EDPS. (2 marks)
c. Enumerate four risk factors. (3 marks)
d. Enumerate two drugs to treat which are safe for infant. (2 marks)

Q10. A 20-year-old daughter was brought by the mother with a complaint that she wants to dress in the clothes typically used by males and resist wearing clothes associated with her. She also wants to be addressed as He.
She strongly preferred to play with children of the other gender in the childhood.
a. Name and define the disorder. (3 marks)
b. Enumerate the possible reasons. (3 marks)
c. How do you address/manage this issue? (4 marks)

ANSWERS

Ans. 1

a. Neuroleptic malignant syndrome (NMS) is a severe condition triggered by an adverse response to medications exhibiting dopamine receptor-antagonist properties or the abrupt discontinuation of dopaminergic medications.
b. Distinctive laboratory findings observed in NMS encompass elevated creatinine phosphokinase (CPK) levels attributed to rhabdomyolysis and the presence of leukocytosis.
c. Medications linked to NMS include haloperidol, fluphenazine, chlorpromazine, and trifluoperazine.
d. Factors such as dehydration, physical fatigue, exposure to high temperatures, hyponatremia, and iron deficiency are associated with the development of NMS.

Ans. 2

a.
- *Mania:* Feeling incredibly "high" or euphoric, delusions of self-importance, high levels of creativity, energy and activity, getting much less sleep or no sleep, racing thoughts, racing speech, and talking over people.
- *Depression:* Feeling sad, hopeless or irritable most of the time, lacking energy, difficulty concentrating and remembering things, loss of interest in everyday activities, and feelings of emptiness or worthlessness.

b. Positive family history, environmental factors such as stress and sleep disruption, and drugs and alcohol may trigger mood episodes in vulnerable people.
c. The prognosis of manic patients is favorable, granted they are adherent to medications and therapy. Some factors associated with a poorer outcome are history of abuse, psychosis, low socioeconomic status, comorbid illness, or young age of onset.

Ans. 3

a. The patient's presentation is suggestive of illness anxiety disorder (formerly known as hypochondriasis).
b. (i) Excessive and disproportionate worry about having a serious medical condition; (ii) preoccupation with having a serious illness despite medical reassurance and negative test results; and (iii) high levels of distress and impairment in daily functioning.
c. Recommend cognitive behavioral therapy (CBT), specifically cognitive restructuring and exposure therapy, which can help the patient modify irrational beliefs and gradually confront her health-related fears.

 Consider pharmacological intervention with selective serotonin reuptake inhibitors (SSRIs) in cases of severe distress or coexisting mood or anxiety disorders.

 Collaborate with the patient's primary care physician to ensure that routine medical evaluations continue and are conducted in a supportive manner that minimizes the patient's distress.

Ans. 4

a. In April 2017, the Mental Healthcare Act was enacted in India, officially came into effect in May 2018.

Psychiatry

b. The purpose of this legislation is outlined as "An Act to provide for mental healthcare and services for persons with mental illness and to protect, promote and fulfill the rights of such persons during the delivery of mental healthcare and services and for matters connected therewith or incidental thereto."

c.
- The Mental Healthcare Act of 2017 endeavors to decriminalize suicide attempts, aiming to provide individuals who have attempted suicide with opportunities for rehabilitation instead of facing legal prosecution or punishment.
- The legislation empowers individuals suffering from mental illness, allowing them to make decisions about their health, provided they possess the necessary knowledge to do so.
- The Act has imposed restrictions on the use of electroconvulsive therapy (ECT), permitting its use only in emergency cases and in conjunction with muscle relaxants and anesthesia.

Ans. 5

a. She is suffering from post-traumatic stress disorder (PTSD)
b. To receive a diagnosis of PTSD, a person must have at least one re-experiencing symptom, at least three avoidance symptoms, at least two negative alterations in mood and cognition, and at least two hyperarousal symptoms for a minimum of 1 month.
c.
- Psychotherapy—CBT such as exposure therapy and cognitive restructuring
- SSRI

Ans. 6

a. Obsessive compulsive disorder
b. Genetics (family history), temperament (reserved behavior), and childhood trauma
c. Psychotherapy, CBT, exposure and response prevention (ERP) therapy; medications—serotonin reuptake inhibitors; and repetitive transcranial magnetic stimulation (rTMS)

Ans. 7

a. Narcotic bowel syndrome
b. Persistent or frequently recurring abdominal pain, when treated with high doses of narcotics, may exhibit certain features, including the pain worsening or incompletely resolving despite continued or escalating narcotic dosages. Additionally, there may be a noticeable exacerbation of pain when the narcotic dose diminishes, followed by improvement upon reinstating narcotics (referred to as "Soar and Crash"). The condition may demonstrate a progression in the frequency, duration, and intensity of pain episodes, and the nature and intensity of the pain cannot be accounted for by a current or previous gastrointestinal diagnosis.
c. In managing narcotic bowel syndrome, the physician–patient relationship plays a crucial role. This involves acknowledging the reality of the pain, engaging in a dialogue with the patient to provide information, discussing the rationale for withdrawal, and implementing a narcotic withdrawal protocol. Specific treatment guidelines may include the use of antidepressants, benzodiazepines, and clonidine.

Ans. 8

a. Trichobezoar refers to the aggregation of hair in the stomach, forming concretions. Typically, trichobezoars are localized within the stomach.
b. Trichobezoars are predominantly observed in females, constituting around 90% of cases, particularly in the age range of 13-19 years. This occurrence is often associated with an undisclosed psychiatric disorder, involving the habit of trichophagia, or the ingestion of one's own hair.
c. Rapunzel syndrome

Ans. 9

a. Postpartum depression
b. Edinburgh Postnatal Depression Scale
c. Young age, economic deprivation, marital violence, and female gender of the infant
d. Sertraline and paroxetine are least likely to be detectable in infant.

Ans. 10

a. Gender dysphoria is characterized by significant and enduring distress, resulting from a misalignment between an individual's gender identity and their biological sex.
b. Genetic connections, variances in neuroanatomy, and exposure to prenatal androgens play roles in shaping gender identity. There is an elevated likelihood of gender dysphoria development with heightened levels of psychopathology in parents and childhood anxiety.
c. Treatment options include nonoperative and operative approaches. Nonoperative interventions concentrate on implementing psychosocial therapy and/or medical management through hormone replacement therapy. Operative procedures span from minor cosmetic interventions to more extensive genital transformation surgeries.

SECTION 20

Biostatistics

QUESTIONS

Q1. A clinician would like to conduct a clinical trial to test the efficacy of the drug used to lower blood pressure in individuals diagnosed with hypertension compared to the standard treatment.

Study details:
- *Sample:* 150 patients diagnosed with hypertension.
- *Procedure:* Half the patients are randomly assigned the new drug, while the other half receive the standard treatment.
- *Duration:* The trial runs for 6 months.
- *Measurements:* Blood pressure readings taken at the beginning and end of the trial for each patient.

Hypotheses:
- *Null hypothesis (H_0):* There is no difference in the effectiveness of the new drug compared to the standard treatment in lowering blood pressure.
- *Alternative hypothesis (H_1):* The new drug is more effective in lowering blood pressure compared to the standard treatment.

a. What statistical test would be appropriate to compare the effectiveness of the new drug to the standard treatment? *(2 marks)*
b. What are the dependent and independent variables in this study? *(2 marks)*
c. Explain type I and type II errors in the context of this study. *(2 marks)*
d. If the *p*-value obtained is 0.03, what can be concluded? *(2 marks)*
e. What sample size calculation might be necessary before conducting such a trial? *(2 marks)*

Q2. A pharmaceutical company has developed a new drug aimed at reducing blood pressure in hypertensive patients. To test its effectiveness, a clinical trial was conducted. 100 patients were randomly assigned to two groups: Group A receiving the new drug and Group B receiving a placebo. After 8 weeks of treatment, their blood pressure was measured.

a. *Hypotheses formulation:* State the null and alternative hypotheses for this study. *(2 marks)*
b. Which statistical test would be appropriate to compare the mean blood pressure reductions between the two groups? Why? *(2 marks)*

c. List assumptions that need to be met for the chosen statistical test. *(2 marks)*
d. If the *p*-value from the *t*-test is 0.03, what does this suggest about the effectiveness of the new drug? *(2 marks)*
e. How would you convey the practical significance of the findings to clinicians and patients? *(2 marks)*

Q3. A diagnostic laboratory has developed a new diagnostic kit (A) for diagnosing disease X. The gold standard for diagnosing the condition is known (B).
a. Name the three different methods used to quantify the diagnostic ability of a test. *(4 marks)*
b. How do you calculate the likelihood ration (LR)? *(2 marks)*
c. Which parameter is affected by the prevalence of the disease and how? *(4 marks)*

Q4. A pharmaceutical company has developed a new drug aimed at reducing blood pressure in hypertensive patients. The company conducted a clinical trial to assess the drug's effectiveness compared to a placebo. The trial involved 200 participants with hypertension, randomly assigned to either the drug group or the placebo group. Blood pressure readings were taken before and after the intervention.
a. What type of study design is most likely used in this scenario? *(2 marks)*
b. What are the independent and dependent variables? *(2 marks)*
c. How would you summarize the blood pressure data before and after the intervention for each group? *(2 marks)*
d. If the mean reduction in blood pressure is greater in the drug group compared to the placebo group, how would you test the hypothesis that the drug is effective? *(2 marks)*

Q5. Suppose you are a researcher investigating the impact of a new teaching method on student performance. You have collected data on two groups of students: One group taught using the traditional method (Group A) and another taught with the new method (Group B).
a. What is the research hypothesis you are testing with a *t*-test in this scenario? *(2 marks)*
b. Why is a *t*-test appropriate for comparing the means of Group A and Group B in this case? *(2 marks)*
c. What are the null and alternative hypotheses for the *t*-test in this context? *(3 marks)*
d. How would you interpret the *p*-value obtained from the *t*-test in this study? *(3 marks)*

Q6. As a medical student, you are involved in a study examining the relationship between a certain genetic marker (present or absent) and the incidence of a specific medical condition, such as hypertension, within a group of patients.
a. What test you would choose to analyze the relationship between the genetic marker and the incidence of hypertension in this medical study? *(2 marks)*
b. Why would you choose this test? *(2 marks)*
c. What would be the null hypothesis (H_0) and alternative hypothesis (H_1) in the context of this study? *(3 marks)*
d. How do you interpret the *p*-value obtained from the test in this genetic marker study? *(3 marks)*

Q7. As a medical student, you are involved in a research project comparing the effectiveness of three different drug treatments for reducing blood pressure in patients with hypertension. The study involves randomly assigning patients to one of the three drug treatment groups.
a. What test would you choose to analyze the effectiveness of the three different drug treatments in reducing blood pressure? *(5 marks)*
b. What are the null hypothesis (H_0) and alternative hypothesis (H_1) for the analysis in this drug treatment study? *(5 marks)*

ANSWERS

Ans. 1

a. A two-sample *t*-test or ANOVA (analysis of variance) could be appropriate for comparing the effectiveness of the new drug and the standard treatment.
b. *Dependent variable:* Blood pressure readings.
   Independent variable: Type of treatment (new drug or standard treatment)
c. *Type I error:* Incorrectly concluding that the new drug is effective (rejecting H_0) when it is not.
   Type II error: Failing to conclude that the new drug is effective (failing to reject H_0) when it actually is.
d. A *p*-value of 0.03 suggests that there is evidence to reject the null hypothesis at a significance level of 0.05, indicating a significant difference between the effectiveness of the treatments.
e. Sample size calculation should consider effect size, desired power, and significance level to ensure adequate statistical power to detect differences between treatments.

Ans. 2

a. *Null hypothesis (H_0):* The mean reduction in blood pressure due to the new drug equals zero.
   Alternative hypothesis (H_1): The mean reduction in blood pressure due to the new drug is greater than zero.
b. An independent samples *t*-test would be appropriate as we are comparing the means of two independent groups (Group A receiving the drug vs. Group B receiving placebo) regarding their blood pressure reductions.
c. Random sampling, normality of the data distributions within each group, and homogeneity of variances between the groups.
d. A *p*-value of 0.03 suggests that there is evidence to reject the null hypothesis at a significance level of 0.05. Thus, it indicates that the new drug likely has a significant effect on reducing blood pressure compared to the placebo.
e. Although statistically significant, the clinical significance should also be considered. Discuss the actual reduction in blood pressure, potential side effects, and whether the observed difference is meaningful in a real-world context for patient health outcomes.

Ans. 3

a. Sensitivity, specificity, positive predictive value, and negative predictive value.
b. LR is really the ratio of sensitivity to (100 – specificity).
c. The predictive values are dependent on the prevalence of the disease being tested. The rarer the prevalence of the disease, the more certain one can be that a negative test result indeed means that there is no disease [i.e., higher negative predictive value (NPV)]. Similarly, the rarer the prevalence of the disease, the less certain one can be that a positive test result indicates the presence of a disease [i.e., lower positive predictive value (PPV)].

Ans. 4

a. The most likely study design is a randomized controlled trial (RCT).

b. The independent variable is the type of intervention (drug or placebo), and the dependent variable is the blood pressure readings.
c. Descriptive statistics such as mean, median, and standard deviation can be calculated for blood pressure readings in both the drug and placebo groups before and after the intervention. This provides a summary of central tendency and variability.
d. A two-sample *t*-test could be employed to compare the means of the two groups. If the difference is statistically significant, it suggests that the drug has a significant effect on reducing blood pressure.

Ans. 5

a. The research hypothesis for the *t*-test in this scenario is that there is a significant difference in the mean performance scores between students taught using the traditional method (Group A) and those taught with the new method (Group B).
b. A *t*-test is appropriate in this case, because we are comparing the means of two independent groups to determine if there is a statistically significant difference between them. The *t*-test helps assess whether any observed difference in performance scores between the two teaching methods is likely due to a real effect or if it could occur by chance.
c. *Null hypothesis* (H_0): There is no significant difference in the mean performance scores between students taught with the traditional method (Group A) and those taught with the new method (Group B).
   Alternative hypothesis (H_1): There is a significant difference in the mean performance scores between the two groups.
d. The *p*-value obtained from the *t*-test represents the probability of observing the observed difference in mean performance scores between Group A and Group B, assuming the null hypothesis is true. If the *p*-value is below a chosen significance level (e.g., 0.05), we would reject the null hypothesis and conclude that there is a significant difference in performance scores between the two teaching methods.

Ans. 6

a. Chi-square test
b. A chi-square test is suitable for analyzing the relationship between two categorical variables, such as the presence or absence of a genetic marker and the occurrence of hypertension. This test helps determine if there is a statistically significant association between these variables, which is crucial for understanding genetic factors contributing to medical conditions.
c. *Null hypothesis* (H_0): There is no association between the presence of the genetic marker and the incidence of hypertension in the population.
   Alternative hypothesis (H_1): There is a significant association between the presence of the genetic marker and the incidence of hypertension in the population.
d. The *p*-value from the chi-square test indicates the probability of observing the association between the genetic marker and hypertension by random chance alone. If the *p*-value is below a chosen significance level (e.g., 0.05), we reject the null hypothesis, suggesting a significant association. In the context of this study, a low *p*-value would imply that the

presence or absence of the genetic marker is associated with a higher or lower incidence of hypertension.

Ans. 7

a. ANOVA is appropriate for comparing the means of more than two independent groups. In this study, we have three drug treatment groups, and ANOVA allows us to determine whether there are any statistically significant differences in the mean reduction of blood pressure among these groups.

b. *Null hypothesis (H_0):* There is no significant difference in the mean reduction of blood pressure among the three drug treatment groups.

Alternative hypothesis (H_1): At least one drug treatment group has a different mean reduction in blood pressure compared to the others.

SECTION 21

Test Yourself

QUESTIONS

Q1. A 48-year-old male presented with increasing swelling in the lateral aspect of the neck for 10 months.

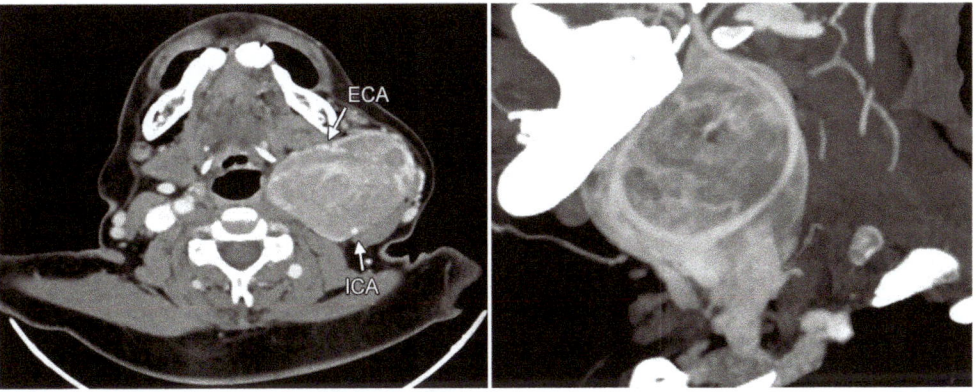

(ECA: external carotid artery; ICA: internal carotid artery)

a. What is the diagnosis? (3 marks)
b. What is the classic sign to diagnose this lesion? (2 marks)
c. What are the other locations of this pathology? (2 marks)
d. What are common differential diagnoses? (3 marks)

Q2. A 46-year-old male presented with acute breathlessness for 2 days.

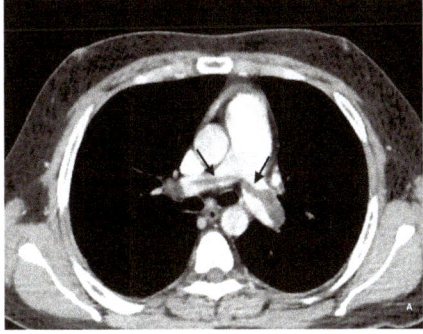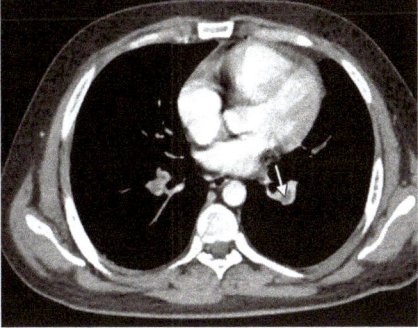

a. What is the diagnosis? (3 marks)
b. What are the imaging features? (2 marks)
c. Name the radiographic signs. (2 marks)
d. What are the radiographic signs of right heart strain? (3 marks)

Q3. A 38-year-old male presented initially with a papulonodular lesion on the dorsal surface of his right hand. Initially, it was red but painless. Over the next few days, several noduloulcerative lesions appeared along the hand, forearm, and arm (Image A). He had a history of (H/O) thorn prick injury acquired while gardening. There were also enlarged and tender epitrochlear and axillary lymph nodes on the right side. The biopsy of the lesions is shown in Image B.

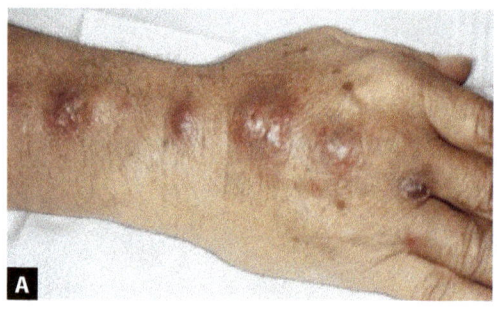
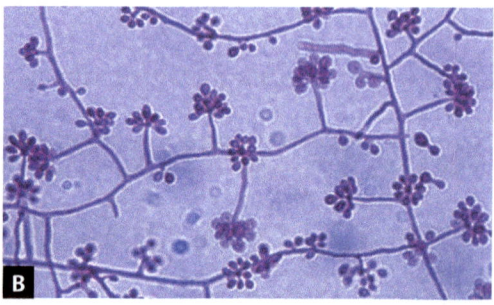

a. What is the diagnosis of this type of skin lesion? (4 marks)
b. Identify the organism. (3 marks)
c. How will you treat this patient? (3 marks)

Q4. Computed tomography (CT) scan images of a 70-year-old man with 2 years history of progressive dyspnea.

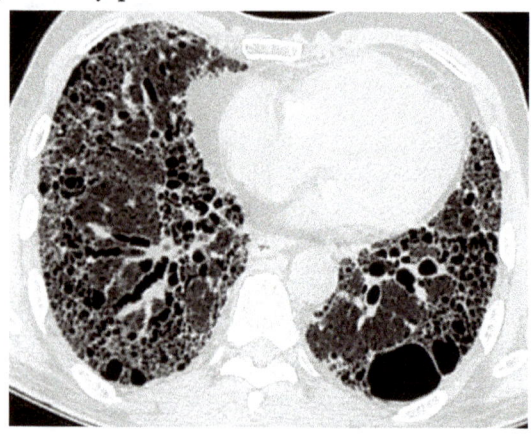
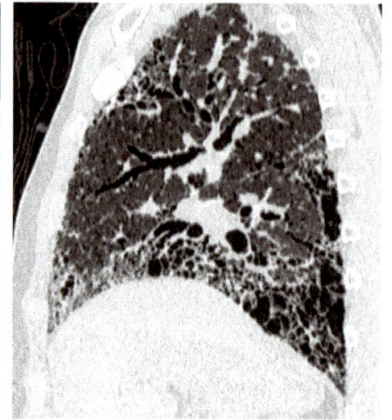

a. What pattern is shown? (3 marks)
b. What are the HRCT features of the pattern shown? (2 marks)
c. What is honeycombing? (2 marks)
d. In view of clinical history, what is the most likely diagnosis? (3 marks)

Q5. A 55-year-old man, a farmer, presented with gradually increasing painless swelling of the dorsum of the nose, forehead, bilateral cheeks, and upper lip resulting in significant facial disfigurement and right-sided nasal obstruction for the last 3 months depicted in image given below. No history of trauma. The swelling was firm to hard in consistency. All other physical examinations were within normal limits. Routine blood examinations showed no abnormality. Histopathology of the endoscopic biopsy of the polypoid growth in the right nasal cavity showed broad thin walled aseptate hyphae enveloped by eosinophilic granular material (Splendore–Hoeppli phenomenon). No vascular involvement was noted.

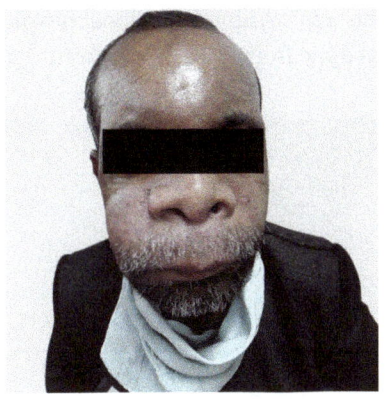

a. What is the diagnosis? *(3 marks)*
b. What is the causative organism? *(3 marks)*
c. How will you treat the patient? *(4 marks)*

Q6. Mrs Gupta, a 58-year-old female, presents with a cluster of painful blisters on her face near her nose. She reports experiencing tingling and burning sensations in the area preceding the appearance of the blisters. Upon examination, you observe erythematous papules that have progressed to vesicles, some of which have ruptured and formed crusts. Mrs Gupta reports a history of occasional cold sores in the past.

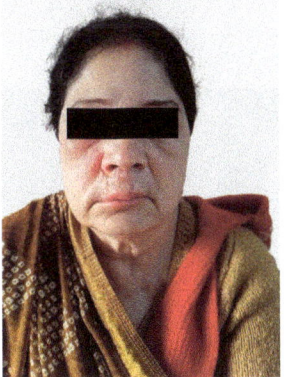

a. What are the typical clinical manifestations and progression of herpes simplex virus (HSV) infection, particularly herpes labialis, in a patient like Mrs Gupta? *(3 marks)*

b. Considering Mrs Gupta's age and the location of her lesions, what potential complications or associated conditions should be taken into consideration during her evaluation and management? *(4 marks)*
c. What treatment options would you recommend for Mrs Gupta to alleviate her symptoms, expedite healing, and prevent the recurrence of her herpes labialis episodes? *(3 marks)*

Q7. A 15-year-old boy resident of Madubani Bihar presented to OPD with this type of skin lesions over ear lobules (Image A), nose, and chin. Three years ago, he had a history of prolonged fever for which he was admitted in a local hospital and was treated with some injections. A slit skin smear was done from the lesion over the ear lobules and examined under a microscope (Image B).

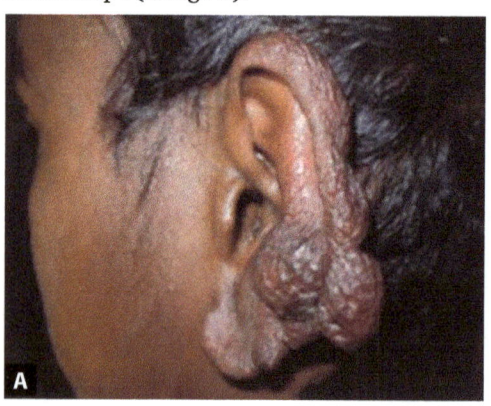
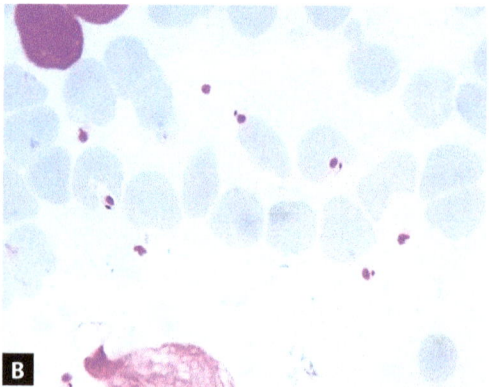

a. What is the diagnosis of the skin lesions shown in Image A? *(3 marks)*
b. Identify the organism shown in the Image B. *(4 marks)*
c. How will you treat the condition? *(3 marks)*

Q8. Describe the X-ray of both feet and tell the diagnosis.
a. What is it? *(3 marks)*
b. Describe the risk factors. *(3 marks)*
c. How you will treat the case? *(4 marks)*

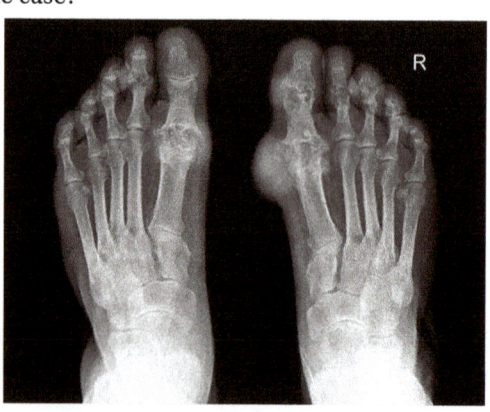

Q9.

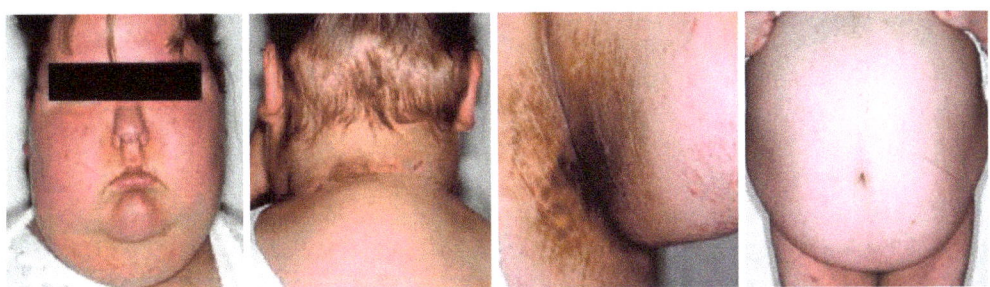

a. Describe the pictures shown above. (3 marks)
b. What is the case? (3 marks)
c. What is the most common cause of this disease? (4 marks)

Q10. A middle-aged male is presented with the following features.

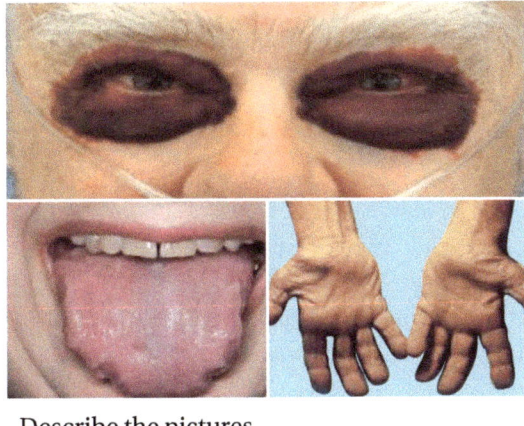
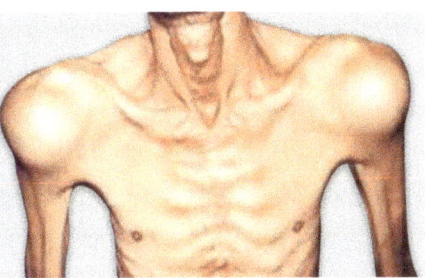

a. Describe the pictures. (3 marks)
b. What is the diagnosis? (3 marks)
c. How do you diagnose the case? (4 marks)

Q11. A 15-year-old boy presented with intermittent right-sided ptosis having diurnal variation and fatigability.

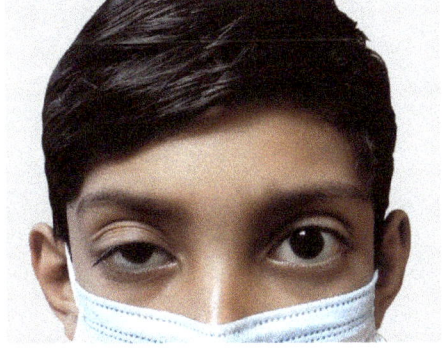

a. What kind of lower motor neuron (LMN) lesion can cause this type of pathology? *(2 marks)*
b. Mention the names of two diseases belonging to this kind of LMN lesion. *(2 marks)*
c. What bedside test is specific for this type of disease? *(2 marks)*
d. Mention the names of the two antibodies most commonly done for diagnosis. *(2 marks)*
e. What are the two electrophysiological tests specific for the diagnosis of this type of disease? *(2 marks)*

Q12. A 22-year-old obese female presented with holocranial headache and transient visual obscurations along with pulsatile tinnitus with the following ophthalmoscopic finding in both eyes.

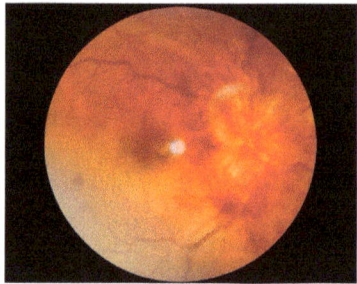

a. What is the ophthalmoscopic finding? *(2 marks)*
b. What is the provisional diagnosis? *(2 marks)*
c. Name two magnetic resonance imaging (MRI) features that can be found in this condition. *(2 marks)*
d. During cerebrospinal fluid (CSF) puncture what specific study must be done for the diagnosis? *(2 marks)*
e. Name one surgical procedure that can be done to treat a fulminant type of this disease. *(2 marks)*

Q13. A 59-year-old hypertensive lady presented with acute onset severe headache with vomiting and neck stiffness and this is her CT scan finding.

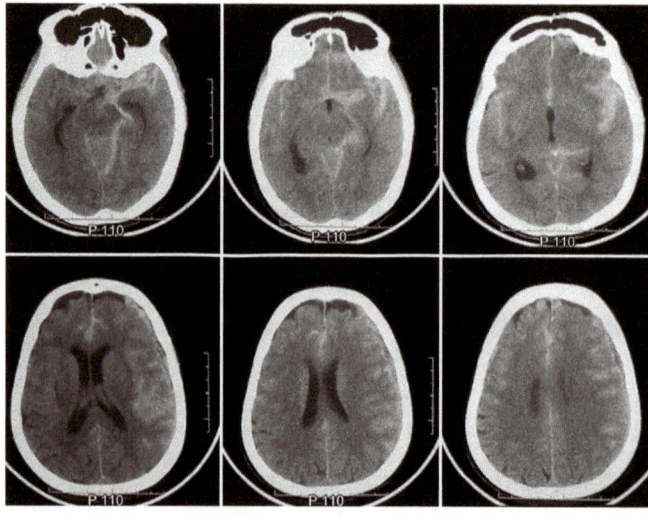

a. What is the diagnosis? *(1 mark)*
b. What is the most common cause of this type of pathology in general? *(2 marks)*
c. Name two grading systems used to classify the severity. *(2 marks)*
d. Name the four most common complications of this type of pathology. *(2 marks)*
e. Name one specific diagnostic entity done before definitive therapy. *(1 mark)*
f. Mention two definitive therapeutic procedures usually done in this type of case. *(2 marks)*

Q14. A 16-year-old male without any contributory family history presented with a gradually progressive ataxia since childhood and history of recurrent sinopulmonary infections.

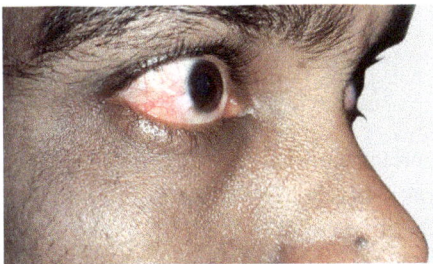

a. What is your diagnosis? *(2 marks)*
b. What is the inheritance pattern? *(2 marks)*
c. Name two other diseases with ataxia linked to deoxyribonucleic acid (DNA) repair defects. *(2 marks)*
d. Name the most common autosomal recessive cerebellar ataxia. *(2 marks)*
e. Name two malignancies associated with this condition. *(2 marks)*

Q15. A 20-year-old female presented with acute onset flaccid quadriparesis for 7 days.

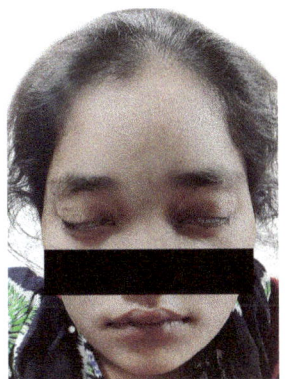

a. Describe the facies. *(2 marks)*
b. Name a few causes of bifacial palsy. *(2 marks)*
c. What variant of Guillain–Barre syndrome (GBS) is usually associated with bifacial palsy? *(2 marks)*
d. How to differentiate bilateral LMN versus bilateral upper motor neuron (UMN) facial palsy? *(2 marks)*
e. Does bifacial palsy prognosticate GBS? *(2 marks)*

Q16. A 20-year-old male presented with low-grade fever with loss of appetite, and nausea with generalized pruritus, his general physical examination shows icterus.

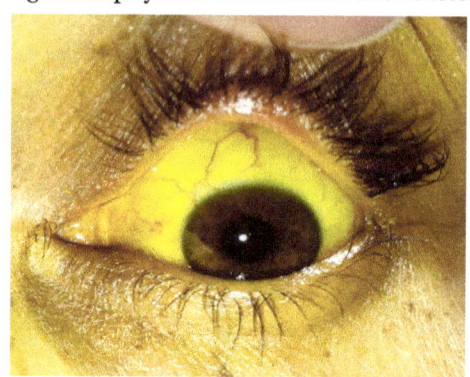

a. Why the sclera is examined for jaundice? (2 marks)
b. Mention the three features of obstructive jaundice. (2 marks)
c. Name bile salts and bile acids. (3 marks)
d. What is Courvoisier's law? (3 marks)

Q17. A 67-year-old male presented in the outpatient department (OPD) with dyspnea on exertion for 1 year increasing progressively. His pulmonary function test results are as below.

PFT report					
FEV_1	FVC	FEV_1/FVC	TLC	RV	DLCO
16%	56%	22%	109%	216%	33%

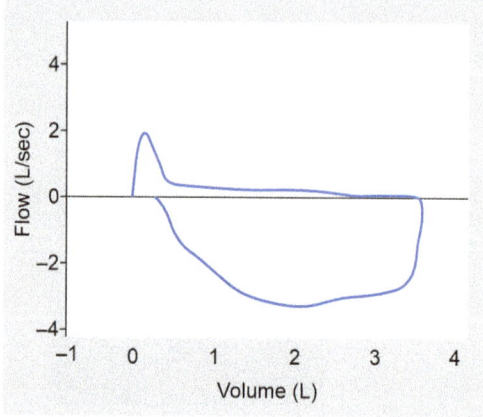

(DLCO: diffusing capacity of the lungs for carbon monoxide; FEV_1: forced expiratory volume; FVC: forced vital capacity; PFT: pulmonary function test; RV: residual volume; TLC: total lung capacity)

a. Discuss the interpretation of the pulmonary function test (PFT). (2 marks)
b. What is cor pulmonale? What is its significance? (3 marks)
c. Discuss the classification of chronic obstructive pulmonary disease (COPD). (3 marks)
d. Name three more investigations for diagnosis. (2 marks)

Q18. A 22-year-old female presented with pain at both wrist joints, headache, and oligomenorrhea with a deep and husky voice.

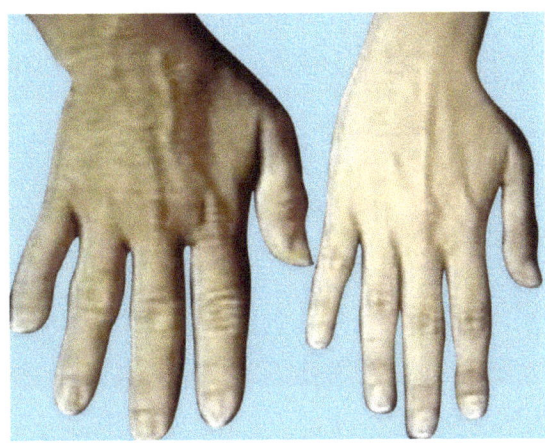

a. What is the probable diagnosis? *(2 marks)*
b. What are the features of acromegaly? *(3 marks)*
c. What is gigantism? *(3 marks)*
d. What is the medical management of acromegaly? *(2 marks)*

Q19. A 68-year-old male patient presented with a chronic cough, cachexia, lymphadenopathy, and hoarse voice. On examination, he is having clubbing and nicotine staining. His chest X-ray is shown below.

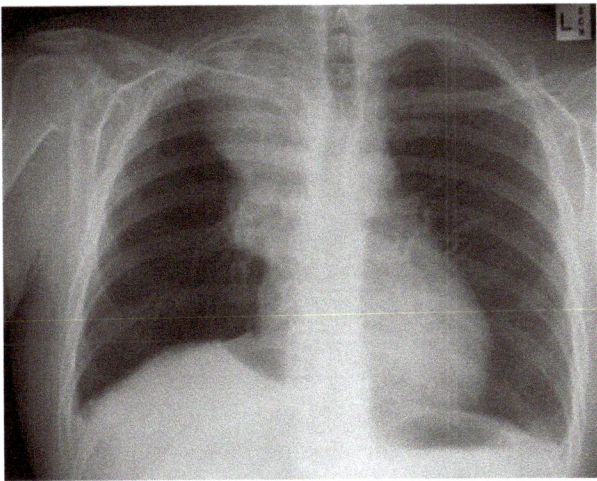

a. What is the probable diagnosis? *(2 marks)*
b. What are the four main histological types of lung cancer? *(2 marks)*
c. Which paraneoplastic syndromes are associated with lung cancer? *(2 marks)*
d. What are the signs of Pancoast's syndrome? *(2 marks)*
e. What are the clinical signs and symptoms of superior vena cava syndrome (SVCO)? *(2 marks)*

Test Yourself

Q20. A 50-year-old patient has had episodes of syncope and chest pain and difficulty in breathing his two-dimensional (2D) echo is shown below.

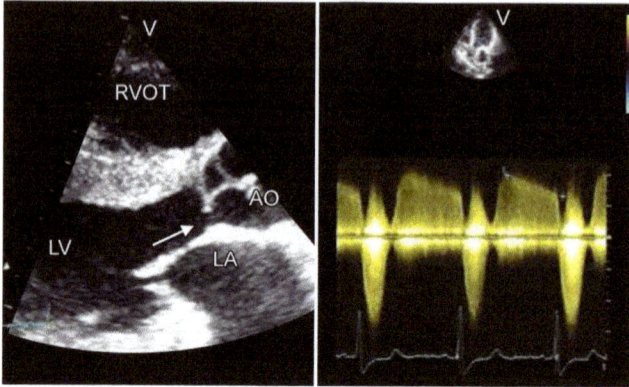

a. What is the probable diagnosis? (2 marks)
b. What are the causes of aortic stenosis (AS)? (2 marks)
c. What are the types of AS? (2 marks)
d. What are the indications for surgery? (2 marks)
e. Why the murmur of AS is midsystolic? (2 marks)

Q21. A 25-year-old man has been experiencing back pain (including pain at night), stiffness, and fatigue. His lumbosacral (LS) spine X-ray is shown below.

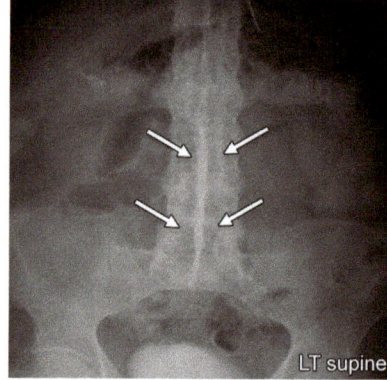

a. What is the probable diagnosis? (2 marks)
b. What are the immunological associations with ankylosing spondylitis? (3 marks)
c. What is the treatment for ankylosing spondylitis? (3 marks)
d. What are the extra-articular manifestations of ankylosing spondylitis? (2 marks)

ANSWERS

Ans. 1

a. Carotid body tumor/chemodectoma/carotid body paraganglioma.
b. Intensely and homogenously enhancing soft tissue density lesion within the carotid space at carotid bifurcation causing splaying of the internal and external carotid artery (ECA). The characteristic splaying of the internal carotid artery (ICA) and ECA is known as a lyre sign.
c. Paragangliomas can occur at any site along the specific locations of paraganglia tissue within the body. In the head and neck, the four most common sites are the carotid body at the common carotid artery (CCA) bifurcation, the jugular foramen, along the vagus nerve, and within the middle ear.
d. The common differentials include nerve sheath tumors, nodal metastasis, glomus vagale tumor, and carotid bulb ectasia.

Ans. 2

a. Saddle pulmonary embolism.
b. Pulmonary embolus that straddles the bifurcation of the pulmonary trunk, extending into the right, and left pulmonary arteries.
c. The signs seen on the chest radiograph are the Fleischner sign (enlarged pulmonary artery), Hamptom hump (peripheral wedge opacity), Westermark sign (regional oligemia), Palla sign (enlarged right descending pulmonary artery, Chang sign (dilated right descending pulmonary artery with sudden cut-off).
d. Signs of right heart strain include dilatation of the right ventricle, straightening or leftward bulging of the interventricular septum, and enlargement of the pulmonary trunk.

Ans. 3

a. Lymphocutaneous sporotrichosis.
b. Oval, spherical, or elongated (cigar-shaped) forms of dimorphic fungus *Sporothrix schenckii*.
c. Capsule itraconazole 100–200 mg/day is given for 2–4 weeks after the complete resolution of all lesions and usually requires 3–6 months for a complete clinical cure.

Ans. 4

a. Usual interstitial pneumonia (UIP) pattern.
b. High-resolution computed tomography (HRCT) features frequently seen in UIP patterns include honeycombing, and traction bronchiectasis/bronchiolectasis, which may be seen with the concurrent presence of reticulation. The typical distribution of UIP is subpleural with basal predominance, although some upper lobe involvement is common.
c. Honeycombing refers to clustered, thin/thick walled cystic spaces usually of similar diameters (3–10 mm, but occasionally larger), in stacks of two or more, usually peripheral. It may also present as a single layer.
d. Idiopathic pulmonary fibrosis (IPF) is the most likely diagnosis. UIP is the hallmark radiologic pattern of IPF.

Ans. 5

a. Entomophthoramycosis—a rare fungal infection.
b. Caused by *Conidiobolus coronatus*
c. Treated by capsule itraconazole (200 mg/capsule), one capsule thrice daily for 3 days then continued as a twice daily dose and gradually increasing the dose of a saturated solution of potassium iodide (SSKI) with a starting dose of five drops thrice daily. Then, gradually increased up to 30–40 drops thrice daily. This combination therapy should be given for several months according to the treatment response.

Ans. 6

a. *Clinical manifestations of herpes labialis in Mrs Gupta:* Tingling, burning, and then erythematous papules progressing to vesicles near her nose.
b. *Considerations:* Increased severity in older adults, potential ocular involvement (herpetic keratitis), and risk of disseminated infection in those with compromised immune systems.
c. *Treatment options for Mrs Gupta:* Oral antivirals (e.g., acyclovir and valacyclovir), topical antiviral creams, pain relievers, and preventive measures, such as identifying triggers and practicing good hygiene.

Ans. 7

a. Post-kala azar dermal leishmaniasis.
b. *Leishman Donovan (LD) body:* Amastigote form of parasite *Leishmania donovani*.
c. Capsule miltefosine, 50 mg twice daily for 12 weeks.

Ans. 8

a. Podagracaused by hyperuricemia. Gout is caused by hyperuricemia and monosodium urate crystal deposition. Uric acid is a waste product of purine metabolism. Monosodium urate crystal formation occurs when the uric acid level exceeds 6.8 mg/dL in the blood.
b. *Risk factors for gout include* genetic predisposition, renal failure, diuretic use, high purine diet, alcohol consumption, myeloproliferative diseases, and diabetes mellitus.
c. Early administration of nonbiologic and biologic disease-modifying antirheumatic drugs (DMARDs) alone or in combination is currently recommended as they induce remission and prevent disease progression [antitumor necrosis factor (anti-TNF) agent, methotrexate, hydroxychloroquine, steroids, leflunomide, azathioprine, sulfasalazine, etc.].
   - Nonsteroidal anti-inflammatory drugs (NSAIDs) and painkillers. *Cold therapy to relieve pain and inflammation*: Ice packs or ice water.
   - *Occupational therapy and rehabilitation:* Orthotic and splint devices, surgical referral for deformity correction.

Ans. 9

a. Truncal obesity with thin limbs, dry and brittle hair, rounded, "moon-like" face, and red cheeks acanthosis nigricans.
b. Cushing's syndrome
c. Iatrogenic

Ans. 10

a. Raccoon eyes.
   - Enlargement of tongue
   - Carpal tunnel syndrome
   - Shoulder pad sign
b. AL amyloidosis
c. Rectal biopsy or abdominal fat stained by Congo red.

Ans. 11

a. Neuromuscular junctional disorder.
b. Myasthenia gravis and Lambert–Eaton syndrome.
c. Ice pack test
d. Antiacetylcholine (anti-ACh) receptor antibody and antimuscle-specific kinase (anti-MuSK) antibody.
e. Repetitive nerve stimulation test and single-fiber EMG.

Ans. 12

a. Grade 5 papilledema.
b. Idiopathic intracranial hypertension.
c. Flattening of posterior sclera, tortuosity of optic nerves, prominent subarachnoid space around optic nerves, and partially empty sella.
d. CSF manometry (opening pressure > 25 cmH$_2$O)
e. Optic nerve sheath fenestration

Ans. 13

a. Subarachnoid hemorrhage
b. Traumatic
c. Huntz–Hess scale, Modified Fisher scale, and World Federation of Neurological Surgeons (WFNS) grade.
d. Intracranial vasospasm, rebleed, hyponatremia, and obstructive hydrocephalus.
e. Digital subtraction angiography (DSA)
f. Clipping or endovascular coiling of the aneurysms.

Ans. 14

a. Ataxia telangiectasia
b. Autosomal recessive
c. Ataxia with oculomotor apraxia 1, 2
d. Friedreich's ataxia
e. Leukemia/lymphoma

Ans. 15

a. Inability to close both eyes, visible sclera, flat nasolabial fold
b. Gullain–Barre syndrome, Lyme disease, sarcoidosis, diabetes, and myasthenia gravis.

c. AIDP
   d. Bell's phenomenon and lagophthalmos in LMN palsy, pseudobulbar affect in UMN palsy.
   e. Bifacial palsy may indicate of impending respiratory failure especially if present with bulbar palsy.

Ans. 16

a. Sclera contains a lot of elastin (bilirubin has a strong affinity for elastic tissue)
b. Urine—deep yellow or mustard oil such as color, stool-pale, and clay-colored and jaundice—greenish yellow bulbar conjunctiva.
c. Bile salts—sodium taurocholate and sodium glycocholate, bile acids—primary—cholic acid and chenodeoxycholic acid and secondary—deoxycholic and lithocholic acid, tertiary—ursodeoxycholic acid.
d. Courvoisier's law—palpable nontender smooth gall bladder in a patient of obstructive jaundice due to neoplastic obstruction of the CBD (usually due to carcinoma of the head of the pancreas) and not due to impacted stone in CBD.

Ans. 17

a. Very severe COPD.
b. Right-sided cardiac dysfunction secondary to pulmonary hypertension. Pulmonary hypertension must be of a respiratory cause (chronic lung disease, pulmonary vasculature disorders, and neuromuscular disease affecting the respiratory system). Untreated cor pulmonale causes right-sided heart failure and death.
c. *Mild:* FEV_1 >80% and *moderate:* FEV_1 50–80%, *severe:* FEV_1 30–50%, and *very severe:* FEV_1 <30%.
d. • Arterial blood gas (ABG) (type 1 or 2 respiratory failure is possible)
   • CXR (hyperinflation, flat hemidiaphragms, bullae, and large prominent pulmonary arteries).
   • Echocardiogram (pulmonary hypertension).

Ans. 18

a. Acromegaly
b. Prognathism, enlarged face, macroglossia, spade-shaped hand, and deep husky voice.
c. Growth hormone stimulates skeletal and soft tissue growth and hypersecretion of growth hormone (GH) before the fusion of epiphysis is known as gigantism.
d. *Bromocriptine:* 10-60 mg daily in divided doses, dopamine agonist—cabergoline 5 mg daily, and somatostatin analogs—octreotide.

Ans. 19

a. Lung cancer
b. Lung cancer can be divided into small-cell lung cancer (SCLC) and nonsmall-cell lung cancer (NSCLC), SCLC comprises 15% of all cases; whereas, NSCLC (adenocarcinoma (35–40), squamous cell carcinoma (25–30%), and large-cell carcinoma (10–15%) account for the remainder of lung malignancies.

c. Cushing's syndrome, syndrome of inappropriate antidiuretic hormone secretion (SIADH), Lambert–Eaton myasthenic syndrome (LEMS), hypercalcemia hypertrophic pulmonary osteoarthropathy (HPOA).
d. Pancoast's syndrome is characterized by an apical lung tumor with the involvement of the brachial plexus and cervical sympathetic nerves; patients may complain of pain in the shoulder/anterior chest wall and arm weakness, and have wasting of the intrinsic muscles of the hand and an ipsilateral Horner's syndrome (ptosis, miosis, anhidrosis, and enophthalmos).
e. Edema of the face, neck, and upper body, prominent neck and chest wall vessels, facial plethora, stridor, and headache (often worse on bending forward).

Ans. 20

a. AS
b. Calcific degeneration (or "calcific AS"), bicuspid valve, rheumatic fever, hypertrophic cardiomyopathy (HCM), congenital (other than bicuspid), and supravalvular stenosis (Williams syndrome).
c. Valvular, supravalvular, and subvalvular
d. Severe stenosis [valve area <1.0 cm^2 on echo, peak arteriovenous (AV) velocity, >4 m/s (corresponding to a mean AV gradient of 40 mm Hg)] Symptoms (angina/collapse/dyspnea/heart failure) with moderate stenosis (valve area <1.5 cm^2 on echo, peak velocity >3 m/s), critical AS = valve area <0.8 cm^2.
e. The pressure gradient between the left ventricle and aorta is greatest in the middle of systole, and this is why the murmur of AS is midsystolic.

Ans. 21

a. Ankylosing spondylitis—Dagger sign, there is ossification of supra spinous and interspinous ligament.
b. Human leukocyte antigen B27 (HLA-B27) positive in >90% of the individuals.
c. Physiotherapy, NSAIDs, paracetamol and weak opioids, corticosteroid injections, TNF-α antagonists, such as etanercept, adalimumab, infliximab, golimumab, and certolizumab pegol.
d.
- *Respiratory:* Restrictive lung defect/reduced lung capacity due to restricted chest wall movement and apical lung fibrosis
- *Cardiac:* Chronic aortitis leading to aortic regurgitation, conduction defects, and cardiomyopathy
- *Neurological:* Atlantoaxial instability/dislocation and cauda equina syndrome
- *Eyes:* Iritis and cataracts
- *Amyloidosis [secondary/amyloid A (AA)]:* Multisystem involvement, including hepatic and renal involvement, and coexistent inflammatory bowel disease is common.

Index

A

Abdominal distension 8
Abscess
　bacterial 234
　brain 246
　cerebral 256
　tuberculous 260
Acanthamoeba 20
Acanthocyte 99
Acanthosis nigricans 84, 316, 319
Acarbose 85
Acetazolamide 260
Achalasia cardia 172, 274
Acid-fast bacilli 274
Acidification test 59
Acidosis 260
Acquired immunodeficiency syndrome 109
Acromegaloid features 326
Acrosteolysis 54
Acute inflammatory demyelinating polyneuropathy 241
Acyclovir 292
Addison disease 69
Adenoma, pituitary 70
Adie's tonic pupil 236
Adrenal insufficiency 68
Adrenocorticotropic hormone 60
Albumin 180
Alkali therapy 133
Allergy 285
Allopurinol 319
Alogliptin 85
Alpha-gal syndrome 41
Alpha-glucosidase inhibitors 85
Alzheimer's dementia 236
Alzheimer's disease 236, 253
Amebic liver abscess 180
Amoxicillin 15, 171, 292
Amphotericin 58
Ampicillin 15
Amyloidosis 355
Androgen replacement therapy 328
Anemia
　congenital hemolytic 97
　sideroblastic 100, 326
Angiotensin-converting enzyme inhibitors 82
Angiotensin-receptor blocker 38
Anhidrosis 355
Anion gap 51
Anisocoria 242
Anisocytosis 100
Ankylosing spondylitis 355
Antiacetylcholine 353
Anti-aquaporin-4 immunoglobulin G 245
Antibiotics 14
　therapy 128
Anticholinesterases 294
Anticyclic citrullinated polypeptide 53
Antiepileptic drugs 246
Anti-hepatitis C virus antibody 16
Antimicrobial agents 129
Antineuronal antibody 234
Antinuclear antibodies 40
Antitubercular drugs 172
Aortic
　dissection 160
　regurgitation 158
Arcus juvenilis 162
Arrhythmia 130
Arrhythmogenic right ventricular dysplasia 157
Arsenic 294
Arterial blood gas 51, 279
Arthralgia 131
Arthritis 131
　mutilans 55
　pattern of 44
Ascites 180
Aspergilloma 304
Aspirin overdose 292
Ataxia telangiectasia 240, 353
Atherosclerotic cardiovascular disease 83
Atlanta criteria 21
Atlantoaxial instability 355
Atrial fibrillation 158, 161
Atropa belladonna 293
Atropine 292, 293
Autoimmune
　disease 58, 132
　polyendocrine syndrome 68
Autosomal-dominant polycystic kidney disease 128, 136, 325
Autosomal-recessive 248, 353
Azathioprine 129, 257
Azithromycin 15
Azzopardi effect 110

B

Balamuthia 20
Bamboo spine 55
Basal cell carcinoma 318
Basal ganglia 237
Basket cell 110
Beck's triad 284
Becker muscular dystrophy 325
Bedaquiline 5, 25
Beevor sign 242
Bell's phenomenon 354
Beta cell depletion 82
Bicarbonate 51
Biguanides 85
Bile salts 354
Bilirubin 180
Biomedical waste guidelines 4
Biopsy 52
Biostatistics 335
Black hairy tongue 316
Bleeding 138
　precautions 325
Blood pressure 51, 335
Bloom syndrome 240
Body mass index 51
Bosutinib 100
Bradycardia 275
Breast cancer 316
Breath, shortness of 7
Breathlessness 279
Bromethalin 294
Bronchial breathing inspiration 276
Bronchiectasis 275
Bronchoalveolar lavage 9
Bronchopleural fistula 274, 278
Bronchorrhea 294
Bronchospasm 294
Bronze diabetes 178
Brouet classification criteria 136
Brugada syndrome 326
Bruns nystagmus 243
Bulging fissure sign 303
Burkholderia pseudomallei 172

C

Calcific degeneration 355
Calcinosis 50
Calcium
　channel blocker nimodipine 236
　pyrophosphate deposition 55

Index

Campylobacter jejuni 241
Canagliflozin 85
Captopril 132
Carbamazepine 242
Cardiac failure 130
Cardiology 139
Cardiomegaly, mild 303
Cardiomyopathy 275
Caroli disease 179
Carotid body
    paraganglioma 351
    tumor 351
Castell's technique 68
Cataract 69
Caudate nucleus 242
Cavernous sinus thrombosis 242
Cefalexin 15
Cefixime 15
Celiac disease 39
Central artery 252
Cerebellar artery, superior 249
Cerebellar signs 2
Cerebellum 256
Cerebral metastases 234
Cerebral venous thrombosis 235
Cerebrotendinous
    xanthomatosis 241
Cerebrovascular accident 48
Charcot's arthritis 53
Chemodectoma 351
Chest
    infection 316
    tube drainage 274
Chilaiditi's sign 306
Chipmunk facies 97
Chi-square test 339
Chloride 51
Chlorpromazine 332
Cholangiocarcinoma 178
Cholecalciferol 294
Cholelithiasis 304
Cholesterol 318
Chordal rupture 163
Chvostek sign 242
Ciclosporin 257
Ciliary dyskinesia, primary 327
Ciprofloxacin 15, 292
Cirrhosis 241
Citrate supplementation 134
Clarithromycin 171
Clindamycin 15
Clofazimine 12
Clonazepam 253
Clopidogrel 132, 328
Cloxacillin 15
Cockroft-gault equation 137
Coeliac disease 68
Cognitive behavioral therapy 332
Colonel's mustache 157

Colubridae group 130
Compartment syndrome 129
Conidiobolus coronatus 352
Coombs test, direct 38
Coronavirus disease 2019 75
Corrigan pulse 158
Cortical bridging veins,
    rupture of 236
Cortical venous sinus thrombosis 239
Corticosteroids 38, 129, 257, 316
Cotrimoxazole 15
Cough 12
Courvoisier's law 354
Coxsackievirus 85
Cranial nerve three palsy 242
Creatinine 60
Critical care medicine 279
Crohn's disease 316
Cruveilhier-Baumgarten
    syndrome 171
Cushing's syndrome 69, 352, 355
Cyclophosphamide 130, 132
Cycloserine 12
Cyst 138
    epididymal 128
    hypoglossal 71
    infection 138
Cystic fibrosis 275
Cystitis 10
Cytomegalovirus 85

D

Dagger sign 355
Dapagliflozin 85
Darier disease 319
Dasatinib 100, 109
Dementia, frontotemporal 253, 256
Demyelination 256
Dentate nucleus 237
Depression 332
    postpartum 334
Dermatomyositis sine myositis 317
Desmopressin 260
Diabetes
    insipidus 260
    mellitus 1, 33
        type 1 39
        type 2 328
Diabetic amyotrophy 252
Diabetic kidney disease 82
Diabetic retinopathy 69
    stages of 84
Diabetology 72
Diarylquinolines 25
Diastolic murmur, long-standing 43
Dietary modification 134
DiGeorge's syndrome 328
Dipeptidyl peptidase 4 inhibitors 85

Disease-modifying antirheumatic
    drugs 45
Disseminated intravascular
    coagulation 98
Dissociated sensory loss 247
Distal arthritis 55
Dizziness 30
Donepezil 236
Dorsal oculomotor vermis 256
Downbeating nystagmus 243
Doxycycline 15
Drowsiness 260
Dry cough 7
Dry gangrene 38
Duke's criteria 317
Dupuytren's contracture 237, 327
Dysautonomia 82
Dysphagia 159
Dyspnea 12
Dysproteinemias 58

E

Ectopic thyroid 71
Eculizumab 97, 130
Edema 51
    pulmonary 158
Edinburgh postnatal depression
    scale 334
Electrolyte disorders 129
Electromyography 71
Embolism 159
Emphysematous bullae 277
Encephalopathy 180
Endocrinology 60
Endoscopic Bougie dilation 172
Enophthalmos 355
Enzyme-linked immunosorbent
    assay 52
Epidemic dropsy 292
Epstein-Barr virus 129
Ergot poisoning 54
Erythema
    multiforme 316
    nodosum 277
Escherichia coli 133, 137, 170
Esophageal dysmotility 50
Esophageal varix 180
Ethambutol 249
Evans syndrome 38
Exner's area 257
Extraocular movements 2
Extremities, paresthesias of 260

F

Facial
    anhidrosis 238
    trauma 285

Fahr's disease 238
Fahr's syndrome 237
Fanconi anemia 97
Fatigue 30
Felty's syndrome 45
Fever 12, 17
 low-grade 9
 rheumatic 253
Fibrates 129
Fibrosis, idiopathic pulmonary 351
Figure of 3 sign 158
Fisher scale, modified 353
Flank pain 10
Fludrocortisone 59
Fluid restriction 133
Fluphenazine 332
Focal cortical dysplasia 306
Follicle-stimulating hormone 60
Fomepizole 293, 294
Foramen ovale 243
Foramen rotundum 243
Francisella 129
Free thyroxine 60
Friedreich's ataxia 353
Fungal infections 260
Furosemide 59

G

Gallbladder 304
Gastric lavage 295
Gastroenterology 165
Genetic anomalies 326
Glasgow coma scale 285
Glecaprevir 180
Gliclazide 85
Glimepiride 85
Glioblastoma 245, 256
Glipizide 85
Glomerular hematuria 135
Glucagon-like peptide-1 82
Glucagonoma 316
Glucocorticoids 68, 109, 130
 therapy 159
Glucose 8
 monitoring, continuous 86
Glyburide 85
Glycopyrrolate 277
Goodpasture syndrome 130
Gottron papules 257, 317
Gout 55
Granulomatosis 131
 eosinophilic 57
Granulomatous amebic
 encephalitis 20
Grave's disease 41, 70
Groin 13
Guillain-Barré syndrome 39, 136, 241, 254

Gumprecht shadows 110
Gynecomastia 327

H

Hallervorden-Spatz syndrome 305
Haloperidol 253, 332
Hard exudates 86
Headache 246
Heart 275
 disease, rheumatic 161
 failure, congestive 157
Heberden's nodes 52
Helicobacter pylori 171
 bacteria 29
Heliotrope rash 317
Hematoma 132, 246
Hematuria 130, 132
Hemithorax 277
Hemochromatosis 178
Hemodialysis 129
Hemolysis, elevated liver enzymes
 and low platelets
 syndrome 130
Hemolytic uremic syndrome 130
Hemoptysis 159
Hemosiderosis, pulmonary 25
Hepatic flexure 306
Hepatitis 241
 B
  surface antigen 18
  vaccination 18
 viral 179
Hereditary hemorrhagic
 telangiectasia 240
Herpes
 labialis 352
 simplex virus 343
Hertel's exophthalmometer 41
High anion gap 284
Hill's sign 158, 161
Hippocampus 237
Hodgkin's lymphoma 109
Homunculus 44
Hormone replacement therapy 334
Horner's syndrome 238, 294, 355
Howell-Jolly bodies 99
Human immunodeficiency
 virus 109
Human leukocyte antigen 355
Human papillomavirus vaccine 18
Humming bird sign 238
Humoral hypercalcemia 110
Hung-up knee reflex 242
Huntington's chorea 242
Huntington's disease 253, 255, 325
Huntz-Hess scale 353
Hydrohemothorax 278
Hydropneumothorax, encysted 278

Hydroxychloroquine 38, 317
Hydroxymethylbilane synthase 327
Hypercalcemia hypertrophic
 pulmonary
 osteoarthropathy 355
Hypercalciuria 59, 134
Hyperdense lesion 246
Hyperemesis 130
Hyperglycemic hyperosmolar
 state 84
Hyperintense signal 303
Hyperosmolar nonketotic
 hyperglycemic state 85
Hyperparathyroidism 54, 58
Hyperpigmentation 316
Hypersegmented neutrophil 99
Hypertension 83, 335
 idiopathic intracranial 353
Hypertensive intracranial
 hemorrhage 234
Hyperthyroidism 70, 85
Hypertrophic cardiomyopathy 161
Hypocalcemia, treatment of 129
Hypochromia 100
Hypocitraturia 59
Hypokalemia 260, 292
Hypoplastic thumb 97
Hypotension 10
Hypothesis
 alternative 335, 338
 formulation 335
Hypothyroidism 242

I

Ice pack test 235
Idiopathic thrombocytopenic 68
Ifosfamide 58
Imatinib 100, 109
Immune thrombocytopenic
 purpura 19
Immunoglobulin 29, 130
Immunology 30
Implantable cardioverter-
 defibrillators 326
Indinavir 292
Infections 85
Infectious diseases 1
Inflammatory bowel disease 171
Insulin
 dextrose 164
 pump 83
 therapy 82
Interferon 85
Intermittent porphyria, acute 327
Interstitial lung disease 131
Intracranial aneurysms 128
Ipratropium bromide 277
Ipsilateral red nucleus 243

Iron
  deficiency anemia 97, 100, 326
  stores depletion 100
Ischemic digital ulcers 40
Isoniazid 249
Isotonic saline 129

J

Jaccoud's arthropathy 52, 53
Janeway lesion 317
Jaundice 354
Joffroy sign 70
Joint pain 30
Juvenile myoclonic epilepsy 244

K

Kartagener's syndrome 327
Kayser-Fleischer ring 178, 248, 327
Ketamine 258
Ketoacidosis
  alcoholic 283
  diabetic 82
Klebsiella pneumoniae 303
Klinefelter's syndrome 328
Knee joint 48
  bilateral 44
Koilonychia 100
Korsakoff psychosis 248

L

Lacrimation 294
Lagophthalmos 354
Lambert-Eaton myasthenic
    syndrome 110, 353, 355
Lead poisoning 99, 100
Ledipasvir 180
Legionella 129
Leipzig score 241
Leishman Donovan body 352
Leukemia 316
Leukocytosis 42
Levetiracetam 258
Levofloxacin 15
Lhermitte's sign 242
Lichenification 316
Linagliptin 85
Lipodystrophy 85
Lips, deviation of 234
Lithium 58, 129, 132, 259
Liver
  abscess 180
  biopsy 180
  cyst 128
  disease, model for
      end-stage 180
  function tests 52

Lung
  abscess 278
      complication of 276
  cancer 354
Lupus nephritis 40
Luteinizing hormone 60
Lymphocutaneous sporotrichosis 351
Lymphocytes 8
Lymphocytic leukemia, chronic 110
Lymphoma 131, 316

M

Magnesium ions 293
Magnetic resonance imaging 325
Malignancy 132, 317
Mandibular nerve 243
Mania 332
Mannitol 129, 246
Marital violence 334
Marsh grading 317
Maxillary nerve 243
McArdle sign 242
McConnell's sign 159
McDonald criteria 242
Meglitinides 85
Memantine 236
Membranoproliferative
    glomerulonephritis 133
Memory loss 250
Meningioma 247
Meningococcal meningitis 20
Menorrhagia 30
Mesangial matrix expansion 82
Mesenteric artery, superior 170
Metabolic
  acidosis 284
  alkalosis 283
Metal phosphides 294
Metformin 82, 85, 129
Methanol 293
  poisoning 294
Methotrexate 317
Methyl alcohol intoxication 283
Metronidazole 15
Microangiopathic hemolytic
    anemia 134
Microcytosis 100
Microfilament tests 84
Midazolam 258
  infusion 258
Middleton's hooking procedure 68
Midfacial hypoplasia 328
Miglitol 85
Miosis 238, 355
Mitral stenosis 161
Mitral valve prolapse 128
Mixed connective tissue disease 54
Moebius sign 70

Molluscum contagiosum 318
Morganella 128
Mosquito control measure 258
Motor disturbances 325
Multiorgan dysfunction syndrome 20
Muscle biopsy 317
Myasthenia gravis 68, 136, 235, 353
Mycobacterium tuberculosis 260
Myeloma
  cast nephropathy 134
  multiple 98
Myeloneuropathy 234
Myoclonus 253
Myotonic dystrophy 71

N

Narcotic bowel syndrome 333
Nateglinide 85
National Tuberculosis Elimination
    Program 238
Necrolytic migratory erythema 316
Necrotic migratory erythema 316
Nephrocalcinosis 58, 59, 132
Nerve conduction test 5
Neural ectoderm 71
Neurocysticercosis 234, 256
Neuroleptic malignant
    syndrome 129, 332
Neurology 181
Neuromuscular junctional
    disorder 353
Neuromyelitis optica spectrum
    disorder 245
Neuropathy, peripheral 131
Nicotinic signs 292
Nilotinib 100, 109
Nixon's maneuver 68
Nodular swelling 48
Noncontrast computed
    tomography 305
Nonglomerular hematuria 135
Nonsteroidal anti-inflammatory
    drugs 52, 129, 316
Nonsteroidal mineralocorticoid
    receptor antagonist 83
Null hypothesis 335, 338, 339, 340

O

Obesity, insulin-resistant 69
Obsessive compulsive disorder 333
Obstructive pattern 278
Obstructive sleep apnea 69, 276
Occupational therapy 352
Ocular telangiectasia 240
Ophthalmic nerve 243
Ophthalmoplegia 248
Organophosphorous poisoning 293

Index

Ortner's syndrome 159
Osler nodes 317
Osler-Weber-Rendu syndrome 240
Osteoarthritis 52
Osteomalacia 178

P

Pachydermoperiostosis 326
Paget's disease 178
Pain 13
    abdominal 279, 333
    epigastric 6
    stabbing 5
Palmar erythema 327
Palpable purpura 317
Pancoast's syndrome 108, 275, 355
Pancreas 304
    multiple calcifications 85
Pantoprazole 171
Paragangliomas 351
Paraplegia 9, 34
Parathyroid hormone 274
Parkinson's disease 236
    idiopathic 249
Paroxetine 334
Paroxysmal hemicrania 259
Paroxysmal nocturnal
    hemoglobinuria 97, 99
Pauci-immune
    glomerulonephritis 133
Pemberton sign 69
Penicillamine 132
Pericardial effusion 160, 275, 284
Pericarditis, purulent 157
Periepithelial lymphocytes 131
Perifascicular atrophy 257
Perihilar consolidation, bilateral 303
Perimysial inflammatory infiltrate 257
Peripheral blood smear 109, 277
Peripheral smear 321
Peritoneal enhancement 135
Peritoneal thickening 135
Petechiae 97
Phenytoin 54, 85, 258
Pheochromocytoma 70
Phosphate 60
Phosphides 295
Photophobia 14
Pigtail drain 278
Pinpoint pupil 293
Pioglitazone 85
Plasma exchange 130
Plasmapheresis 136
Plasmodium vivax 100
Plummer-Vinson syndrome 172
Pneumatocele 278
Pneumothorax 277
Poikilocytosis 100

Poisoning 286
Polyangiitis 131
    viral 55
Polycythemia rubra vera 108
Portal hypertension 180
Postcricoid dysphagia 100
Posterior reversible encephalopathy
    syndrome 239
Post-kala azar dermal
    leishmaniasis 352
Postsplenectomy 97
Post-traumatic stress disorder 333
Potassium 51
    citrate 133
Pott's paraplegia 238
Prednisolone 244
Presynaptic voltage-gated calcium
    channel 110
Pretibial myxedema 41
Prognathism 354
Propofol 258
Proteins 8
Prothrombin time 180
Proton pump inhibitors 129
Providencia 128
Proximal muscle group 61
Pseudomonas 128
Psoriatic arthritis 46, 55
    classification criteria for 46
Psychiatric disorder 334
Psychiatry 330
Psychotherapy 333
Ptosis 238, 355
Puerperal sepsis 130
Pulmonary embolism, saddle 351
Pulsus paradoxus 284
Purple urine bag syndrome 170
Purpura fulminans 285
Pyelonephritis, emphysematous
    133, 137
Pyogenic infections 260
Pyrazinamide 249
Pyrimethamine 234

Q

Quadrantanopia 250
Quadriplegia 245
Quadruple therapy 29

R

Raccoon eyes 353
Radioablation 71
Radio-active iodine 69
Ranson's criteria 21
Rapunzel syndrome 334
Raynaud's phenomenon 50
    primary 38

Reed-Sternberg cells 109
Rehydration 130
Renal artery stenosis 134
Renal disease, end-stage 69
Renin-angiotensin system 83
Repaglinide 85
Respiratory rate 51
Restless legs syndrome 253
Reticulocytes 99
Rhabdomyolysis 110, 129
Rheumatoid
    arthritis 42, 53, 54, 58
    factors 42
Rheumatology 42
Rickets 303
Rifampicin 17, 249
Rituximab 130, 132, 257
Roflumilast 277
Rosenbach's sign 70
Rosiglitazone 85
Rosuvastatin 329
Rubella 85

S

Sacroiliitis, bilateral 56
Salivation 294
Salmonella 129
Sarcoidosis 274, 278
    pulmonary 276
Saxagliptin 85
Scadding staging 277
Schmidt syndrome 68
Sclerodactyly 50
Scleroderma 58
Sclerosing cholangitis 178
Sclerosis
    amyotrophic lateral 256
    systemic 35, 58
Scrotum 13
Sebaceous hyperplasia 318
Seizure 7, 8, 130
    disorder 237
    focal 253
    gyratory 245
Selective serotonin reuptake
    inhibitors 332
Sengstaken-Blakemore tube 170
Sensitivity 338
Sensory examination 2
Sertraline 334
Serum protein electrophoresis 98
Shingles vaccine 254
Sinusitis, treatment of 246
Sitagliptin 85
Sjögren's syndrome 58, 131, 133
Skin biopsy 316
Slit-lamp examination 14
Smudge cell 99, 110

Sodium 51
  channel blockers 244
  monofluoroacetate 294
  valproate 258
  valproic acid 244
Sodium-glucose transport protein 82
Sofosbuvir 180
Solitary brain metastasis 246
Somogyi phenomenon states 84
Spider angioma 317
Spinal digital subtraction
      angiography 245
Splendore-Hoeppli phenomenon 343
Spondyloarthritis 55
Squamous cell carcinoma 97, 318
Staghorn calculi 128
Staphylococcus aureus 129, 278
Statin-associated musculoskeletal
      symptom 329
Statins 38, 129
Stellwag sign 70
Stenosis, severe 355
Steroids 85, 244
Still's disease, adult-onset 52
Streptococcus pneumoniae 129, 157
Streptomycin 249
Stroke, ischemic 303
Struchnine 294
Subarachnoid hemorrhage 246,
      325, 353
Subdural hematoma 236
Sulcus tumor, superior 275
Sulfadiazine 234, 292, 319
Sulfonamides 316
Sulfonylureas 85
Superior cerebellar artery 242
Supine palpation technique 68
Swan neck deformity 53
Sweet syndrome 316
Swelling 13, 341
Syndrome of inappropriate
      antidiuretic hormone
      secretion 138, 355
Synpharyngitic nephritis 130
Syringoma 318
Syringomyelia 247
Systemic lupus erythematosus 33,
      38, 130

T

Tachycardia 284
Tachypnea 284
Tacrolimus 257
Telangiectasia syndrome 50
Tendon xanthoma 241
Tension pneumothorax 276, 277, 304
Tetrabenazine 253

Thalamic infarct 253
Thalassemia 100, 326
  minor 326
Theophylline 129, 277
Thiamine 236, 248
Thiazides 85
  diuretics 135
Thiazolidinediones 85
Thiopentone 258
Thromboembolism, pulmonary 305
Thrombolytic therapy 238
Thrombotic microangiopathy 130
Thyroid
  disease 68
  function test 70
  profile 65
  scintigraphy 69
  stimulating hormone 60
Thyrotoxicosis 70
Thyroxine 85
Tiotropium 277
Toluene toxicity 58
Tolvaptan 326
Topiramate 260
Touraine-Solente-Gole syndrome 326
Toxicology 286
Toxins 129
  withdrawal of 59
Toxoplasma gondii 235
Transjugular intrahepatic
      portosystemic shunt 179
Traube's space percussion 68
Tremor 253
Trichobezoar 334
Trifluoperazine 332
Trigeminal neuralgia 242
Triglyceride 318
Tropheryma whipplei 39
Trousseau sign 242
Tru-cut kidney biopsy needle 132
Tubercular meningitis 25
Tuberculoma 256
Tuberculosis, pulmonary 5, 17
Tubular basement membrane 136
Tumor
  lysis syndrome 130
  pituitary 259
  solid 132
Tyrosine kinase inhibitor 109, 100

U

Ulcerative colitis 316
Ultrasonography 304
Ultrasound abdomen 305
Umbilicus 3
Urea 60
Urea-splitting organism 59

Urinalysis 51
Urination 294
Urine
  anion gap 59
  myoglobinuria 110
  protein-creatinine ratio 128
  routine examination 133

V

Vasculitis 130, 249
Velpatasvir 180
Vena cava
  inferior 161
  superior 109
Ventricular tachycardia 139
Verapamil 259
Vesicular breath sound 147
Vestibulocerebellum 256
Vibratory sensation 82
Video-assisted thoracoscopy 274
Vildagliptin 85
Viperidae group 130
Viral syndrome 100
Vitamin
  B_{12} deficiency 234
  D 328
Voglibose 85
Vomiting 3, 130, 246
von Graefe sign 70
von Willebrand disease 100

W

Waldenström's
      macroglobulinemia 98
Watershed infarct left anterior cerebral
      artery territory 245
Weight 260
  loss 12, 17
Wernicke encephalopathy 244, 248
West Haven criteria 253
Whipple disease 39
White blood cell 30
Wilson's disease 179, 241, 327
Wing-beating tremor 327
Wolff-Parkinson-white syndrome 159

X

Xanthelasma 162

Z

Z deformity 53
Zidovudine 129
Ziehl-Neelsen stain, wet mount
      modified 16

EU GSPR Authorised Reprsentative
Logos Europe, 9 rue Nicolas Poussin
1700, La Rochelle, France
Phone: +33 (0) 6 67 93 73 78
E-mail: contact@logoseurope.eu